Lehmanns Media

Cardiac Surgical Operative Atlas

edited by

Th. Wahlers, Th. Wittwer, Cologne
and
D. H. Adams, New York, USA

Contributors:

D. H. Adams, New York, USA
J. M. Albes, Bernau
J. Cremer, Kiel
U. F. W. Franke, Stuttgart
J. Gummert, Leipzig
W. Harringer, Braunschweig
H. H. Sievers, Luebeck
H. H. Scheld, Muenster
Th. Wahlers, Cologne
O. Wendler, London, UK
Th. Wittwer, Cologne
H. R. Zerkowski, Basel, Switzerland
G. Ziemer, Tuebingen

Including 300 high-quality operative photographs.

Cardiac Surgical Operative Atlas

Printed in Germany by AZ Druck und Datentechnik, Kempten

Published by Lehmanns Media, Berlin, Germany

Editors: Thorsten Wahlers
Thorsten Wittwer
David H. Adams

Cover- and Interior Designer: Annett Zebrowski, krea.tif-design
www.krea.tif-design.de

2008: First Edition

ISBN: 978-3-86541-220-1

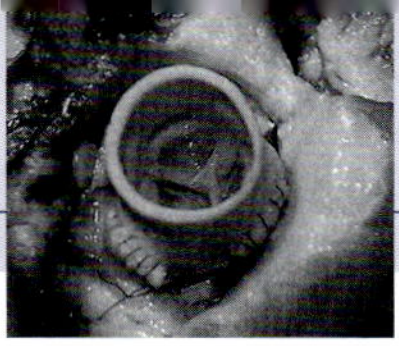

Contents

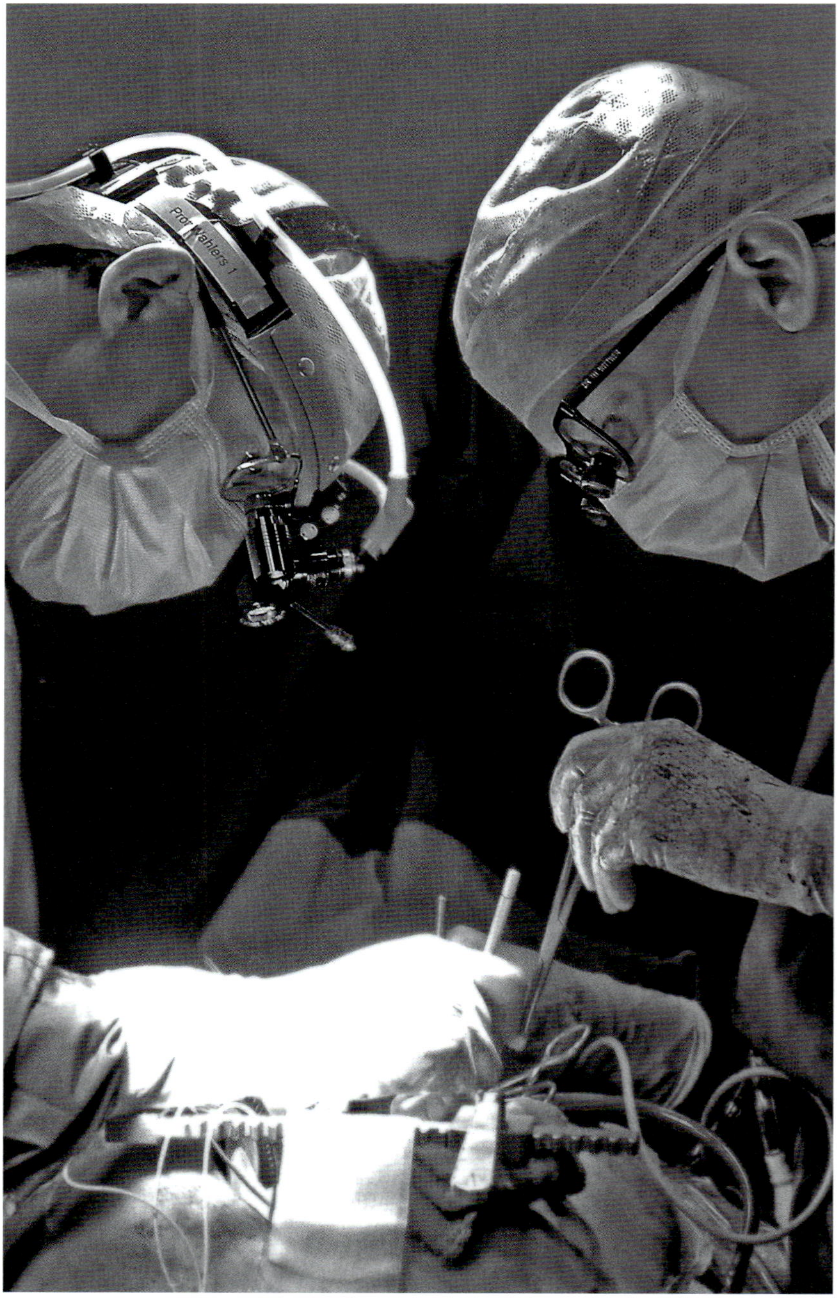
Prof Wahlers 1

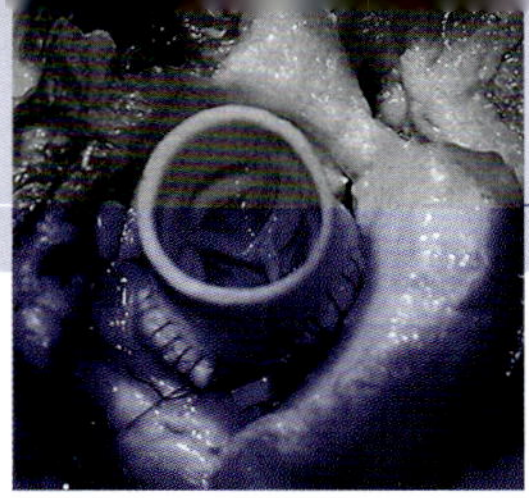

Foreword

Th. Wahlers, Th. Wittwer, D. H. Adams

There is nothing quite like the pleasure of "passing on" the lessons of surgery from one generation to the next. As experienced cardiac surgeons, all of us remember the trainee phase in our specialty when we tried to acquire all of the available Operative Atlases we could find and studying from them to prepare for the next day of teaching in the operating room. However, written chapters and drawings are different as compared to real surgery. To overcome this limitation, we developed together the second edition of this new-concept operative atlas.
When our co-editor, the New York Professor of Cardiac Surgery, David H. Adams, first received a copy of the German Cardiac Surgical Operative Atlas edited by Thorsten Wahlers and Thorsten Wittwer, with a request to provide an additional chapter on Tricuspid Valve Repair for this first English edition, he was struck by the simplicity and obvious utility of this book. He considered it not hard to understand why the total first German Edition sold out in a matter of months.
In the second International Edition of the Cardiac Surgical Operative Atlas, the beginning surgeon can review very basic techniques and maneuvers such as cannulation strategies and internal mammary harvest. In other chapters, cardiac surgeons of all levels can review complex procedures such as valve sparing or reconstructive operations, captured step by step with high-quality operative photographs. As good as the art work is in a typical Operative Atlas, original pictures from an actual surgical procedure provide the student of surgery with a depth and clarity not possible in a drawn picture. The accompanying concise legends provide the reader with the key points and "take home messages" to learn from each photograph. We have no doubt there is something in this Atlas for every student of cardiac surgery, from the surgical resident at the beginning of his training over the more experienced surgeon "on-call" being confronted with a complex case in the middle of the night to the expert surgeon wanting to learn an advanced technique.
Operative Atlases have been an essential part of surgical training since the beginning, and this particular edition is designed to be helpful for young cardiac surgeons and is hopefully a valuable addition to anyone´s collection.

Cologne/New York, January 2008

Thorsten Wahlers Thorsten Wittwer David H. Adams

STANDARD CANNULATION TECHNIQUE

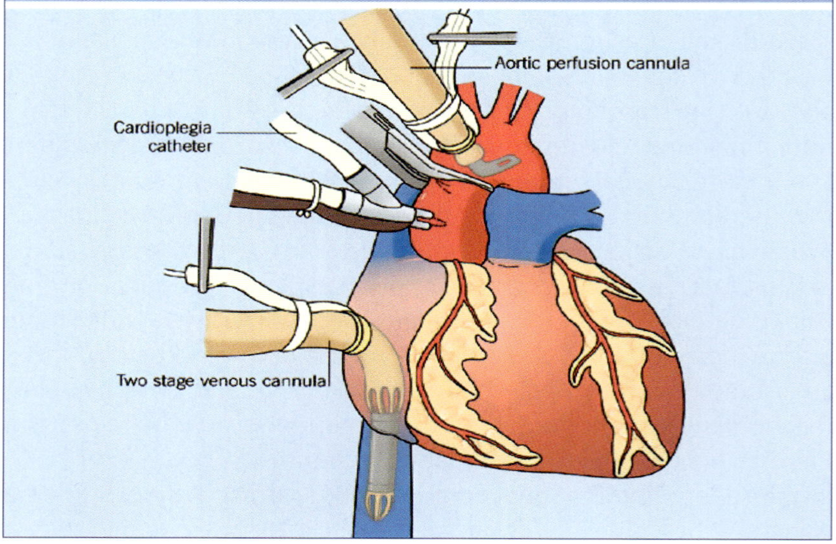

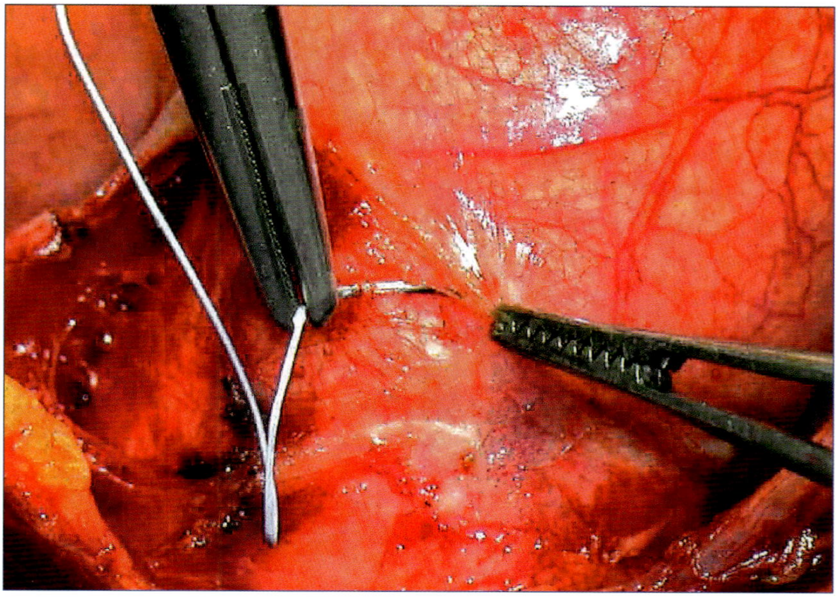

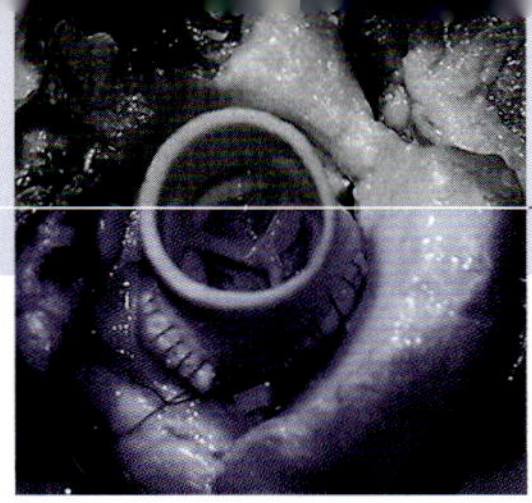

H.-R. *Zerkowski*

"A standardized routine for cardiac operations is essential: An established routine makes every operation more efficient and in case of emergency provides a means for speed and accuracy."(D. B. Doty)

Set up for on- pump cardiac surgery.
Intra-thoracic standard cannulation techniques.

These comprise cannulation of the ascending aorta as well the proximal aortic arch, application of the cardioplegia delivery cannula as well as cannulation for venous return in its versions "single-stage cannula" as well as "separate cannulation of the superior and inferior venae cavae" (via right atrium or distant, near to their atrial orifice).
For understanding it is mentioned that all photographic representations in this chapter differ slightly from the usual surgeon's view of the heart standing at the right side of the open chest of the supine patient. The photographs are taken from the observers view, its "observing eye" some 30 degrees more cranial, between the patient's and the surgeon's head.

Purse-String Aorta – "Life-line" for arterial cannula.

The appropriate site for aortic cannulation is identified by careful palpation of the anterior third of the vessel circumference near the pericardial reflection to exclude regions with calcified plaque formation thus preventing embolization when inserting the cannula.
The purse-string (diameter 3–4 mm larger than cannula) is placed stitch by stitch strictly avoiding penetrating the inner layers of the aortic wall (stay intramurally!); a second purse-string is placed 2–3 mm from the first one, the intramural course of the stitch alternating to inner string. Tourniquets are placed on the purse-string stitches, inner string's orientation to the left, outer one's to the surgeon.

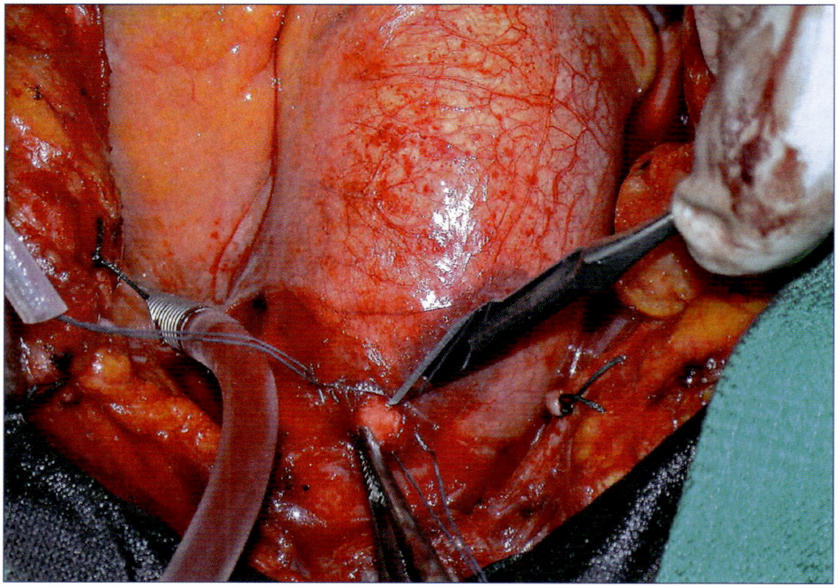

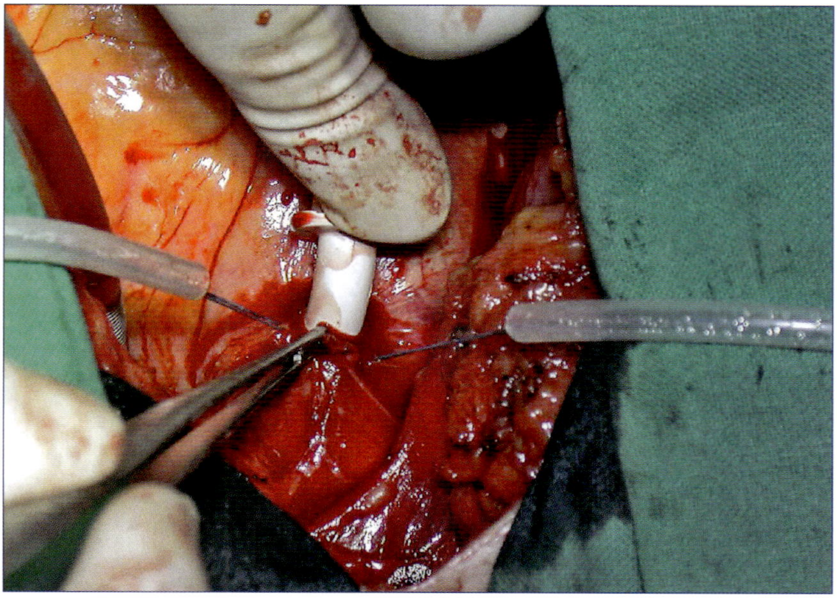

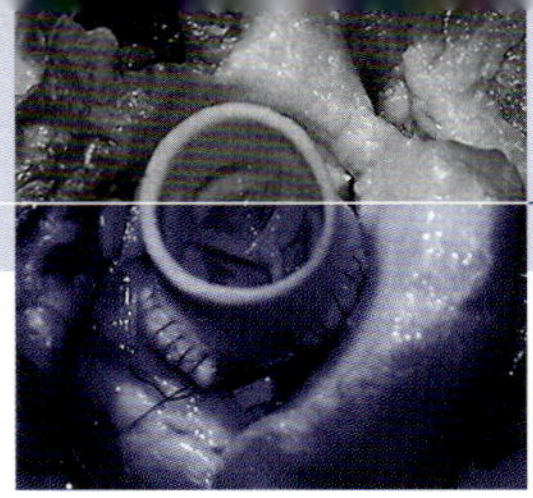

Incision – Opening of the Aorta

The pericardial layer inside the purse-string is incised to form a small flap. This flap is lifted and the aortic wall is incised horizontally using a scalpel with a resulting incision which should be 1–1.5 mm larger than the diameter of the chosen aortic perfusion cannula.
The incision is controlled by the flap or by the surgeon's thumb.

Insertion of Arterial Cannula

By lifting the pericardium-adventitia flap the cannula is placed into the lumen in a proximal direction using its convex shape. Then it is turned easily by 180 degrees to a cranially orientated direction. The aortic blood must easily reach the end of the cannula.
In rare cases with doubts concerning the correct position, the orientation of the cannula can easily be controlled by palpating the uncalcified aorta between thumb and index finger.

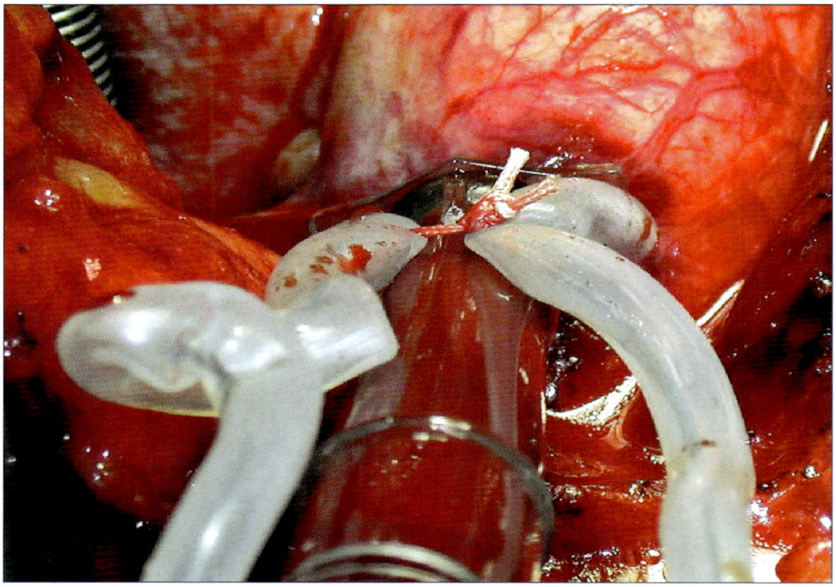

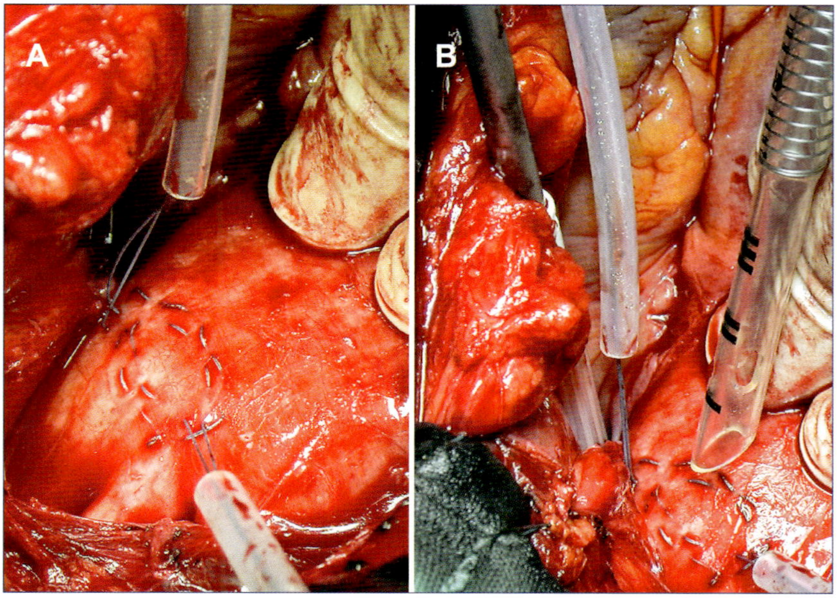
A
B

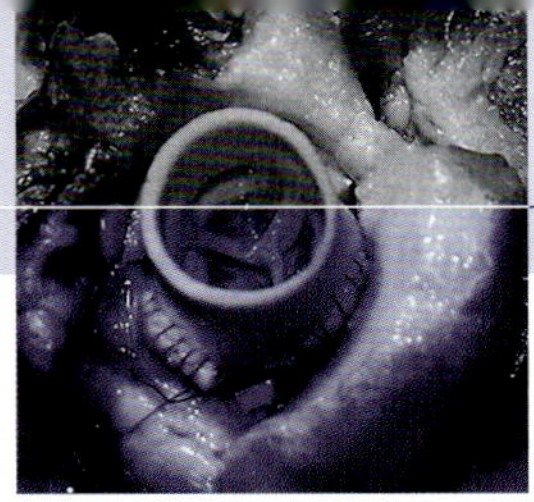

The purse string sutures are tightened, secured by using small mosquito clamps and ultimatively fixed to the perfusion cannula by ligature as close as possible to its tip.
When choosing the insertion site of the (double-purpose) cardioplegia delivery cannula (we use it for venting and de-airing as well) it should be mentioned in case of CABG surgery that this place must be suitable for a central graft anastomosis.

Proximal aortic arch

In case of aortic dilatation, calcification of the proximal aorta, intended proximal replacement or desired cross-clamping in the proximal arch, specific cannulation of the proximal arch is feasible following the same basic principles (Figure 2–5). However, a different perfusion cannula should be used in order to avoid a "jet-shape" isolated perfusion of the brachiocephalic trunk. Therefore, in our group a cannula with different types of "side-holes" is preferred in cases with proximal aortic arch cannulation (B).

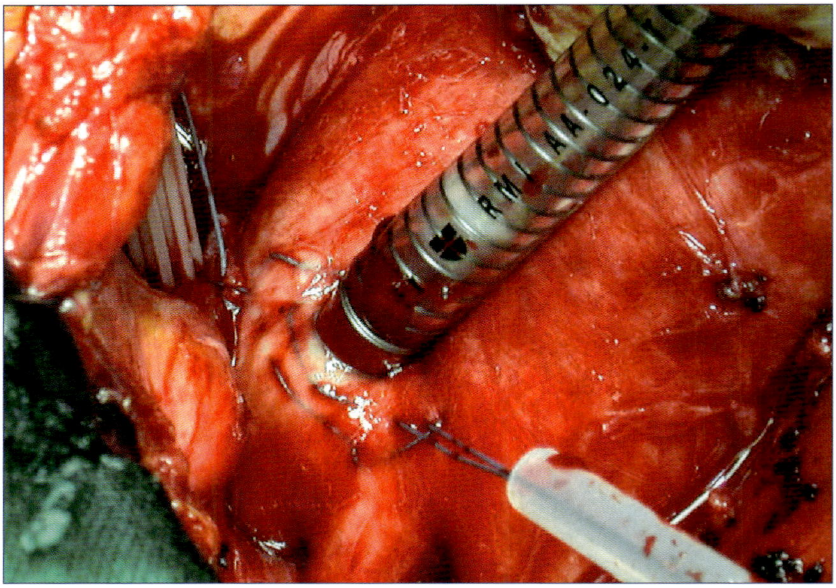

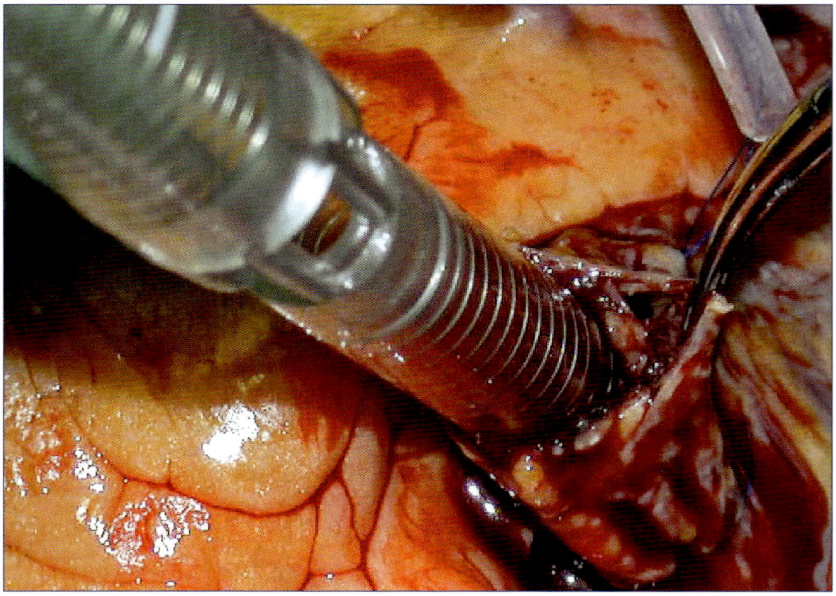

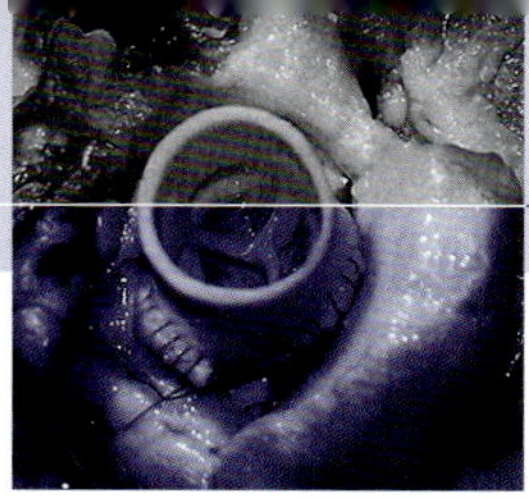

The cannula is inserted in a way that under orthograde flow conditions regular flow to arch and all supra-aortic vessels is provided.

Venous return by two-stage cannula (single-bore cannula according to Cooley)

A purse-string suture is placed at the base of the right atrial appendage. The appendage is amputated (or incised) in a way that the resulting orifice matches the largest diameter of the chosen venous cannula. Remember: Atrial myocardium is less elastic and tends to tear!
The cannula is inserted directly towards the orifice of the inferior vena cava without any resulting resistance. Care must be taken not to enter the coronary sinus. The cannula is inserted down to the second marking which generally places the side-holes in the middle of the atrium (digital control!) with the tip of the cannula in the caval funnel. Selective cannulation of large liver veins by inserting the cannula in a too deep fashion has to be avoided.

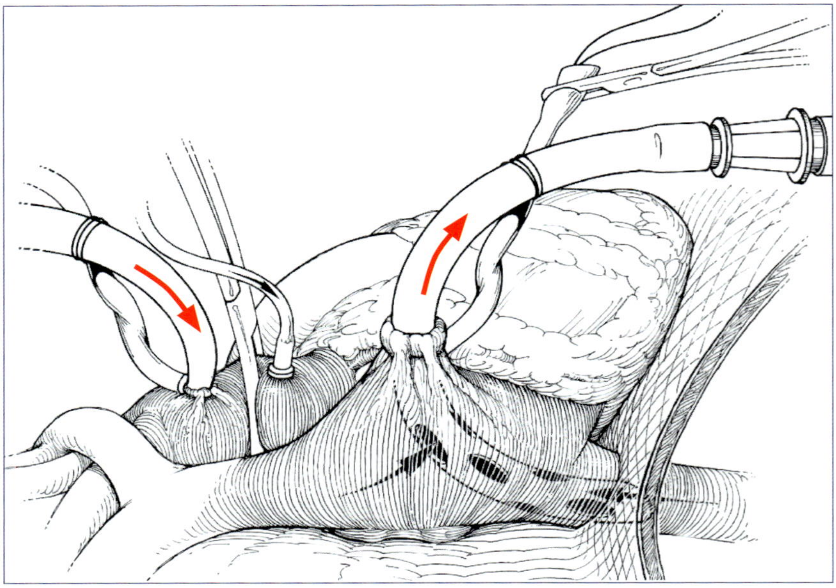

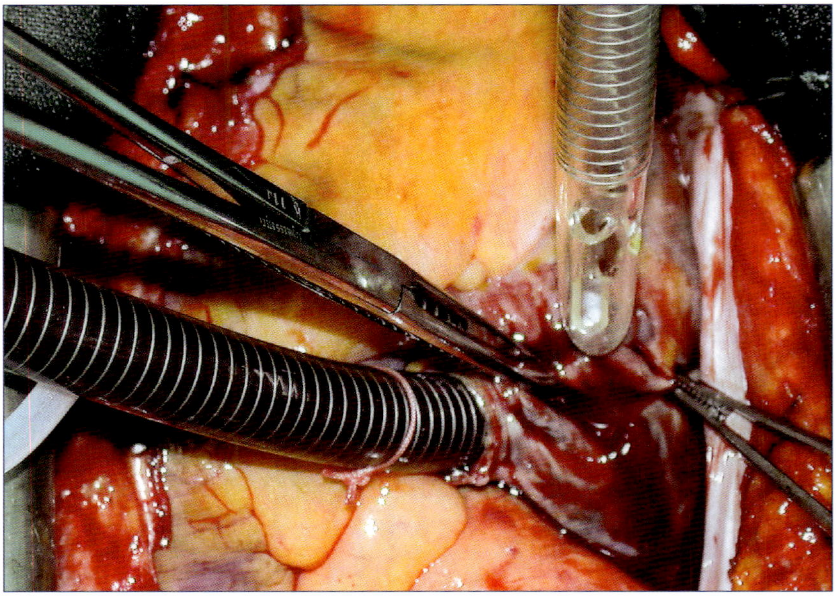

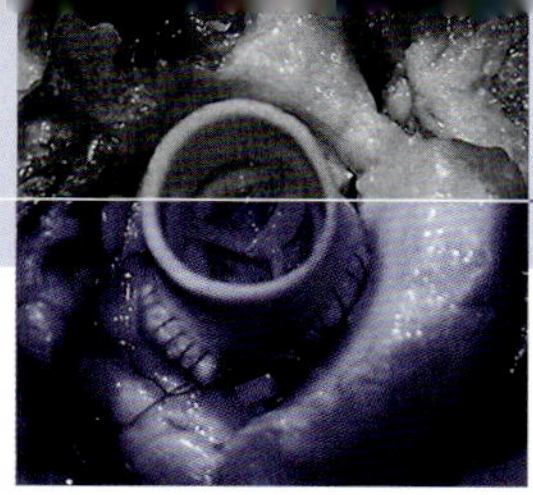

Positioning of Two-Stage Cannulas

Irrespective of the product used in your institution take care that free orthograde flow from the inferior vena cava to the cannula and via side-holes from the superior vena cava and right ventricle, respectively, is ensured.

Entering of the coronary sinus, damage of the tricuspid valve as well as occlusion of parts of the liver veins must be strictly avoided by gently insertion.

Venous Double-Cannulation through right atrium

The straight venous cannula for venous return from the inferior vena cava is inserted as described for two-stage cannulation. Some centimeters dorsally and distally to its insertion a second purse-string suture is placed for the cranial cannula which is inserted into the superior vena cava. The purse string sutures in the atrial wall should be placed intramurally in a region where the muscle looks brighter (i.e. the atrial wall is thicker!).

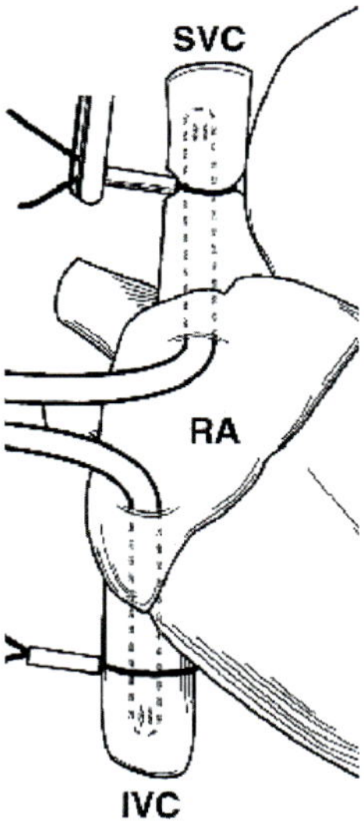
SVC
RA
IVC

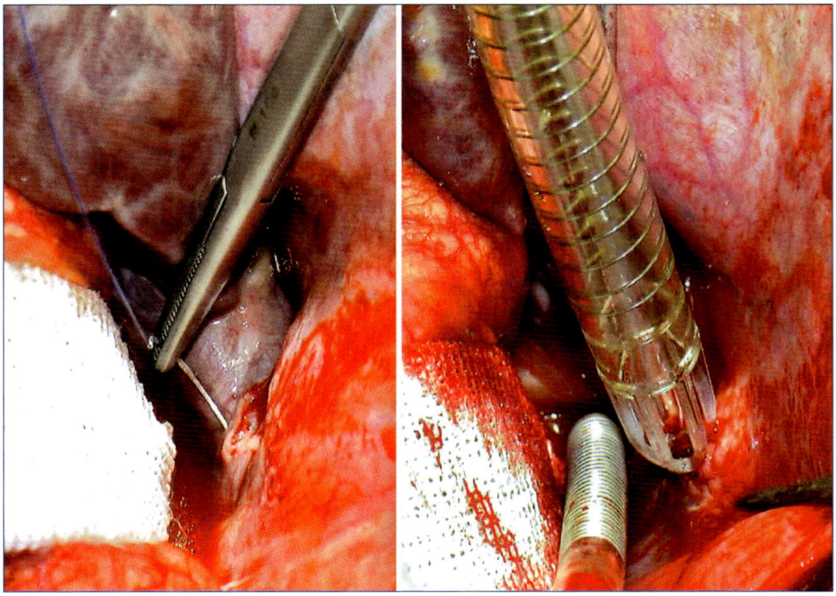

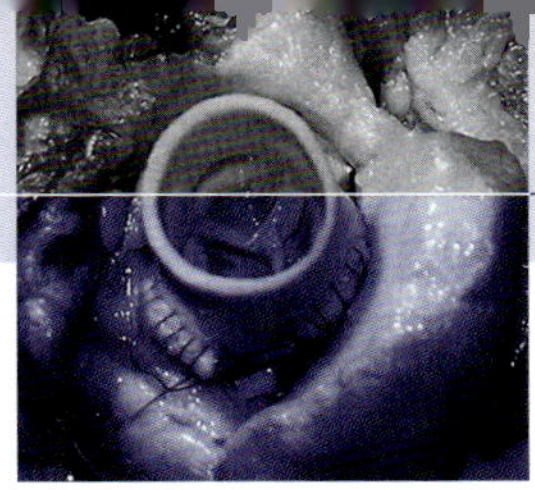

1 2 3 4 5 6 7 8 9 10 11 12 13 14 15

Total cardiopulmonary bypass

A right angle clamp is passed behind the superior and the inferior cava, respectivly, and the cannulae are secured by snaring vessel loops or umbilical bands under slight traction.
Central venous or pulmonary artery catheters should be temporarily displaced cranially in order to avoid damage or constant leakage of blood to the operative field.superior

Venous double cannulation for transplantion or extensive trans-atrial surgery

The superior vena cava is exposed clearly proximally from the sinus node region, and a purse-string suture is placed on the anterior (ventral) aspect of the vessel. After gentle mobilization und incision a 90-degree angled (ring-enforced) cannula is inserted with the same caution as used in atrial cannulation.

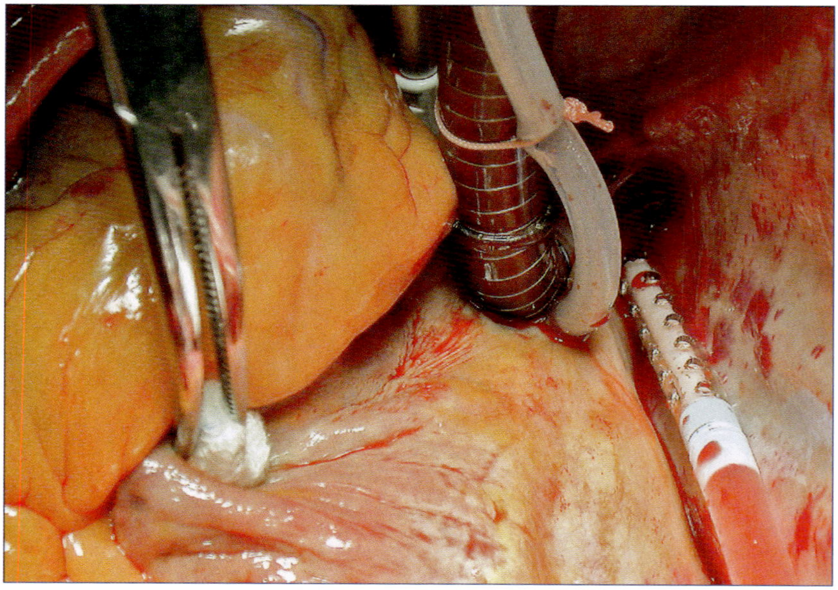

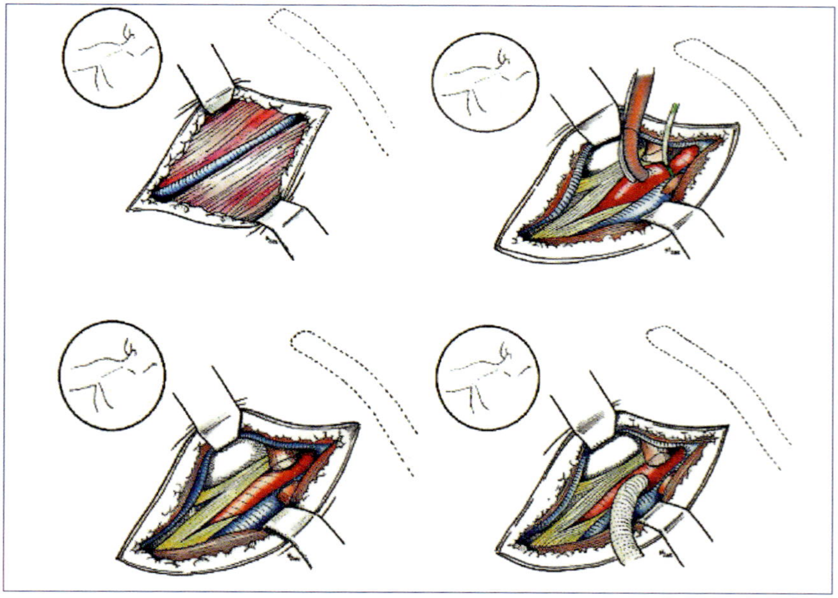

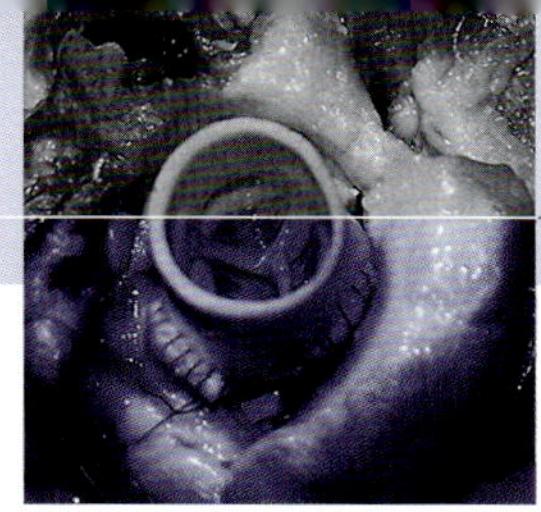

For cannulation of the inferior vena cava a region of the right atrial wall is chosen somewhat cranially the pericardial reflection of the inferior caval funnel, i. e. that region where white-gleaming is indicating more stable fibrotic tissue. A purse-string suture is placed, a horizontal incision is made and the angled cannula is inserted strictly into the center of the inferior vena cava!

Cannulation via Arteria subclavia according to Hetzer

In cases of extremely calcified ascending aorta or acute aortic dissection it might be helpful to connect CPB via the subclavian artery.

A transverse incision is made below the clavicle to expose Mohrenheim's groove. Both the subclavian artery as well as the subclavian vein are dissected and and secured using vessel loops.

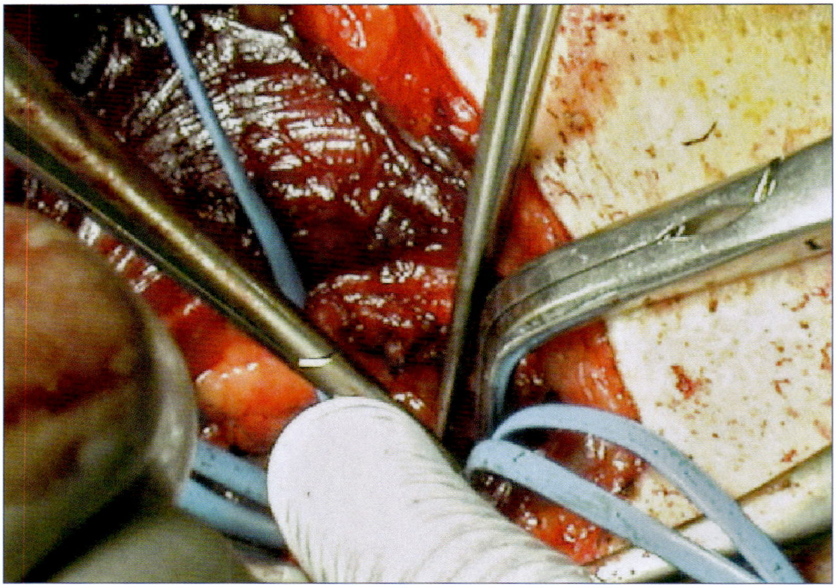

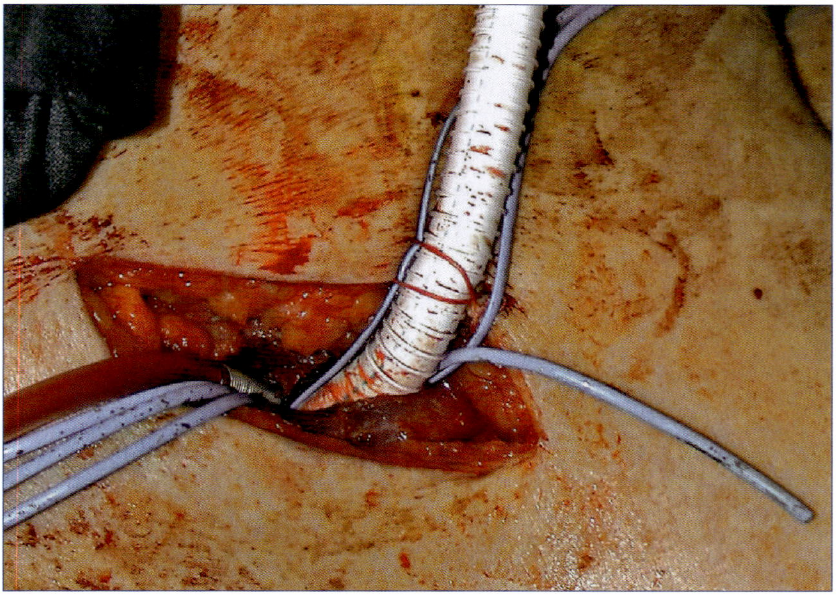

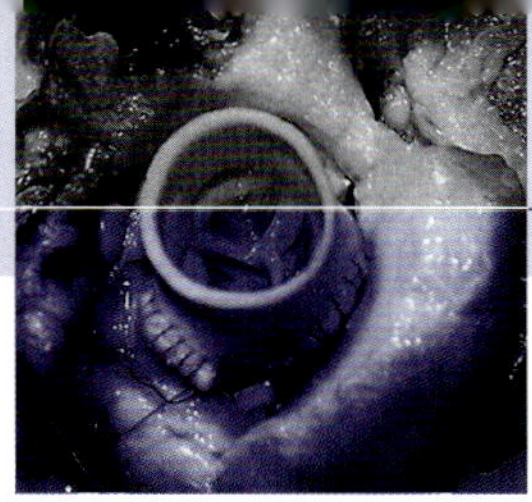

1 2 3 4 5 6 7 8 9 10 11 12 13 14 15

Subclavian artery cannulation via graft (Basel approach)
In our institution the following technique is preferred: The subclavian artery is opened between vessel clamps and a ring-inforced Goretex-graft is anastomosed to the vessel. Cannulation and connection to the CPB is done via this graft.

Option for intraoperative switching of the arterial cannulation site (arterial perfusion via A. subclavia is changed to ascending aortic graft)

Primary insertion of a Y-shaped connector between the subclavian artery cannula and the arterial pump line facilitates a potential connection of another arterial cannula to the aortic prosthesis at later time points intraoperatively.

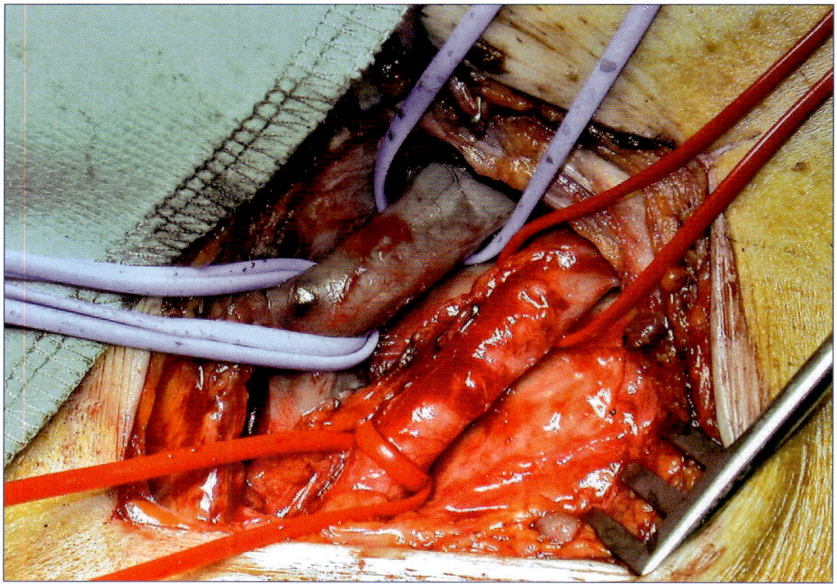

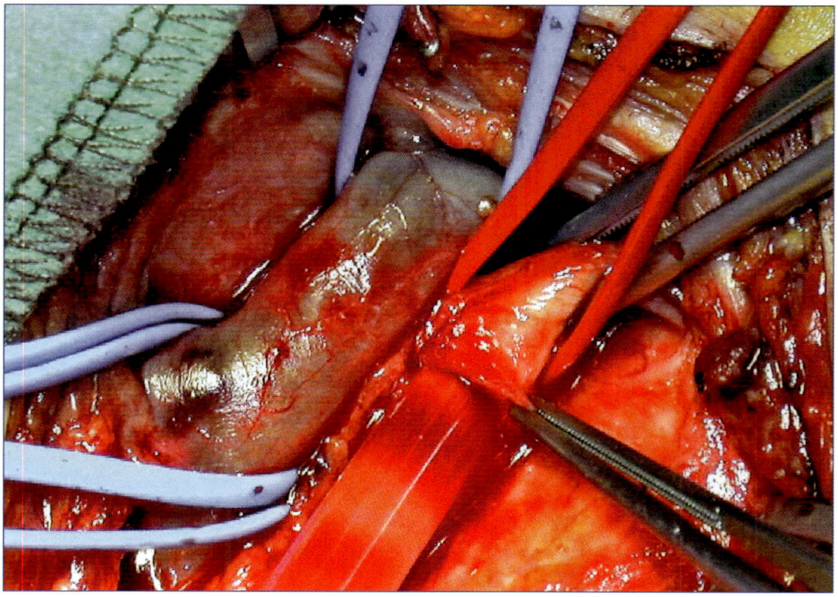

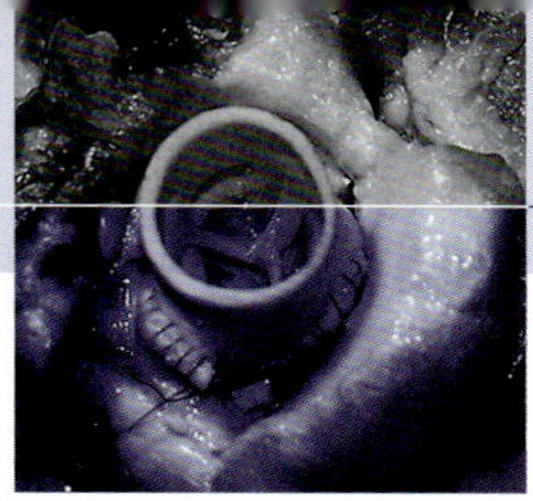

Standard Femoral Cannulation

Common femoral artery as well as femoral vein are dissected and exposed in the groin and secured with vessel-loops.

After incision of the artery the vessel is carefully dilated using an Overholt clamp, and a short arterial perfusion cannula is inserted. The cannula is secured by fixation to the skin.

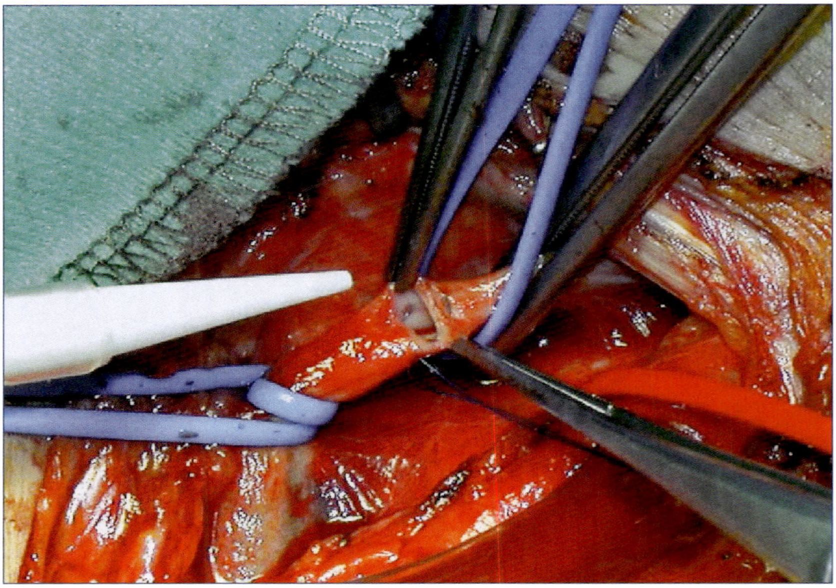

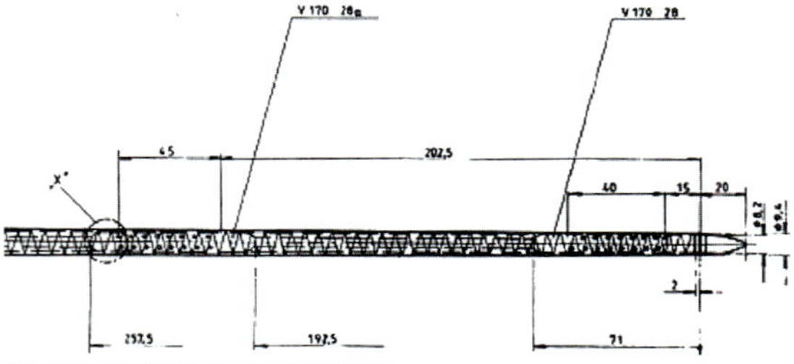

Abb. 1: Intrakorporaler Anteil des venösen Leistenkatheters

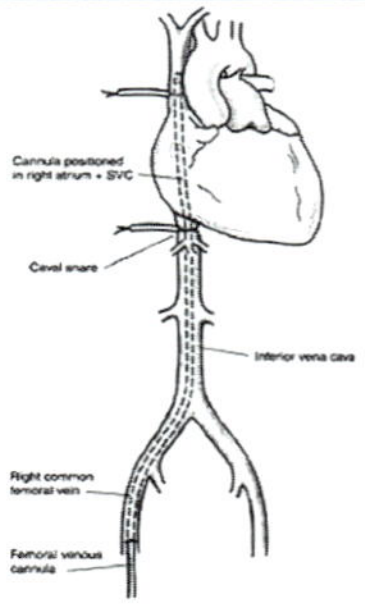

Merke: Das betroffene Bein nimmt „funktionell" nicht am Kreislauf teil.

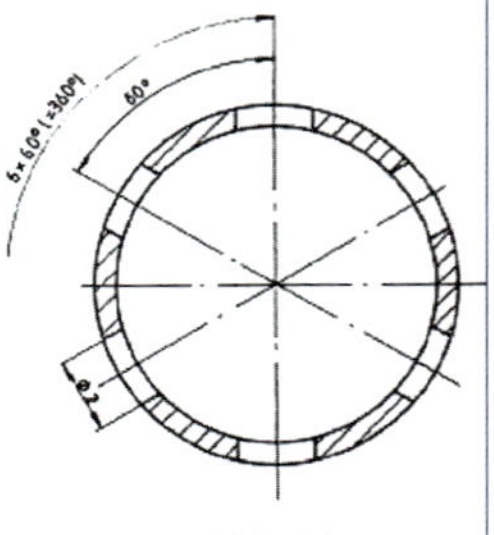

Doetsch et al. *Die extrathorakale venöse Kanülierung*

Aus der Abteilung für Thorax- und Kardiovaskuläre Chirurgie, Herzzentrum der Universität Essen

Die extrathorakale venöse Kanülierung

N. Doetsch, H.-R. Zerkowski, G. Roth, H. Schmidt, N. Sauerland, H. Hees, J. Graban

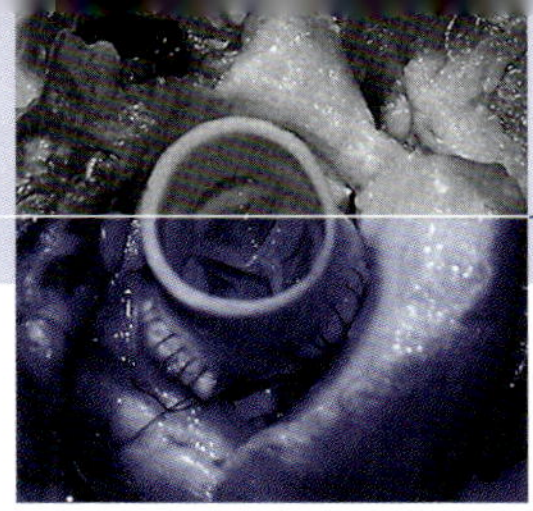

The femoral vein is incised identically. In our institution a 900-mm-standard cannula is inserted (the new Smart-cannula according to von Seggesser is an excellent alternative) using the specific dilatator and introducer set.
If there is any resistance in the pelvic region, the cannula has to be rotated by some degrees prior to further attempts. Usually it is possible to pass the iliac veins easily.
The resulting correct distance from the insertion site to the right atrium should be measured "on the surface" before cannulation.

For ideal venous return and decompression of the heart the tip of the venous cannula should be placed directly in the caval funnel (i.e. the orifice to the right atrium.

Important note for the perfusionist:
Even in the case of perfect positioning of all arterial and venous cannulae, studies have shown that it is impossible to reach the normal calculated "100%-flow" values (under normothemic conditions) with femoral cannulation.

1
2
3
4
5
6
7
8
9
10
11
12
13
14
15

Cannulation Techniques

H.-R. Zerkowski

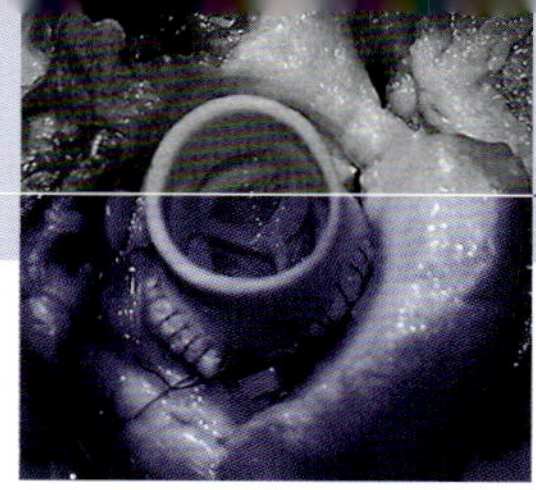

References

1. Kron JL, Smith CD. Cardiopulmonary bypass: access and technical options. in: Gardner TJ, Spray TL. Operative cardiac surgery, 5th ed., Arnold, London, 2004
2. Klövekorn WP, Meisner H, Sebening F. Technische Voraussetzungen der Herzchirurgie. In: Borst HG, Klinner W, Oelert H. Herzchirurgie. 2. Aufl., Springer, Berlin-Heidelberg-NewYork, 1991
3. Cooley DA. Techniques in cardiac surgery, 2nd ed., WB Saunders, Philadelphia, 1984
4. Pasic M, Schubel J, Bauer M, Yanhah C, Kuppe H, Weng Y-G, Hetzer R. Cannulation of the right axillary artery for surgery of acute type A aortic dissection. Eur J Cardio-ThoracSurg 2003; 24:231-36.

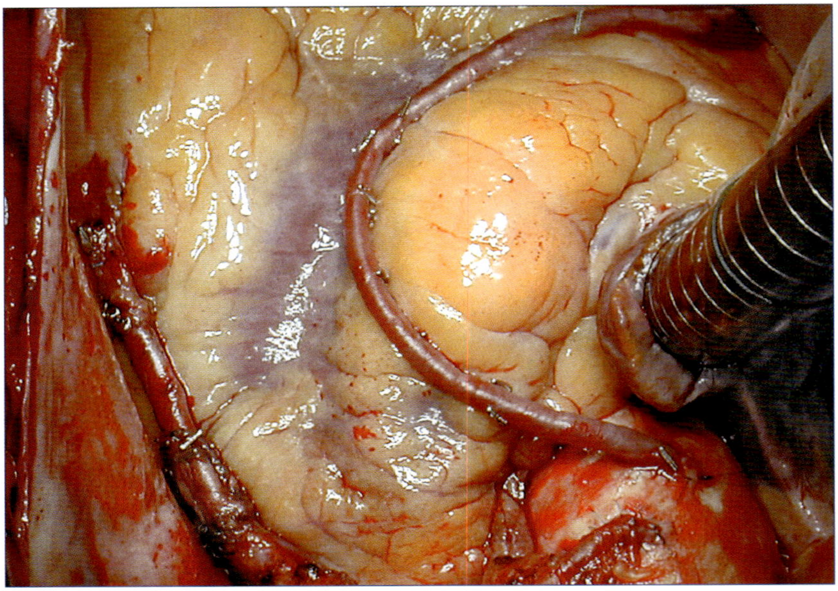

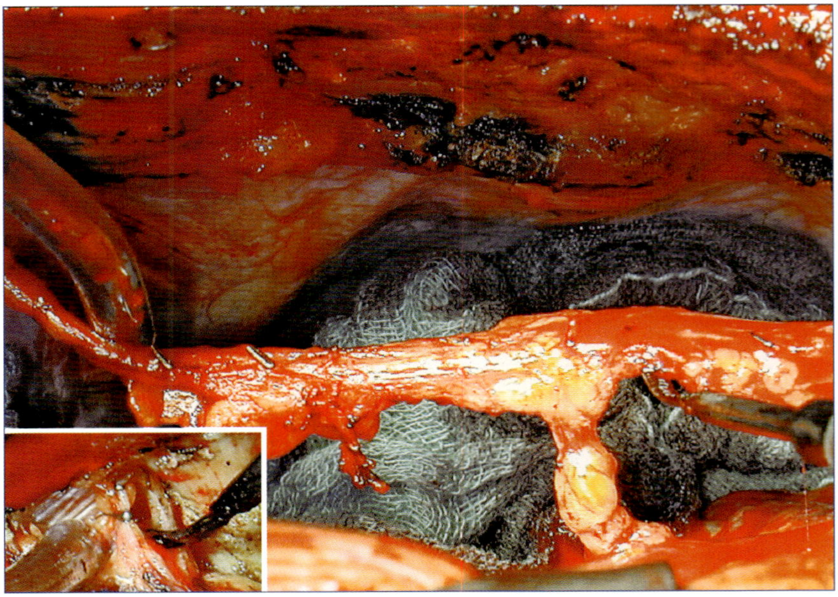

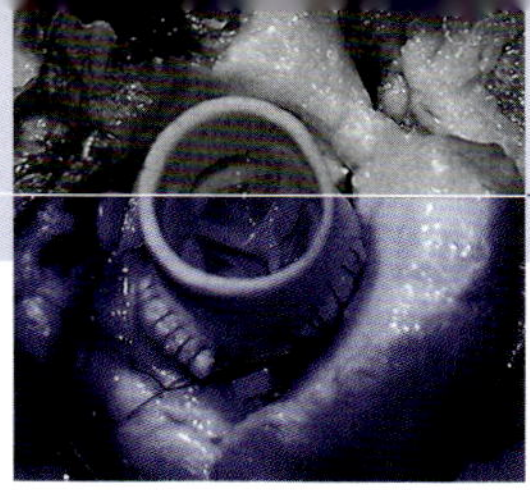

Standard Coronary Artery Revascularisation

J. M. Albes

Standard aorto-coronary bypass surgery utilizing the left internal mammarian artery (LIMA) as well as vein-grafts is still the most widely used revascularisation procedure. However, new strategies are being constantly incorporated into the established technique. Nowadays, the technique of coronary anastomosis, handling of grafts as well as detection and choice of appropriate anastomotic sites are all relevant for novel measures such as MIDCAB, OPCAB, or total arterial revascularisation and therefore represent an important armamentarium for the cardiac surgeon.

After median sternotomy the left internal mammarian artery (LIMA) is prepared with the electro-coagulator. This can be accomplished by preparing a so-called pedicle i.e. inclusion of the parietal pleura, the muscle fascia, and the accompanying veins. Side-branches to the thoracic wall require clipping or coagulation. Attention: Deep coagulation can damage the intercostal arteries, which are of paramount importance for blood supply of the left sternal half. Preparation can be performed either with the pleura open or closed. Evidence concerning an advantage of one particular technique over the other does not exist.

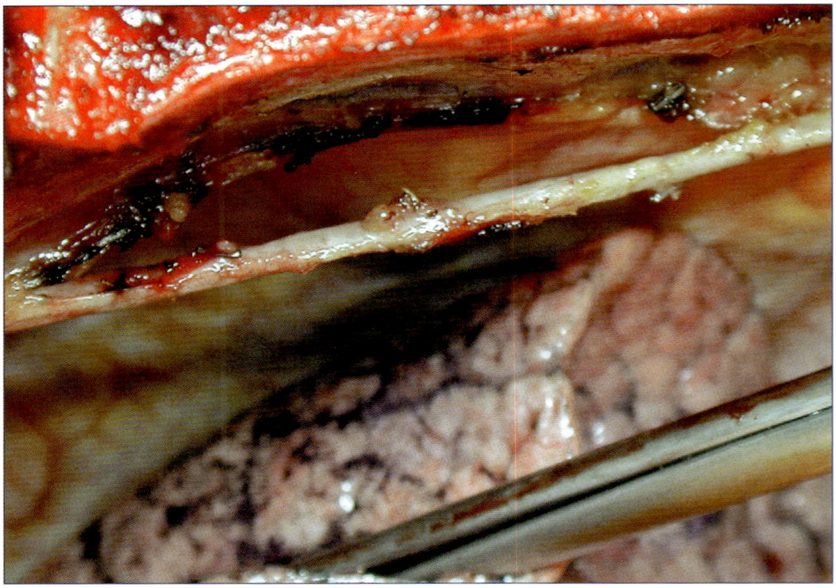

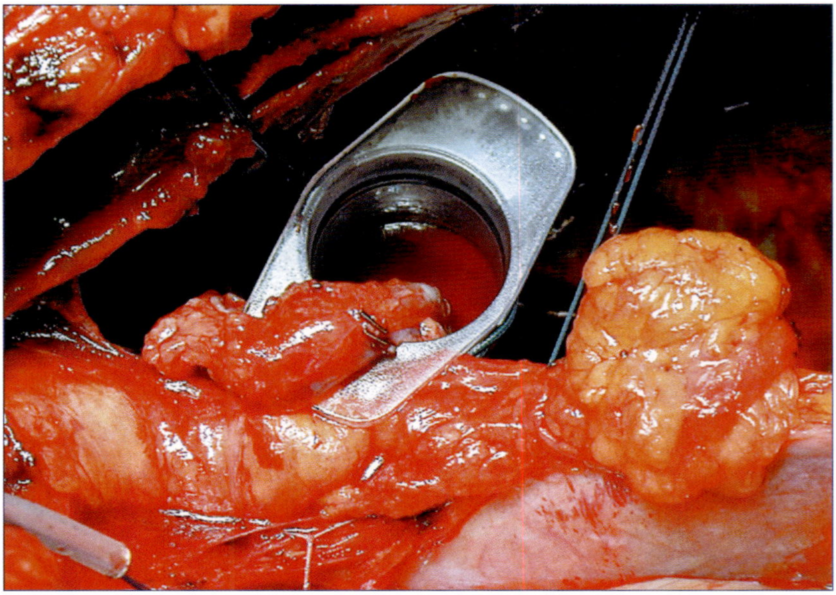

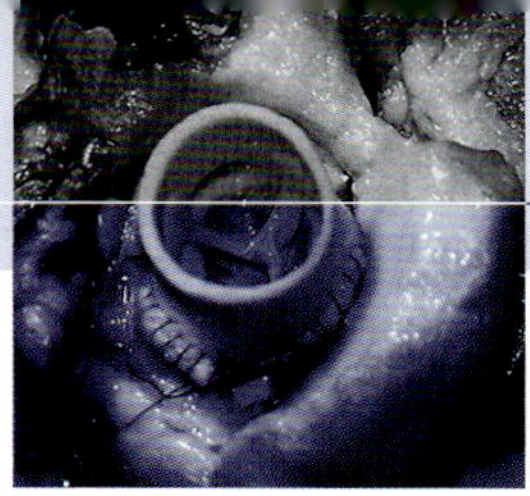

As an alternative, the LIMA can be prepared in a skeletonized fashion. The advantage is the resulting excessive length of the graft as well as a non-traumatic treatment of the thoracic wall, which may reduce sternal healing problems (sufficient evidence, however, does not exist). Attention: The skeletonized take-down needs to be subtle, because of the absence of the "cordon sanitaire" of the pedicle. A hot coagulator-knife for example can produce a thermal damage of the LIMA, which, if transmurally, can destroy the vessel.

After application of heparin (400 IE/kgBW) the LIMA is distally transsected, distally closed with a clip and submersed in a 20cc plugged syringe filled with . Other techniques of conditioning are clearly also feasible such as injection of Papaverin into the pedicle in close vicinity to the LIMA. An instillation of Papaverin directly into the vessel may damage the intima while a Papaverin-soaked compress wrapped around the pedicle does not provide sufficient dilation. Other vasodilating agents are also used. Papaverin, however, is preferred. Non-treatment of the LIMA is not recommended because it can result in spastic reaction and consecutive early flow-limitations.

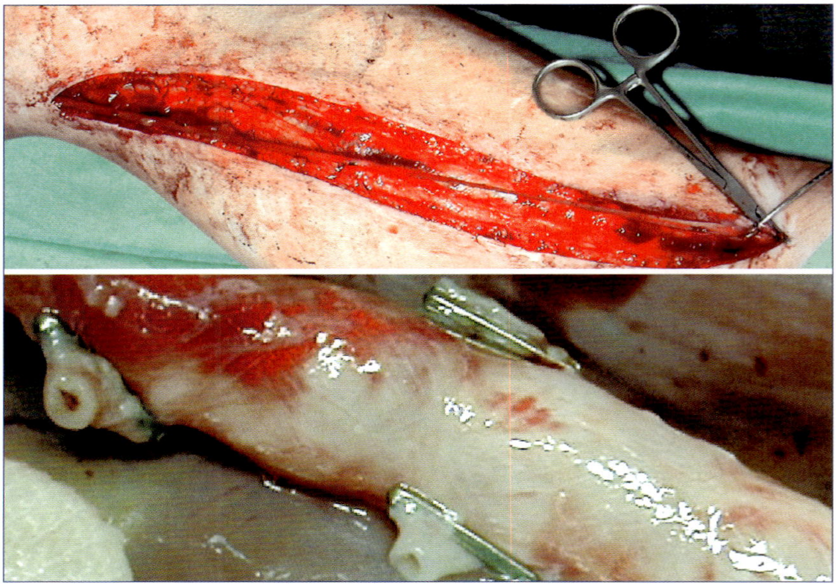

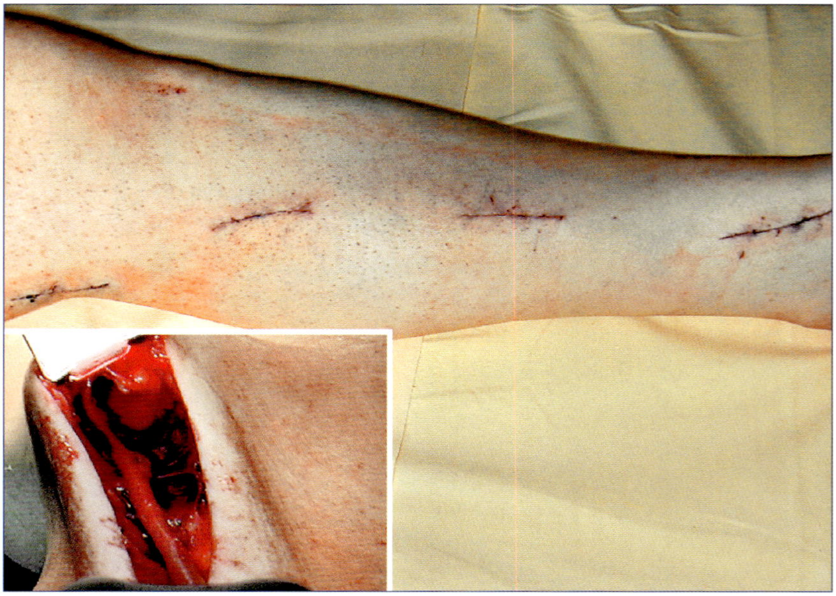

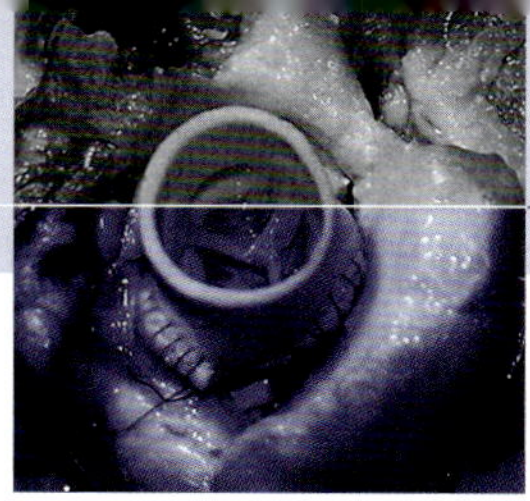

Vein-graft retrieval is carried out simultaneously. In the conventional, open technique the saphenus nerve can be clearly identified and spared. The vein must not be filled with more than physiological pressure of max. 150mmHg. Physiologic saline is favored over a blood/heparin-mixture (Evidence, however, does not exist). Utilization of a blunt cannula with an olive is recommended. The side-branches of the vein can be ligated (6/0 non-resorbable, braided thread) or clipped. Clips facilitate removal considerably. Two clips are better than one and reduce the danger of a slip-off. Attention: Clips must not be positioned too close to the vessel in order to avoid an "ourglass" stenosis.

As an alternative, less-invasive vein-graft removal can be performed by means of interrupted incisions. This can be accomplished entirely without any special instruments utilizing a Zenker-retractor and a headlight. Healing of the leg is enhanced after such a technique in contrast to the open approach. Attention: Avulsion of the side-branches underneath the skin-bridges can occur. The vein is an important graft and must not be destroyed because of negligence. An otherwise necessary removal from the contralateral leg can thus be avoided facilitating an eventual redo-procedure.

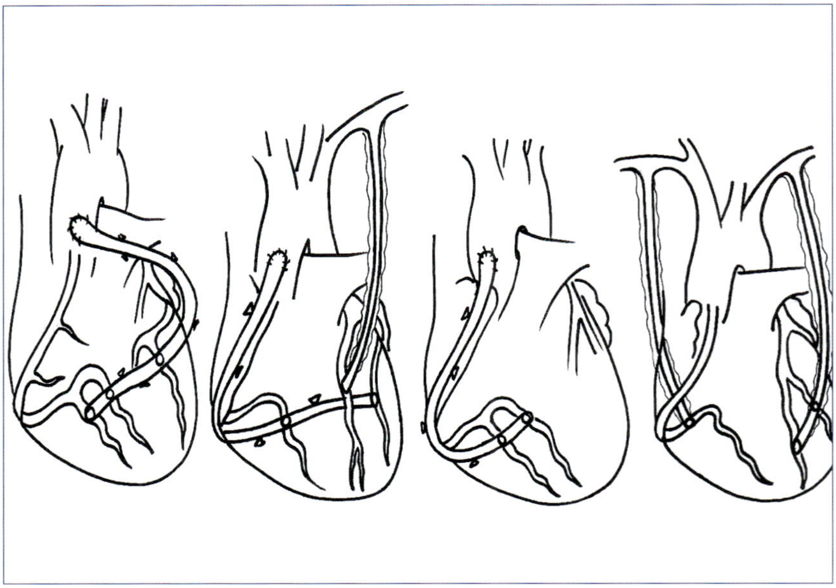

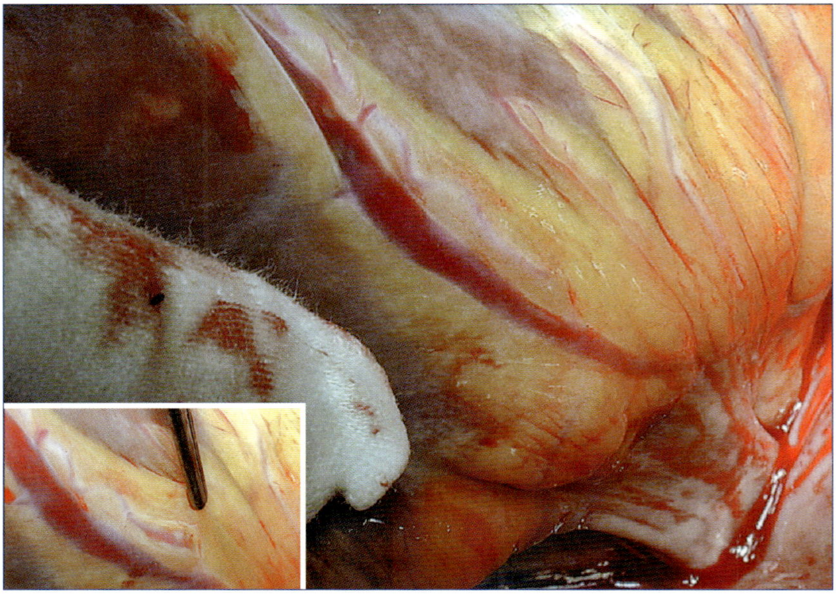

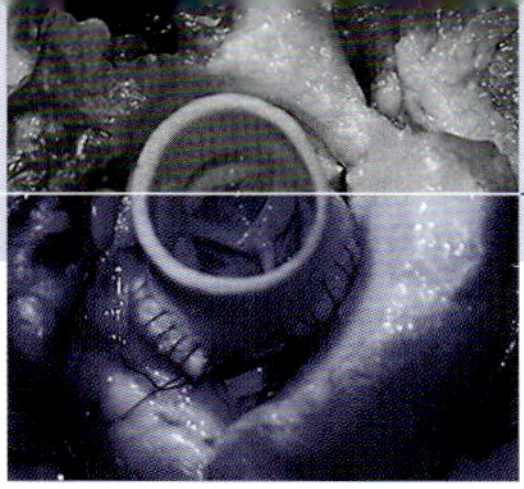

Strategies of revascularisation are manifold. It is, however, generally understood that the LIMA needs to be anastomosed to the most important vessel owing to the far superior long-term patency of the LIMA in contrast to all other material. Typically, the LAD is the leading vessel. As an exception, a large marginal branch may be chosen. So-called jump-grafts (LIMA to LAD end to side and diagonal branch side to side) can not be readily recommended, because the optimal positioning of the LIMA is jeopardized for the purpose of Revascularisation of a subsidiary vessel.

Vein grafts can clearly be anastomosed entirely in an end to side fashion for every single coronary vessel. Sequential grafts, however, have their merits. They require less length and usually allow higher flows. Attention: One poor anastomosis can jeopardize the entire construction. Distortion of a side to side anastomosis with flattening and kinking is not rare. Single vein grafts are more robust in this regard. The region of the proximal anastomosis should be chosen carefully already at the beginning of the procedure. The cardioplegic cannula can already define one of the future sites.

Preparation of the vessels is a prudent task. Epicardial exposition is much safer while the heart stands still because unpleasant lateral lesions of the coronary artery as well as lacerations of the accompanying vein do occur every so often when preparing under beating conditions. An orienting inspection of the vessels, however, can be made prior to cardioplegic arrest while the heart is still beating.

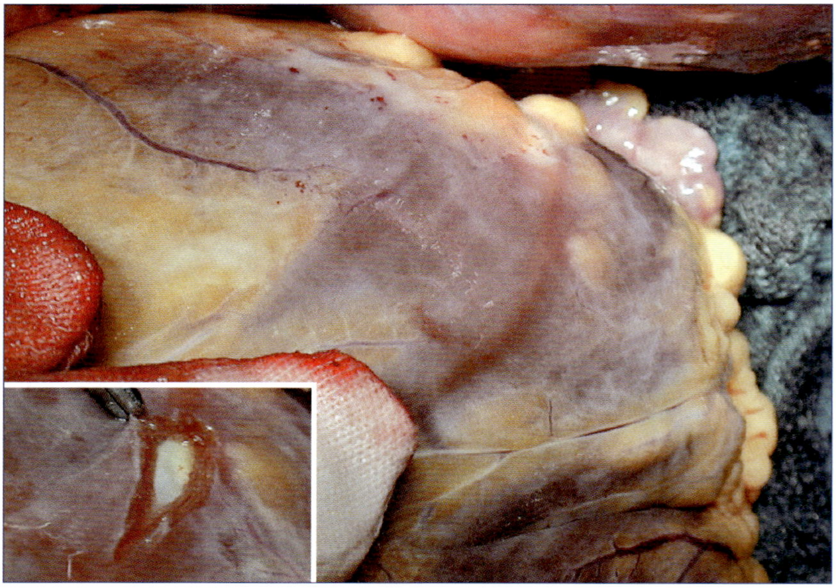

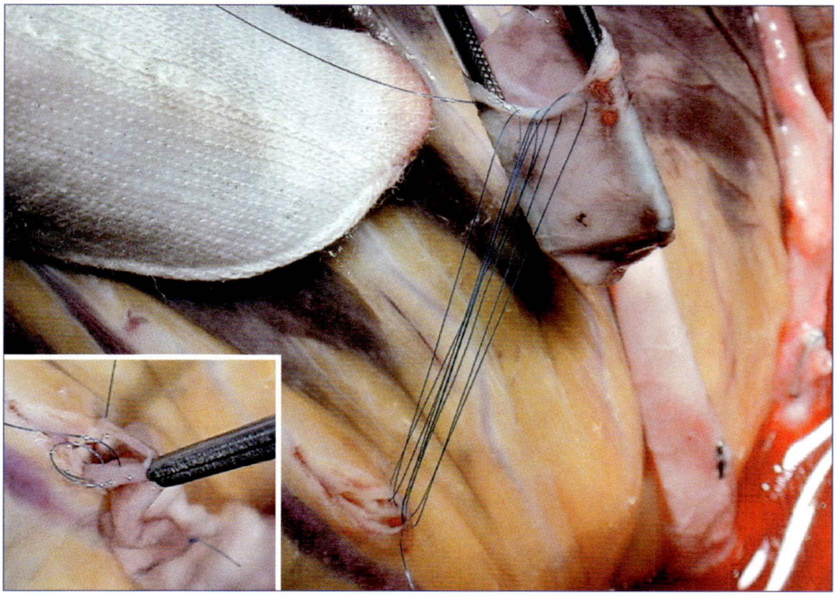

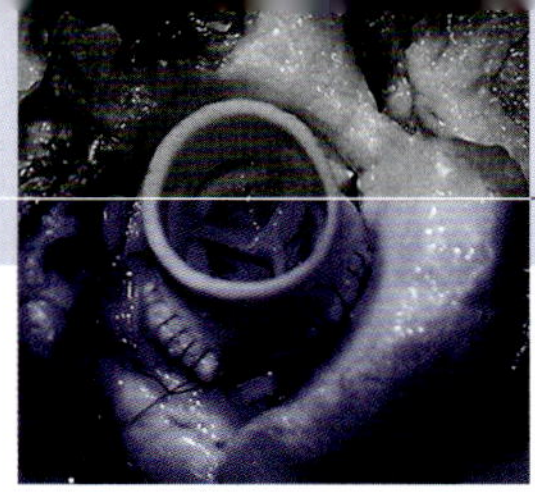

In some cases the coronary vessels exhibit an intramyocardial course. In these instances, it is absolutely mandatory to prepare these vessels during arrest. The myocardium of the suspected site is incised with utmost care until the anterior wall of the vessel is reached. Attention: Intramyocardial coronary arteries often show a much thinner wall than typical epicardial vessels.

The end to side anastomosis is performed with a 7/0 polypropylene suture in a running fashion. After longitudinal incision of the coronary vessel the first assistant stabilizes the vein-graft with two forceps. 5–6 sutures are passed around the heel of the vein-graft and the proximal pole of the incision in a distant fashion. Thereafter, the vein-graft is lowered onto the coronary artery by gently pulling the sutures. The sutures are then tightened. The anastomosis can now be completed. It is recommended to pass the needle always from the inside to the outside of the coronary vessel in order to avoid dislocation of calcified plaque material into the coronary lumen. As a consequence, a redirection of the suture is necessary in case of a change of the needle. Completion of the anastomosis around the toe needs to be meticulously performed. The concavity of the needle can be used as a sled. Sliding on the posterior wall of the vessel with free-floating tip of the needle can securely pass the coronary wall from inside to outside avoiding accidental pick-up of the posterior wall. Careful probing prior to completion of the anastomosis with a 1mm probe is valuable to ensure adequate maintenance of the inner lumen. A well-performed end to side anastomosis exhibits an angle of 30°.

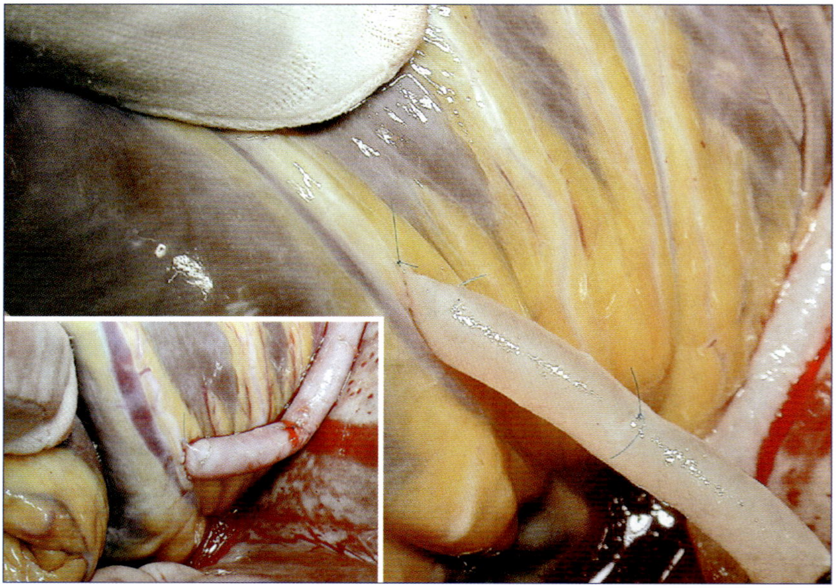

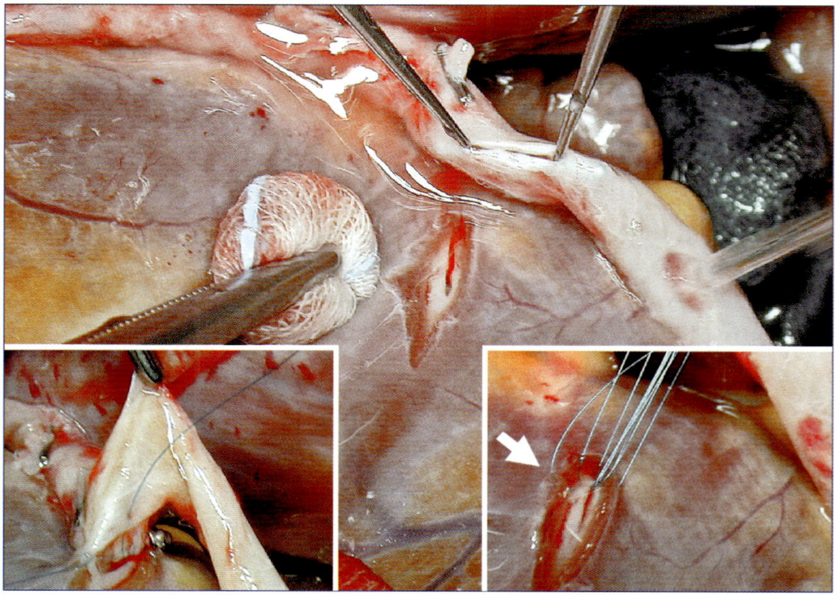

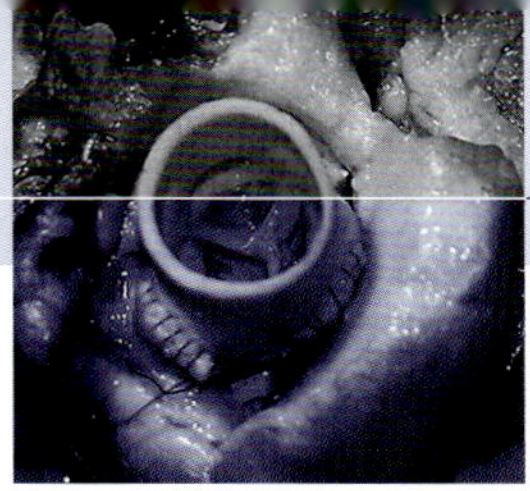

Testing of patency and tightness is carried out with physiologic saline. If the anastomosis is tight under these conditions it will certainly be tight if perfused with blood. During the next cardioplegic shot the heart is lifted gently in order to verify tightness. In case of doubt tightness can be tested using blood-cardioplegia applied directly via the graft with adequate perfusion pressure. Attention: The perfusionist must be provided with the information of an isolated vein-graft perfusion to be carried out.

A side to side anastomosis of a sequential graft is performed in a diamond-shaped fashion. Attention: Do not incise too liberally (rule of thumb: 2/3 of the length of an end to side anastomosis) in order to avoid flattening. The first assistant ideally stabilizes the vein with two nerve-hooks while hovering 3 to 4 cm above the field. The first 5 stitches are carried out on distance (1 lateral length of the incision of the vein equals the circumference of the heel of the coronary vessel). After approximation the suture will be completed. Attention has to be turned to the toe of the anastomosis. Pick-up of adjacent epimyocardium improves tightness of the lateral parts of the anastomosis. Control does not only verify tightness and patency but also lumen-congruent positioning. A marked flattening can not be tolerated. If the anastomosis is to be preserved two strategies are worthwhile. Accomplishment of a functional end to side anastomosis: The vein graft will be double-clipped distally and transsected. The distal part of the graft carrying the end-to side anastomosis then need to be extended. Alternatively, the vein can be incised directly above the anastomosis and can be augmented with a vein-patch plasty. Attention: excoriating the adventitia of the vein-graft with a preparation knife or dissection of fibers with coronary scissors can provoke secondary rupture.

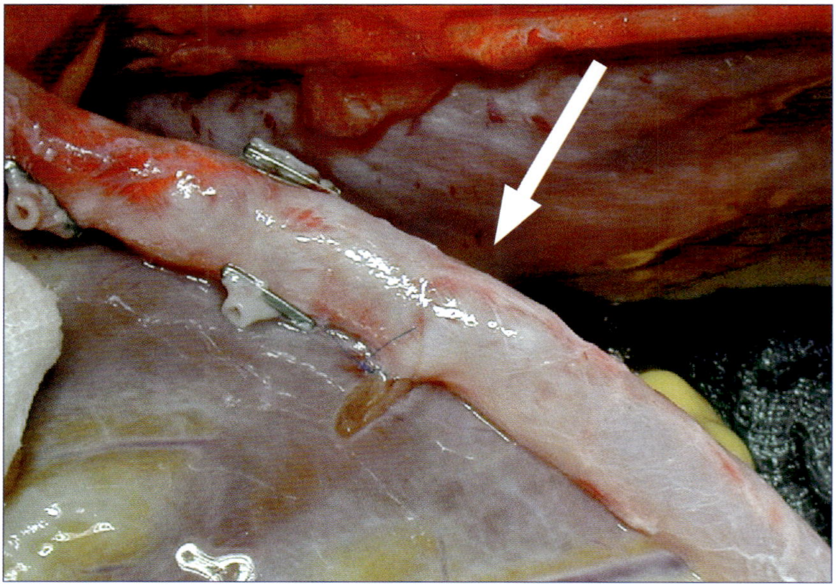

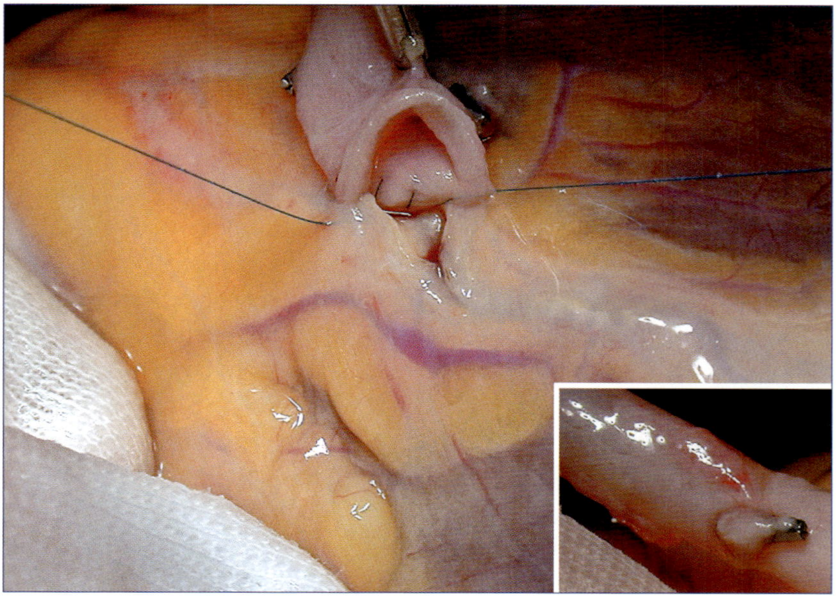

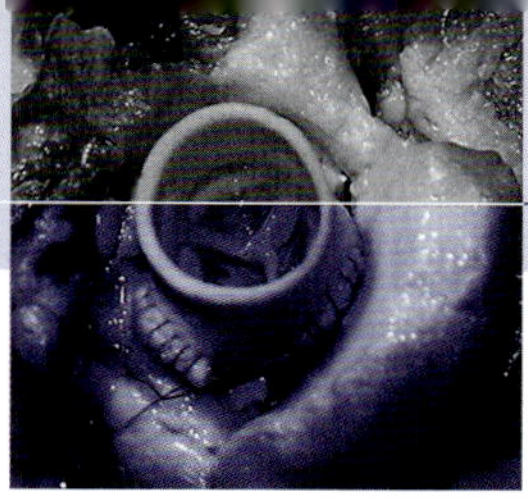

Testing for tightness and patency as well as congruent positioning.

The diagonal branch should only be incorporated into a sequential graft as an exception, because the anastomotic site of the diagonal branch differs much from the marginal branches provoking a kinked course of the sequential graft. An end to side anastomosis of a vein-graft with the diagonal branch can be performed with ease. An underlying towel is helpful for proper exposition. Because of the exposition and the rather subordinate importance of the diagonal branch such an anastomosis can very well be performed by a junior resident to enhance motivation.

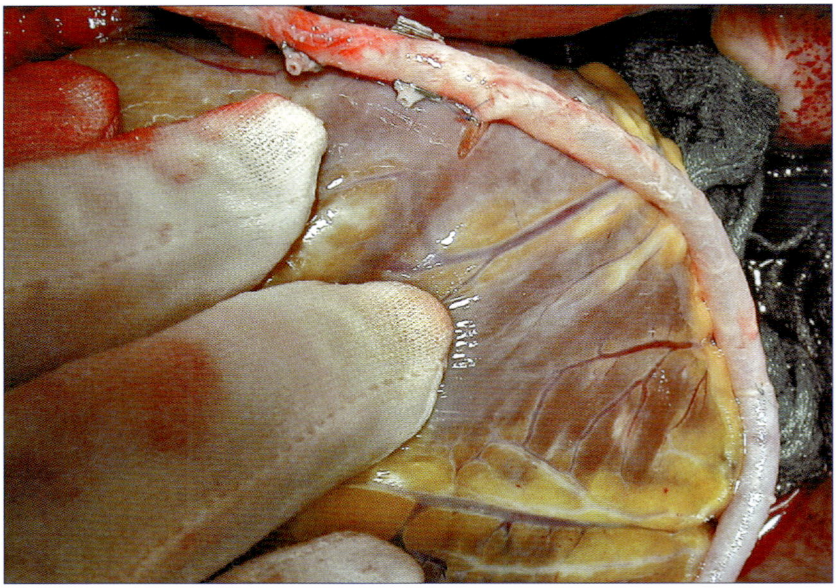

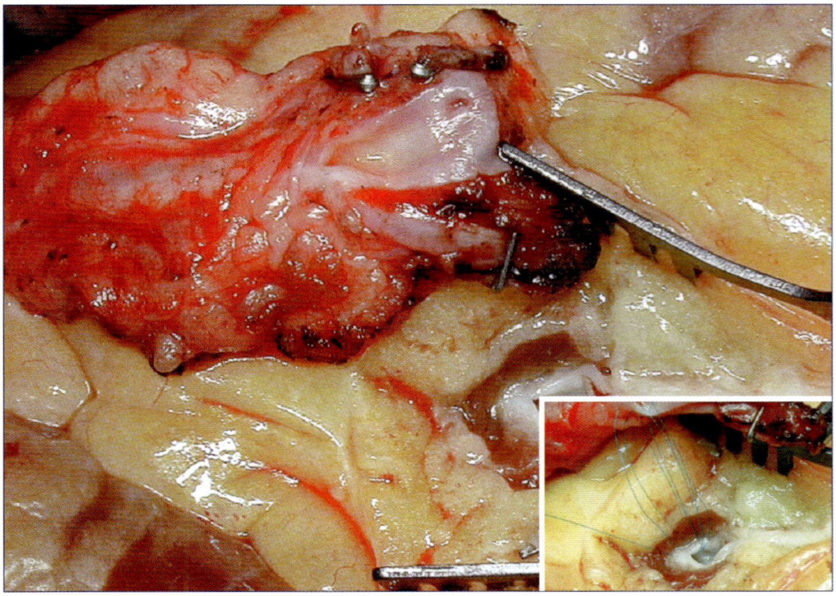

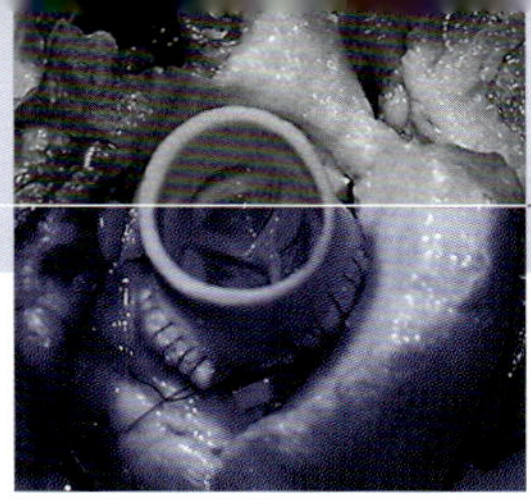

Control of the entire sequential graft is carried out with slightly luxated heart in order to mimic the regular filling state. A slight excess of length is acceptable. A significant excess, however, can provoke kinking. This can be avoided by fixing the graft with fibrin glue in a meandering fashion.

After exposition of the LAD typically in the middle portion (in case of an intramyocardial position of the vessel use of a small fat-retractor is recommended {figure}). The LIMA is taken out of the syringe, the distal portion of the pedicle with the clip in place is transsected and discarded. Flow through the LIMA should now be excellent. The LIMA is temporarily closed with a bulldog-clamp. Thereafter, the LIMA is incised longitudinally. This incision can by all means be performed on the anterior wall of the vessel opposite to the fascia, because only little excessive tissue need to be prepared. The LIMA can tolerate a half-twist around the longitudinal axis without any problem. The anastomosis is carried out in a subtle manner with 7/0 or 8/0 polypropylene suture in a running fashion. The heel will be sutured first at distance.

1
2
3
4
5
6
7
8
9
10
11
12
13
14
15

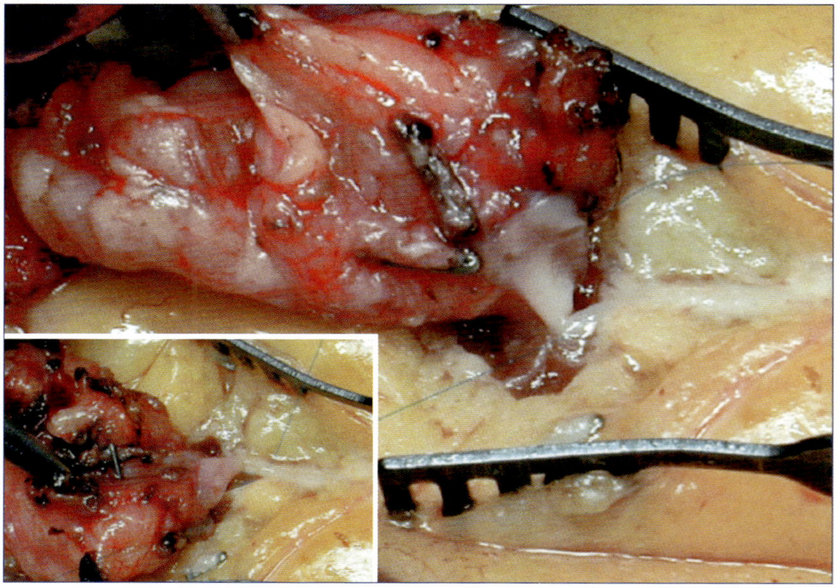

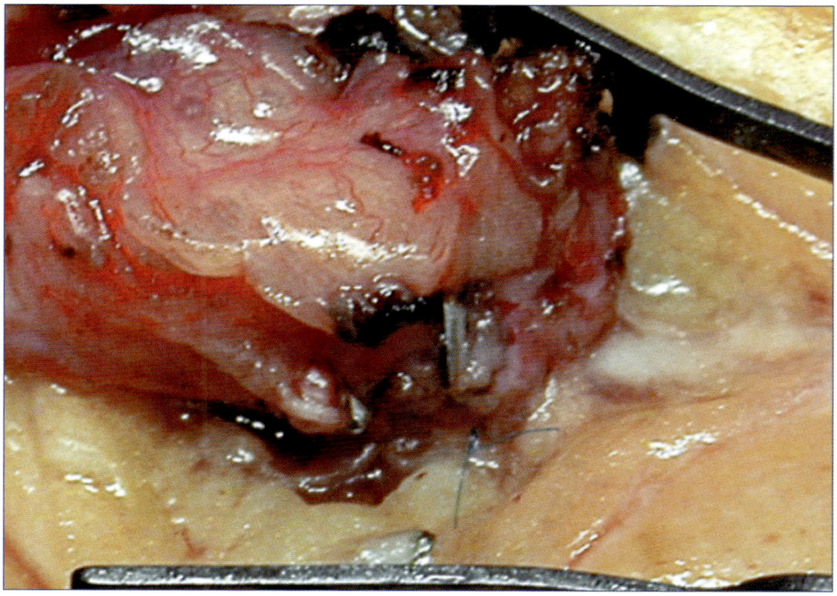

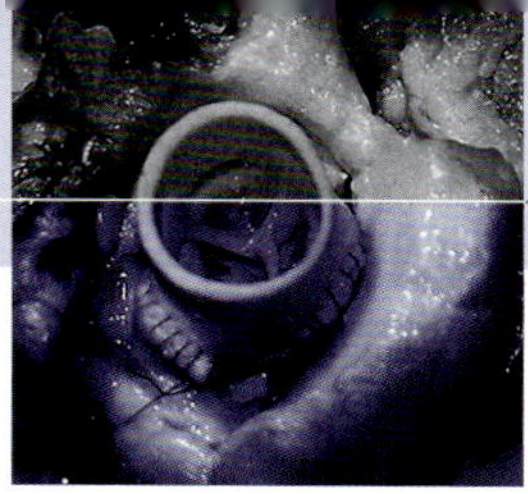

Thereafter the LIMA is approximated and the suture is completed. Prior to knotting the bulldog-clamp is removed in order to verify unimpeded inflow.

Only now the sutures are knotted thereby verifying tightness by observing cessation of oozing. The pedicle should be attached to the epicardium with two 5/0 polypropylene sutures in order to avoid torsion.

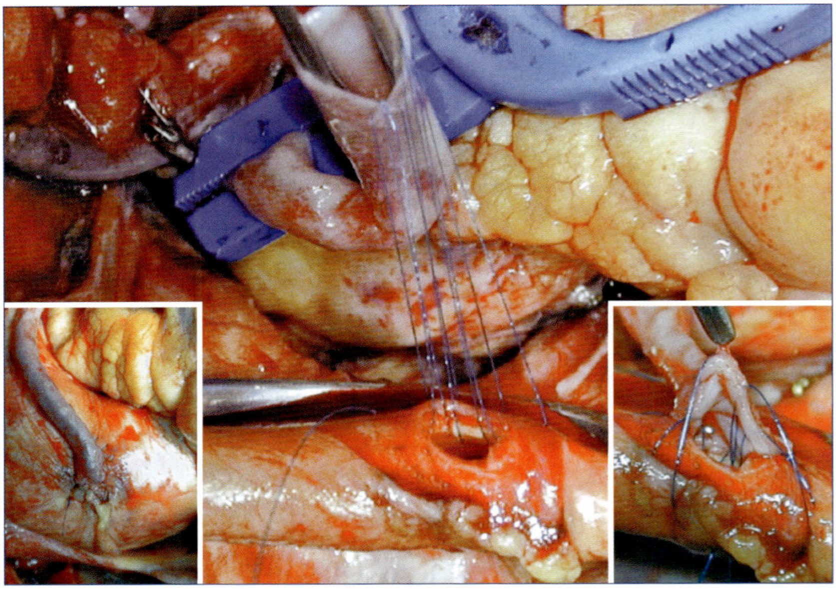

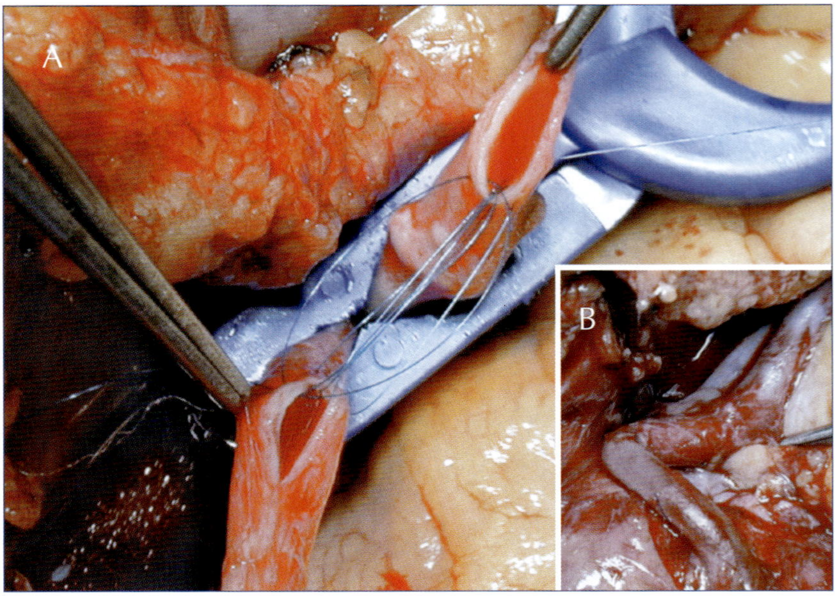
A
B

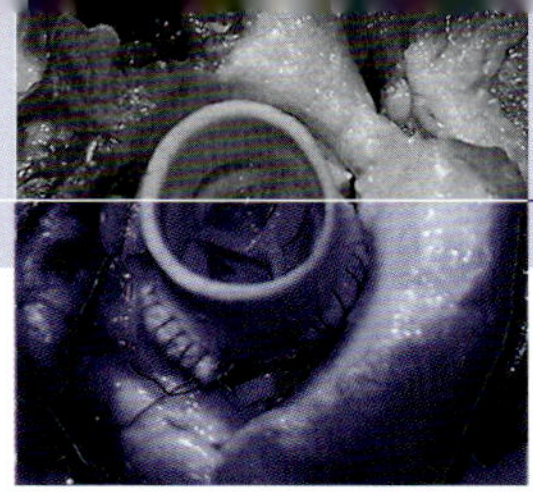

After removal of the X-clamp the length of the vein-graft is measured. In case of uncertainty concerning the diameter of the pulmonary artery the heart is temporarily filled by reducing venous drainage. The length can then be securely verified, the vessel is shortened and incised longitudinally. Only now side-clamping and punching of the wall is performed. The vein-graft is anastomosed to the aorta with 6/0 polypropylene sutures in a running-fashion. The first 5 stitches are carried out at distance. The vessel is approximated and the anastomosis is completed. Prior to removal of the bulldog-clamp the graft is deaired with a small needle. Air bubbles can be easily visualized through the translucent wall of the vein-graft. Thereafter the Bulldog-clamp is removed. A perfect proximal anastomosis should resemble a cobra head.

Sometimes the graft happens to be too short for a tension-free anastomosis. In these instances a Y-anastomosis is recommended. The already anastomosed graft is again closed with a bulldog-clamp and incised longitudinally. The short vein-graft is also incised. An end to side anastomois is then performed with 7/0 polypropylene running suture. The heel is stitched at distance. After approximation the anastomosis is completed. The entire graft is again deaired (both arms!) and the bulldog-clamps are released. Such a Y-anastomosis can also be useful if the ascending aorta is calcified and space for another proximal anastomosis is limited. Finally, all anastomoses will be inspected while the pump is still running.

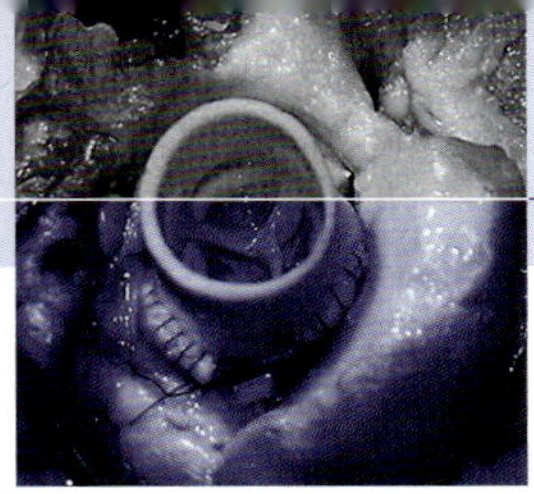

References

1. Kolessov VJ. Mammary artery-coronary anastomosis as a method of treatment for angina pectoris. J Thorac Cardiovasc Surg 1967; 54:535
2. Vavaloro RG. Saphenous vein autograft replacement of severe segmental coronary artery occlusion. Ann Thorac Surg 1968; 5:334
3. Green GE. Rate of blood flow from the internal mammary artery. Surgery 1971; 70:809
4. Berger PB. et al. BARI-Trial - Survival after CABG > PTCA-2 and 3-Vessel disease, LAD-involvement, LV-Dysfunction. J Am Coll Cardiol 2001; 38: 1440–9
5. Van Dijk D. et al. OPCAB vs. CABG – comparable results. Circulation 2001; 104: 1761–6
6. Abizaid A. et al. ARTS-Trial. CABG > PTCA in diabetic multivessel patients. Circulation 2001; 104: 533–8
7. Smith KM. et al. Octogenarians do profit from CABG CMAJ 2001; 165: 759–64
8. Vural KM. et al. Long-term patency of sequential and individual saphenous vein coronary bypass grafts. Eur J Cardiothorac Surg 2001; 19: 1040–4

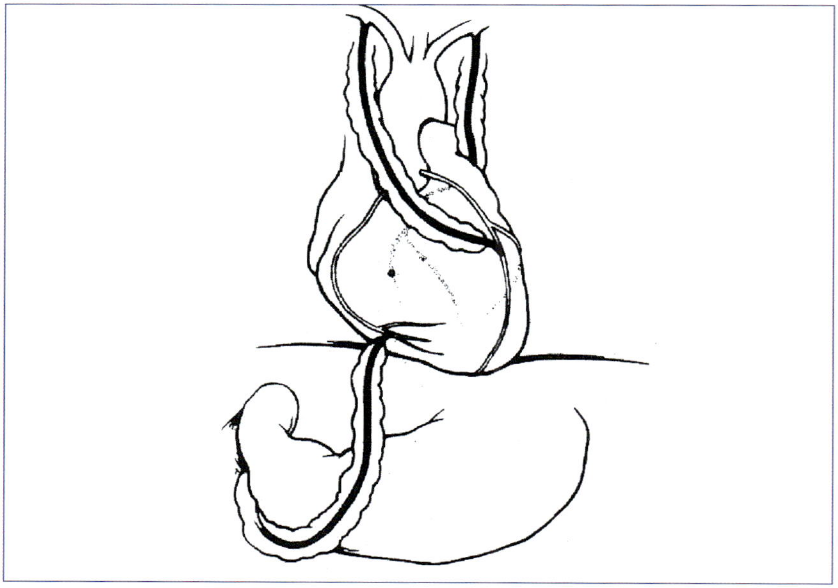

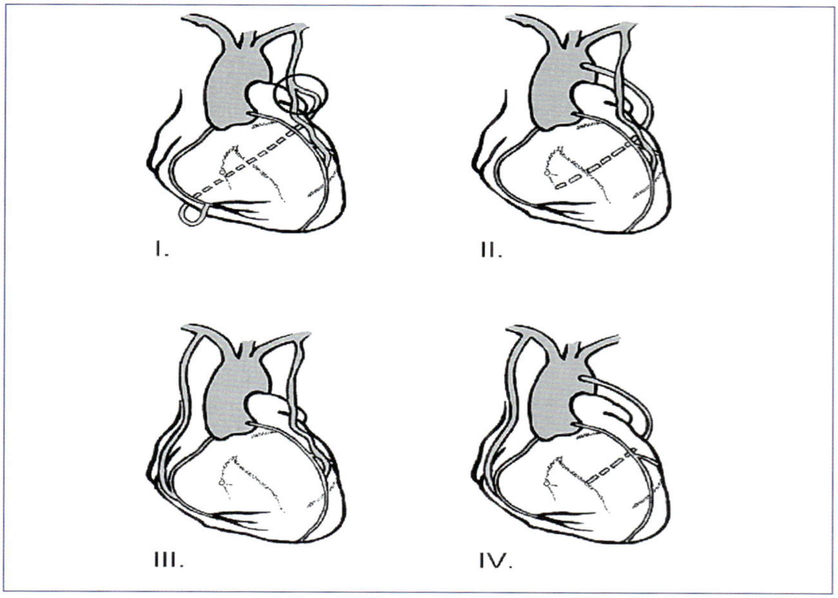
I.
II.
III.
IV.

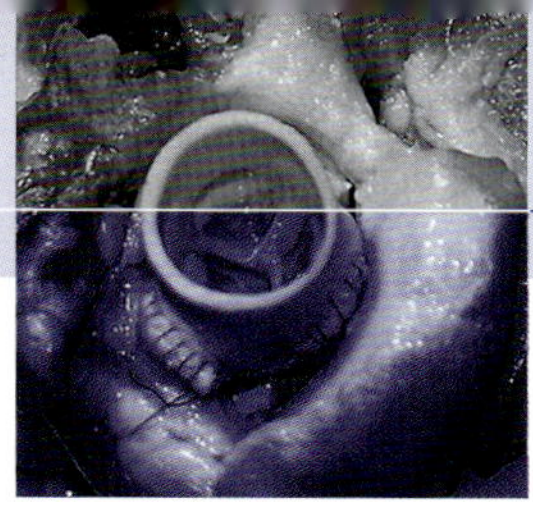

Total Arterial Revascularisation

Ch. Rajakaruna • O. Wendler

Coronary artery bypass grafting (CABG) using arterial conduits (gold standard is the internal thoracic artery/ITA) has been shown to result in improved long-term results. The indication for total arterial revascularisation is seen to be of prognostic benefit in patients with a life expectancy of more than 10 years (patient age ≤70 years) or in the presence of missing appropriate venous conduits. Complete arterial revascularisation can be achieved using multiple arterial conduits (picture above) or using two arterial grafts (picture below). Although the gastro-epiploic artery has the advantage that it can be used in a pedicle fashion, the radial artery (RA) is the preferred additional arterial graft by most surgeons, due to its advantages: 1. No laparotomy. 2. No risk of post operative abdominal angina. 3. The long-term results of the RA are discussed less controversially.

At present there is no consense about which of the two surgical techniques (multivessel vs. two vessel) can be recommended. The operation using multiple arterial conduits (figure above) has the disadvantages of: 1. Longer operation time. 2. It leaves fewer arterial conduits for potential repeat operations. 3. It makes an anastomosis of free arterial grafts to the ascending aorta more likely. 4. The right ITA often crosses the ascending aorta. Using two arterial conduits, with both ITAs or ITA and RA, a complete arterial revascularisation is feasible. However, the total flow in the bypass grafts with the "T"-graft configuration (picture I) is dependent on the blood flow in the left ITA, which can be a potential disadvantage. We describe the operation using a "T"-graft technique in detail as it is the most recent surgical innovation.

1
2
3
4
5
6
7
8
9
10
11
12
13
14
15

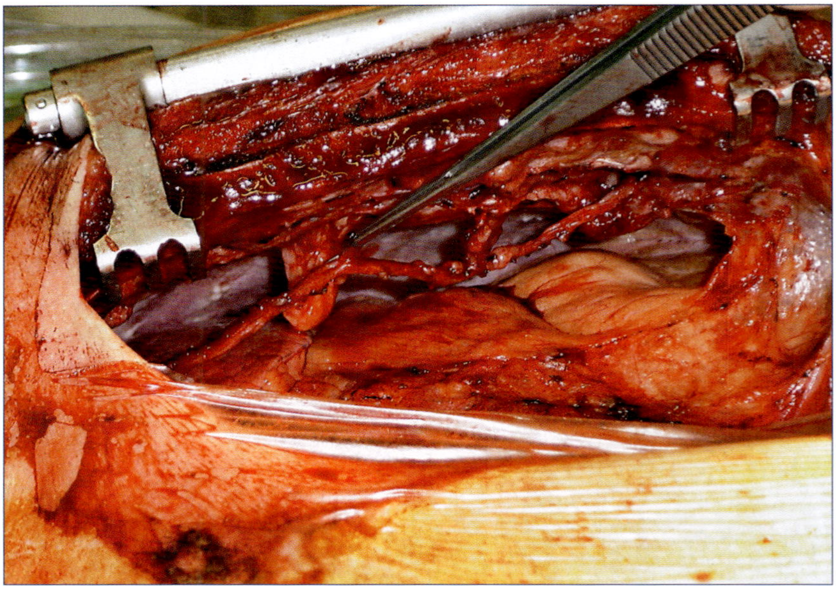

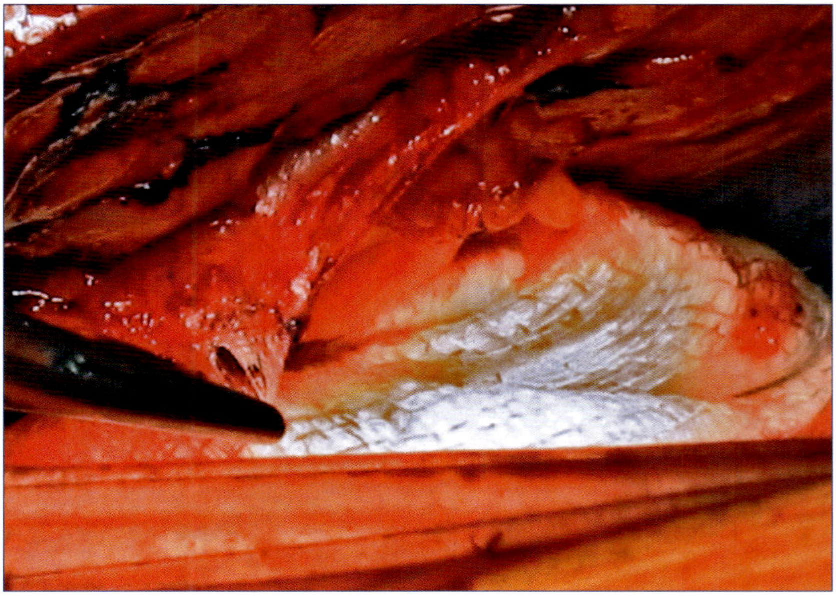

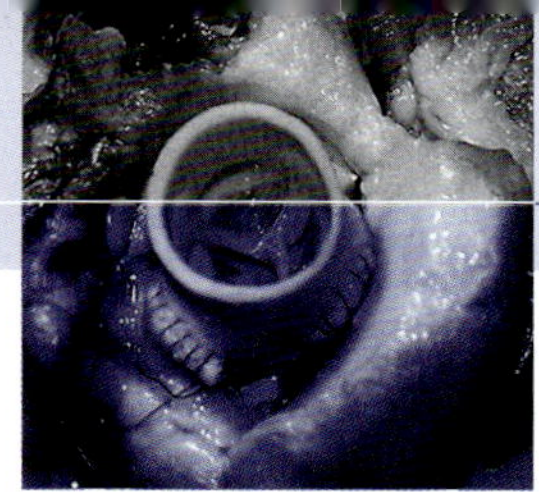

Low peri-operative morbidity and mortality are the basis for improved long-term results after total arterial revascularisation. It is considered, that the skeletonized harvesting technique of the ITA (dissecting the artery out of it's surrounding tissue as shown in the picture) can reduce the risk of sternal wound infections and improve respiratory recovery, particularly in patients where both ITAs are harvested and who are diabetic. Compared to the conventional harvesting technique, the skeletonized ITA offers: 1. more length. 2. greater diameter. 3. Maximized free blood flow. This is of advantage in patients with "T" grafts and makes the construction of sequential anastomosis, technically more feasible. The long-term results do not differ between the two techniques.

To achieve reproducible results with skeletonisation it is mandatory to have a standardised surgical technique. After the parietal pleura is dissected from the endothoracic fascia (the pleura can be kept closed) the quality of the ITA can be assessed. The endothoracic fascia is now opened in the 3rd intercostal space, approximately 5–8mm medial to the internal thoracic vein. This incision extends proximally to the subclavian vein and distally into the bifurcation of the ITA. If the diathermy is used, the energy should be reduced and some distance should be kept from the ITA to avoid the risk of thermal damage. Now, the internal thoracic vein can be pushed upwards, behind it, the ITA can be seen and it's surrounding connective tissue can be opened using a fine scissors. This exposes the anterior and dorsal branches of the ITA.

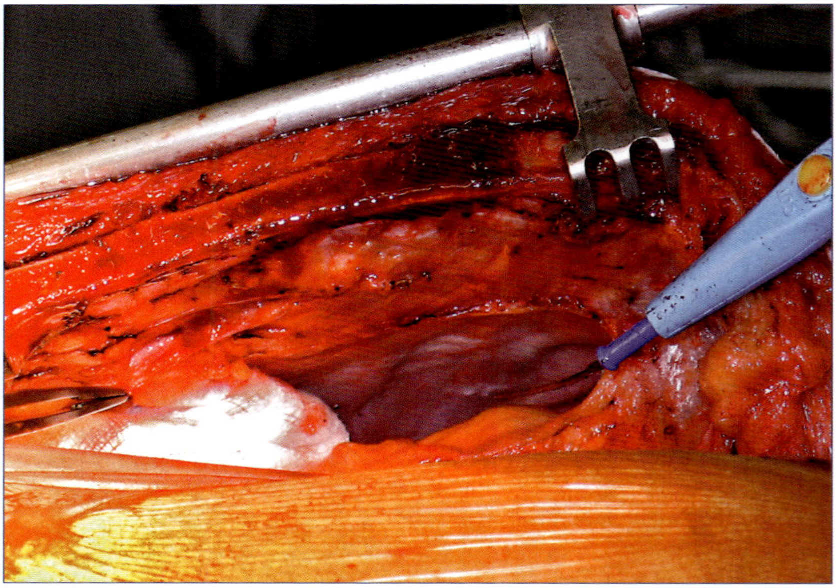

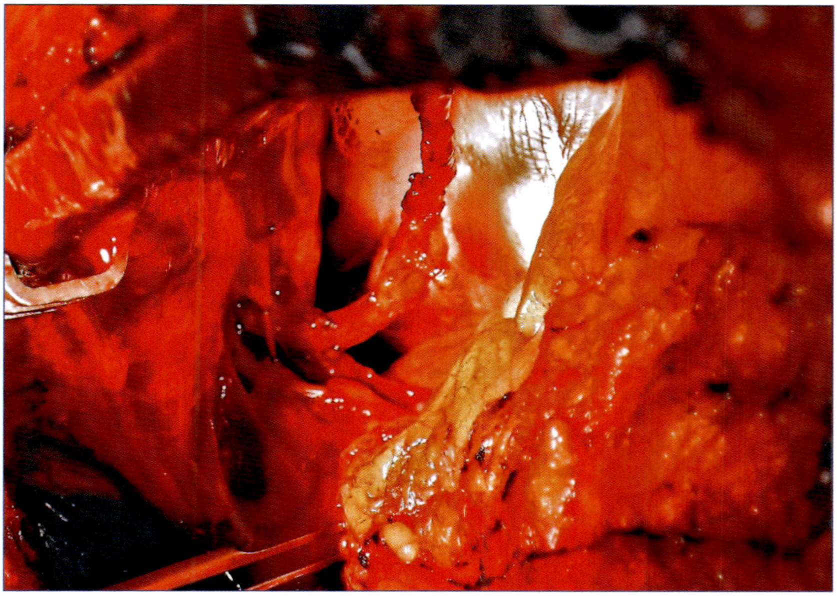

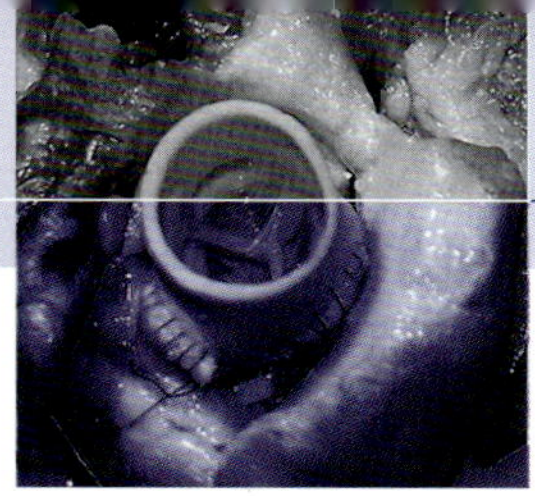

Using forceps the endothoracic fascia, which is still attached to the ITA, is now pulled away from the chest wall, exposing the side branches of the ITA better. These then can be dissected using fine scissors and ligated with hemoclips. If the ITA has previously become detached from the fascia, it is possible to use forceps to push the ITA downwards exposing the branches. The ITA should never be directly grasped with the forceps to prevent trauma to the vessel and reduce the risk of vasospasm. Proximally the internal thoracic vein crosses the ITA (normally anterior to the ITA). After this vein is dissected it becomes much easier to identify the proximal ITA.

Particular attention has to be paid to the phrenic nerve (normally dorsal and medial to the proximal ITA). The risk of damage is even higher on the right ITA because it crosses the phrenic nerve more distally compared to the left. Proximally the dissection should go beyond the subclavian vein, enabling ligation of the first pericardial and intercostal branches which is important to maximize free blood flow through the conduit. This extended preparation moves the left ITA closer to the left side of the mediastinum, where tension caused by the inflating lung is avoided consequently reducing potential vasospasm.

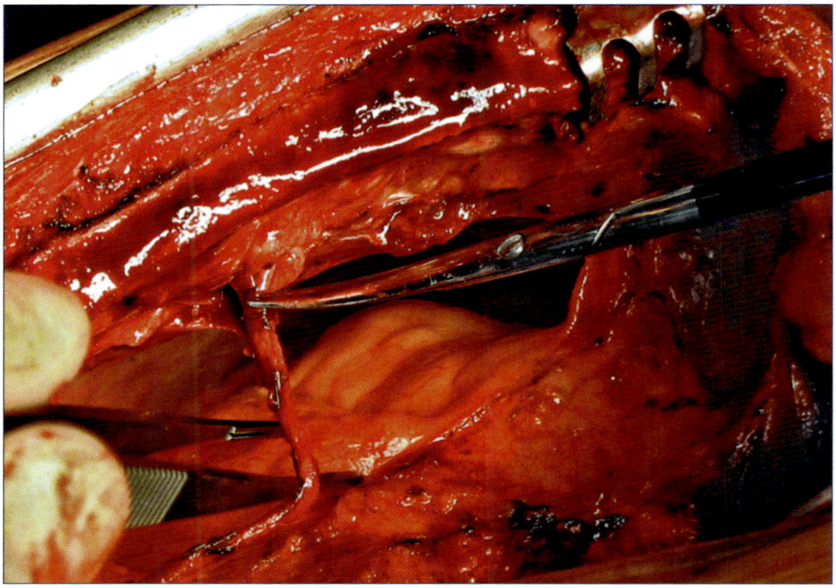

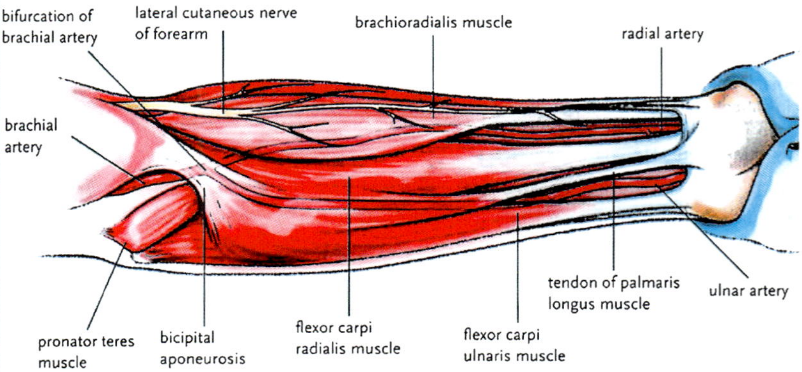

"Reprinted from Buxton B. Ischemic Heart Disease - Surgical Management. 1st Edition 1999, Mosby Ltd., with permission from Elsevier"

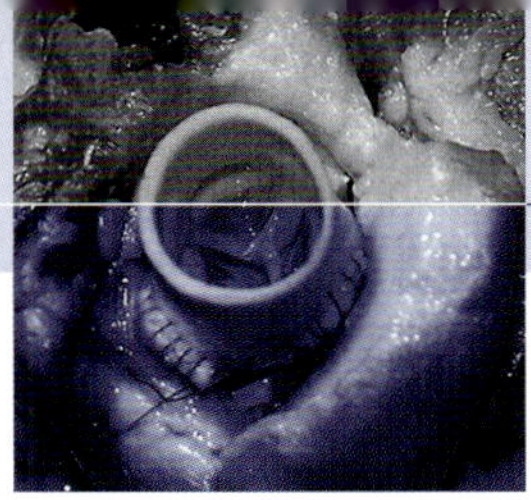

The preparation can now be extended distally using the same technique by pulling on the endothoracic fascia or pushing the ITA away from the thoracic wall, as shown in the picture. The distal preparation should go beyond the bifurcation of the ITA which is ligated using hemoclips. The free blood flow can now be assessed, and diluted Papaverin (50mg/20ml of heparinized blood) is introduced into the lumen of the ITA using an atraumatic cannula. A hemoclip is applied to the distal end and the full length of the wall of the ITA can now be assessed. It is important to make sure that the pulsation of the ITA extends into it's periphery, as no pulsation can be a sign of endothelial damage or dissection.

The RA is more often used as a second graft in this kind of "T"-graft revascularisation. Before the RA is suggested as an arterial conduit an appropriate collateralisation of the suggested hand has to be documented. The Allen's Test has been found to be most practical and by far the cheapest examination technique and is therefore favoured against more technical based investigations. Although the Allen's Test is dependent on the experience of the examiner, there is excellent correlation with the clinical results. Morbidity and mortality after harvesting of the RA has been found to be extremely low. Therefore, some surgeons use the RA's of both arms, although usually the non-dominant arm is preferred. After the patient is anaesthetised, the arm is exposed on an arm board positioned in pronation.

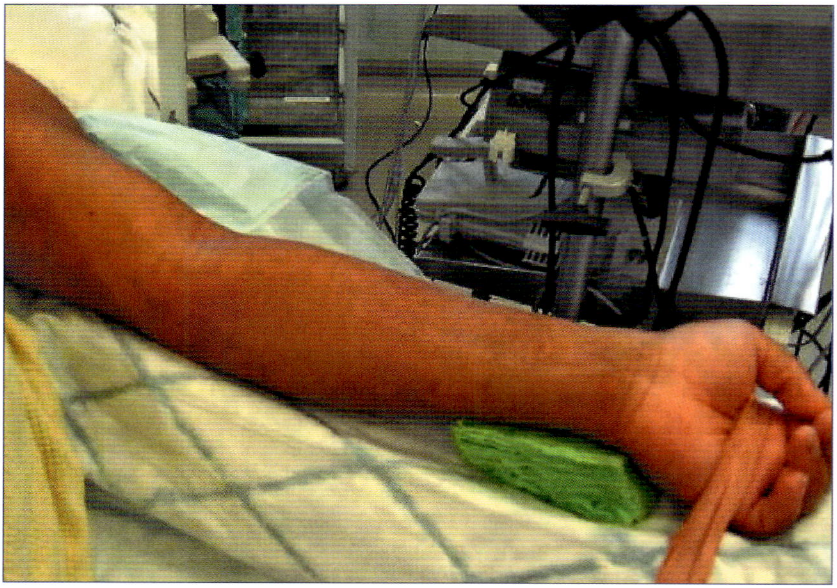

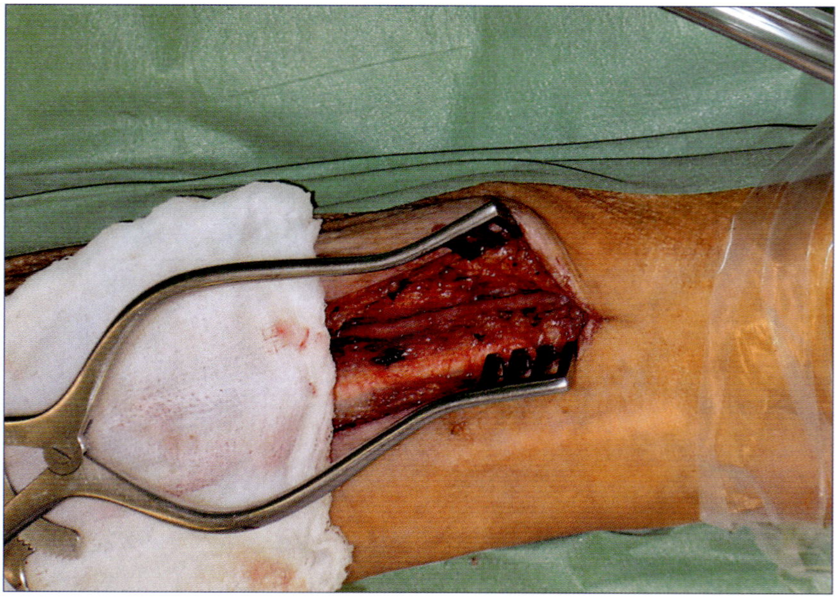

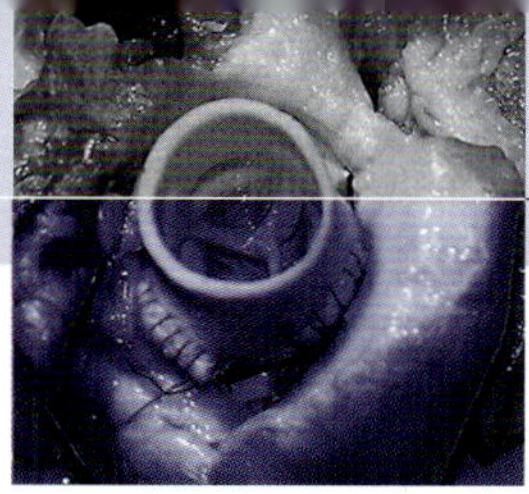

Care should be taken when positioning the arm so that the angle of abduction is less than 90° to reduce the risk of damage to the brachial plexus. The hand should be fixed in slight dorsi flexion as seen in the picture. Before skin incision, the pulse of the RA should be identified and the incision is made 1cm proximal to the head of the radius and 1cm medial to the RA pulse. This more medial incision makes the damage to the lateral cutaneous nerves less likely and reduces post-operative paraesthesia in the thumb.

The distal RA can now be assessed for quality through a limited skin incision of 4cm (if it is not usable only a small incision has been made). To reduce the risk of vasospasm it is important to avoid direct grasping of the arterial vessel with forceps. If the RA is of acceptable size and wall quality (exclude severe calcifications) the skin incision is extended proximally to the insertion of the biceps muscle. In patients who had some kind of previous intervention of the RA (heart catheterisation, arterial line) the very distal part of the RA can be sclerotic.

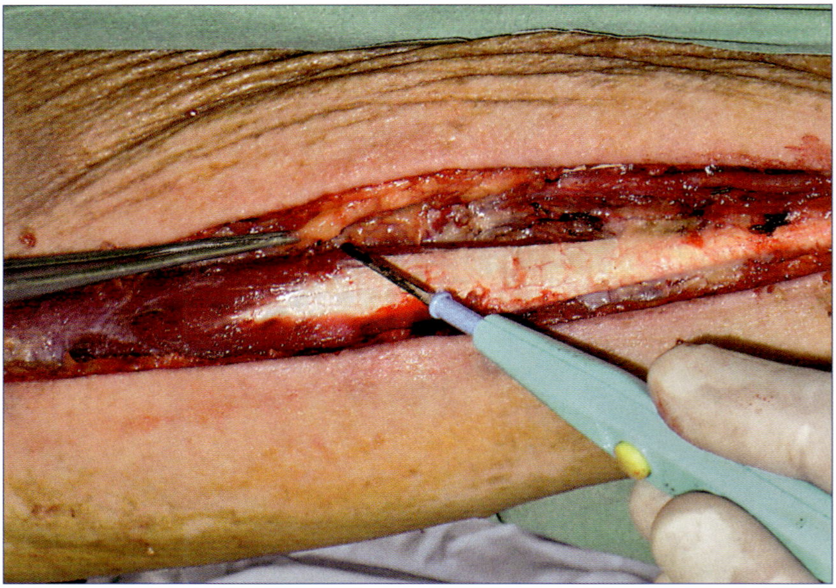

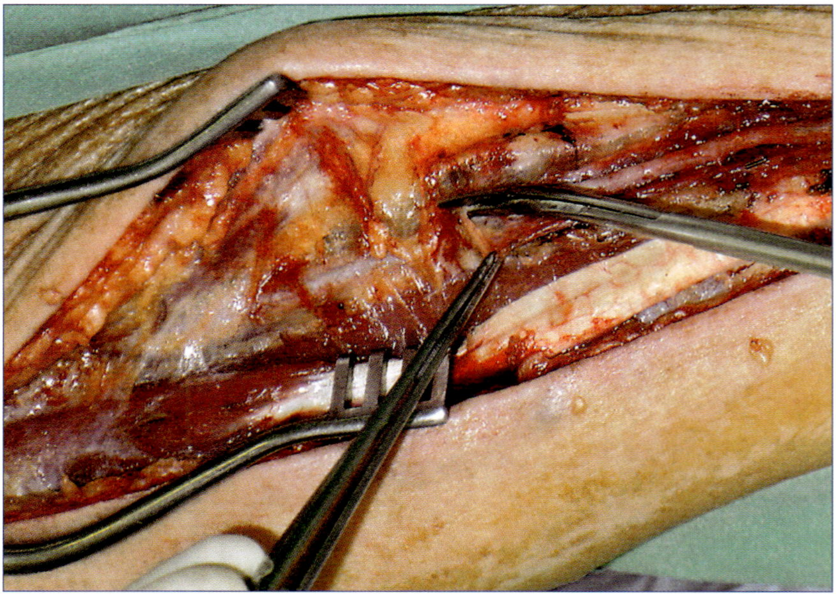

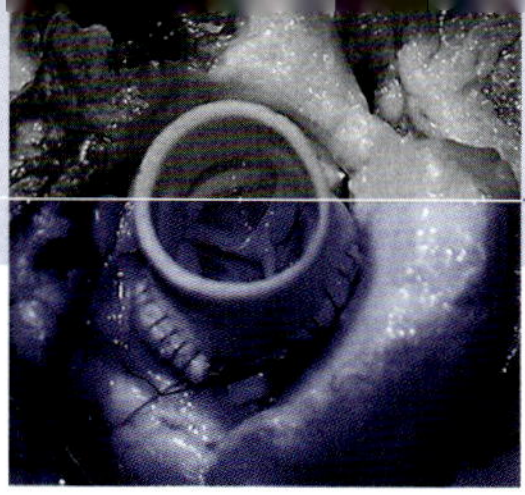

Next the subcutaneous tissue and fascia between brachio-radialis muscle and flexor carpi radialis muscle is opened. This is done using the diathermy or scissors on top of a finger, inserted under the fascia as a guide. The opened tissue exposes the RA with its accompanying vein.

The connective tissue which covers the RA is now opened with fine scissors. It is important that the scissors are guided directly on top of the surface of the vascular wall. The risk of damaging branches of the RA can be reduced if staying on top of the vessels wall, because branches are usually located on the side and posteriorly. In the areas where the covering fascia is opened, the side branches can be easily identified (see picture), ligated with hemoclips and dissected with fine scissors. The RA, should never be grasped directly with forceps to reduce the risk of trauma and vasospasm. A safe technique is to take the RA between two fingers and pull it in different directions to identify its branches and mobilise from the accompanying vein.

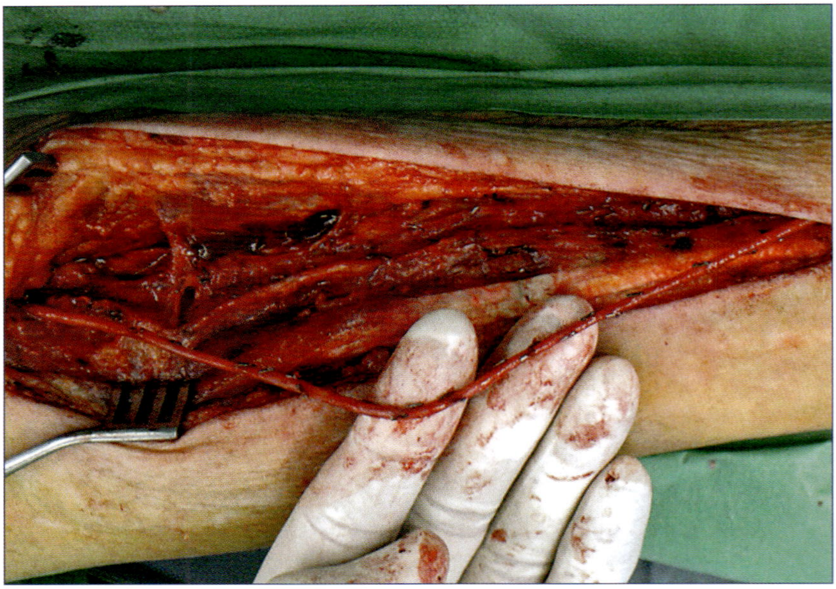

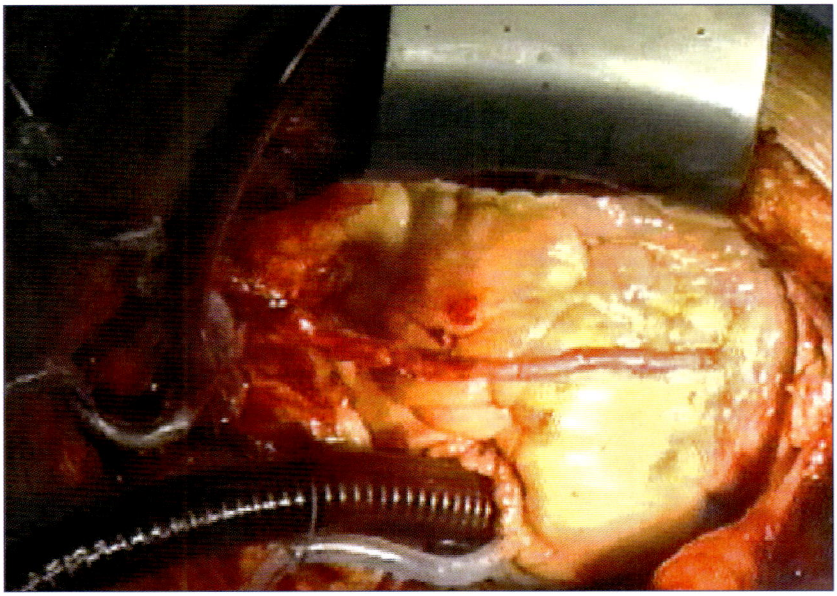

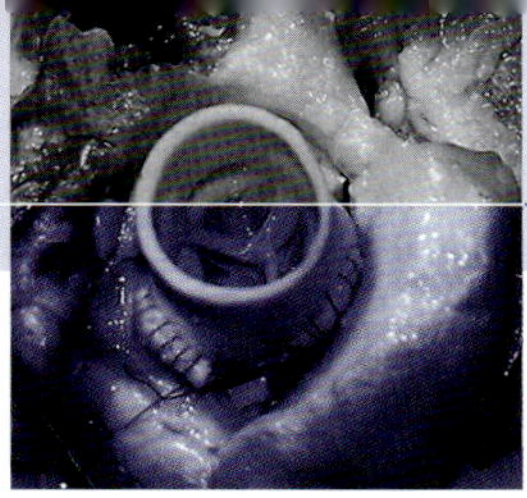

After the RA is freed from its branches it should be occluded with two fingers to assess if a retrograde pulse fills it from the deep palmar arch. The RA then can be ligated distally with two hemoclips and dissected. The free blood flow of the vessel is often reduced at this time due to vasospasm. After diluted Papaverin is introduced intra-luminally, the RA can be assessed regarding its quality (wall hematoma, side branches). In addition diluted Diltiazem (20mg/20ml of saline) is topically applied while the RA is lying in the operated forearm still connected to the pulsatile arterial inflow. Directly before the RA is used for the distal anastomosis to the coronary artery, it is ligated using two hemoclips beyond the bifurcation with the ulnar artery. The forearm is closed using absorbable sutures after hemostasis, drain placement is usually unnecessary.

After the two arterial conduits are assessed regarding their quality, it is important to reflect if the "T"-graft approach is still suitable given the biological material you harvested (no compromise). If there is any doubt it is time to change to a multivessel approach (bilateral ITA's + RA's). The most important pre-condition for a working "T"-graft is an excellent quality of the left ITA due to free blood flow, adequate length and size. The risk of a post-operative hypoperfusion syndrome of the "T"-graft is increased in patients with left ventricular hypertrophy, dilatation and severe main stem stenosis, in combination with right coronary artery (RCA) occlusion. The length of the arterial conduits can be measured on the beating heart to optimize the length of the graft in order to avoid tension of the grafts after the operation, which can induce vasospasm.

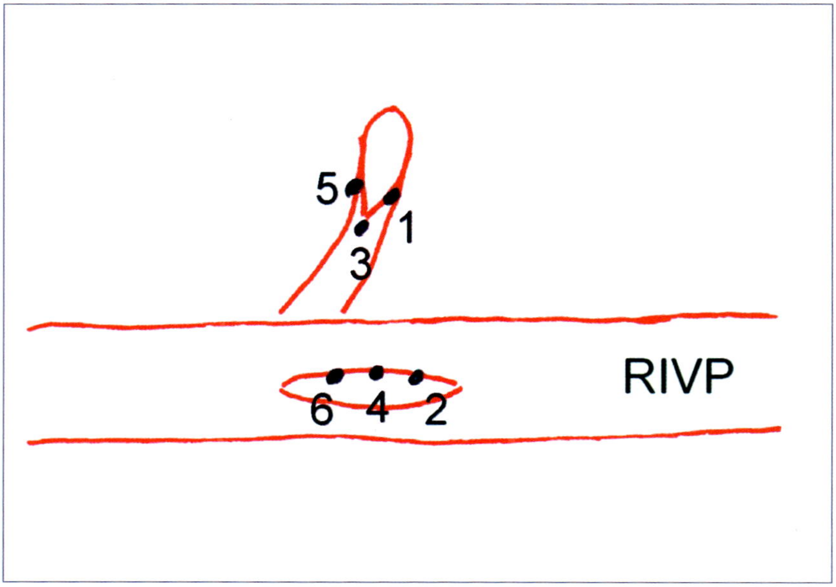
5
1
3
RIVP
6
4
2

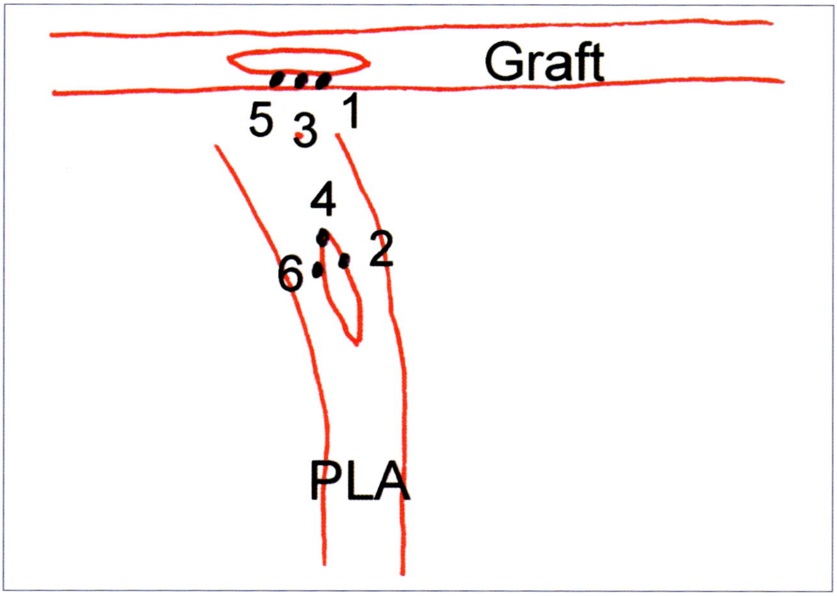
Graft
5
3
1
4
2
6
PLA

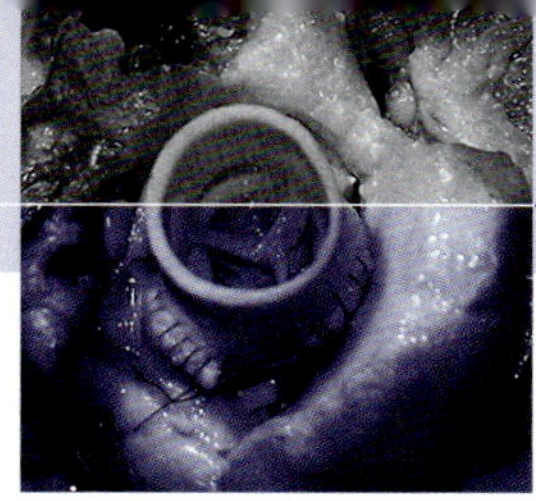

1 2 3 4 5 6 7 8 9 10 11 12 13 14 15

After the coronary arteries are identified, cardioplegia is given if the revascularisation is done in ischaemia. Antegrade cold blood cardioplegia is recommended to improve myocardial protection and to increase ischaemic tolerance. The heart can be lifted out of the pericardium and the PDA opened. The second arterial conduit is now anastomosed to the PDA using 7/8-0 Prolene sutures in an end to side 90° anastomosis. The suture starts to go into the graft from the outside and is followed by a stitch from the inside to outside of the coronary artery (see picture). After completing the anastomosis, the graft is positioned over the postero-lateral wall of the heart to measure the distance to the next side-to-side anastomosis. Attention has to be paid to prevent the graft from twisting.

The side-to-side anastomosis with the left ventricular branch of the RCA or the branches of the circumflex coronary artery, are usually performed in a diamond shape fashion. This means that after the coronary artery is opened, the longitudinal incision on the graft is placed at appropriate distance (more length better than less!). The surgical assistant takes the adventitia of the arterial graft with forceps opposite the coronary incision and, as shown in the picture. The needle of the 7/8-0 Prolene suture is placed from the outside to the inside of the graft. The suture is continued on the inner side of the coronary artery as shown in the picture. The configuration and length of the graft between the two anastomoses should be re-assessed after the anastomosis is finished which is facilitated if cardioplegia is given at the same time and if there is retrograde filling into the bypass grafts.

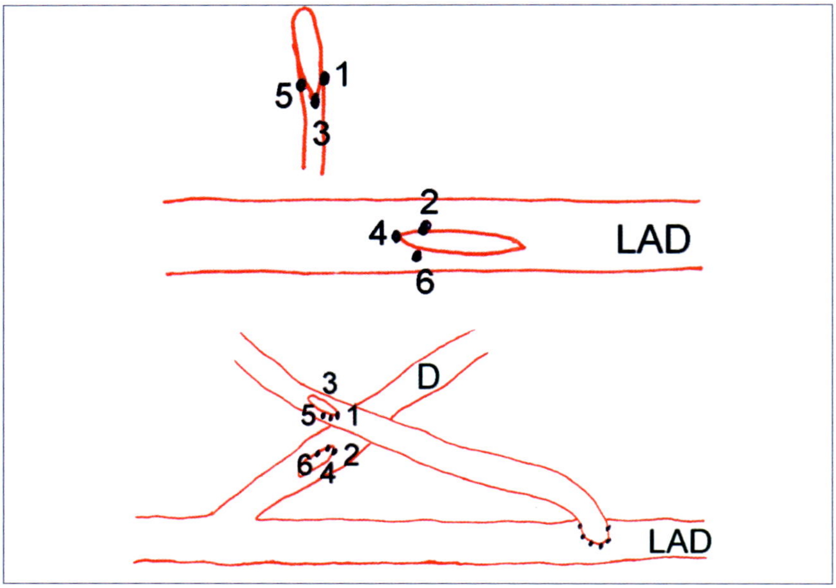
5
1
3
2
4
LAD
6
3
D
5
1
6
2
4
LAD

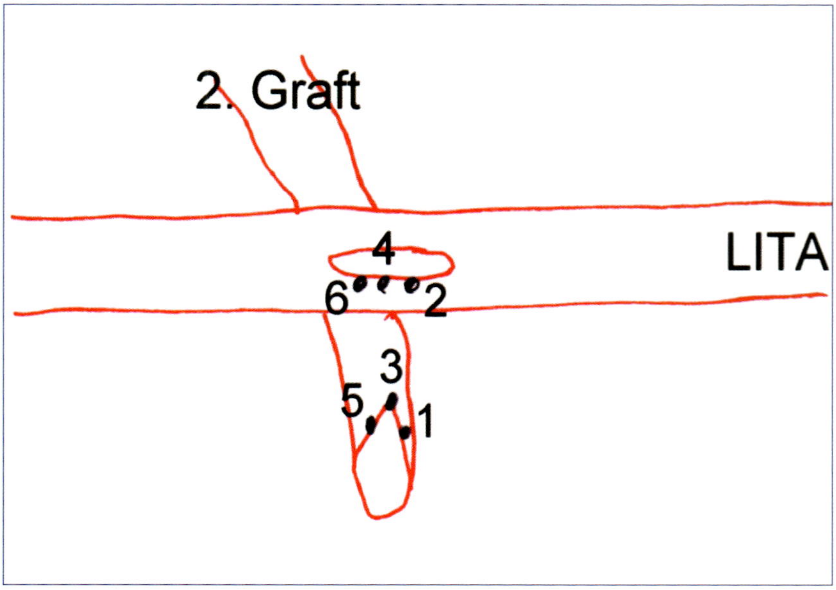
2. Graft
4
LITA
6
2
3
5
1

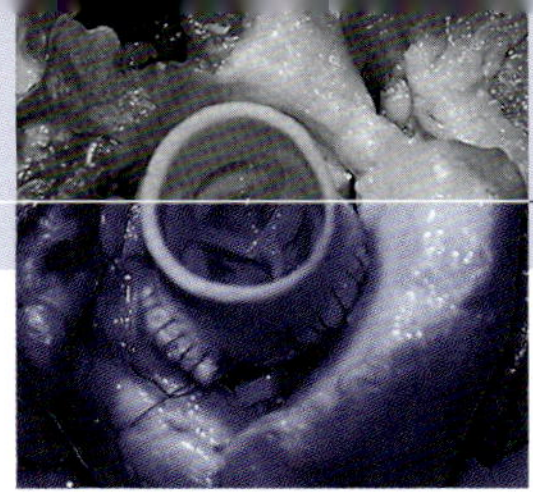

The left ITA can be now pulled into the pericardium (incision above the phrenic nerve, on the level of the pulmonary artery). The distal hemoclip on the ITA is removed and the free blood flow re-assessed. The vessel is occluded with a temporary soft arterial clip and the end-to-side anastomosis with the LAD is performed using 7/8-0 Prolene suture. The ITA should be opened briefly to see its configuration under blood filled condition. The diagonal branch can now be opened in longitudinal fashion and the left ITA is opened with a longitudinal incision in its corresponding area. This side-to-side anastomosis is performed in a parallel fashion using 7/8-0 Prolene suture, while the first assistant grasping the left ITA with forceps places it above the incision of the diagonal branch.

After completion of all distal anastomoses cardioplegia is administered again. The grafts are usually filled by retrograde inflow and it is possible to re-assess length and configuration of the conduits. The "T"-anastomosis should be performed close to where the left ITA enters the pericardium. The adventitia of the left ITA is grasped by the assistant with forceps at the level of the longitudinal incision and placed above the end of the second graft. The second graft is trimmed and incised longitudinally and anastomosed using 7/8-0 Prolene suture in a "T"-configuration (if the second graft is extremely short, a "T" is preferred over an "Y" angled configuration). Directly before the last two stitches on the anastomosis, the temporary clip on the left ITA is removed, which fills the "T"-graft and guarantees appropriate de-airing.

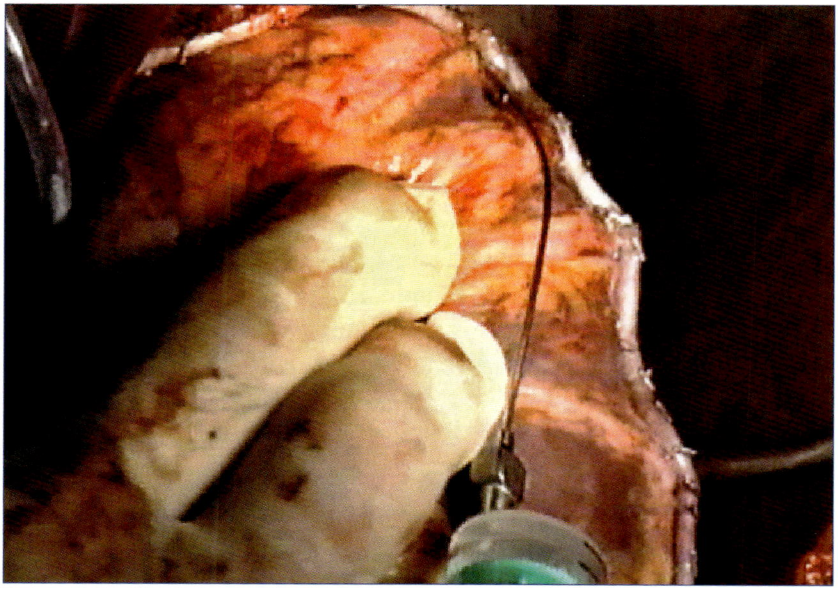

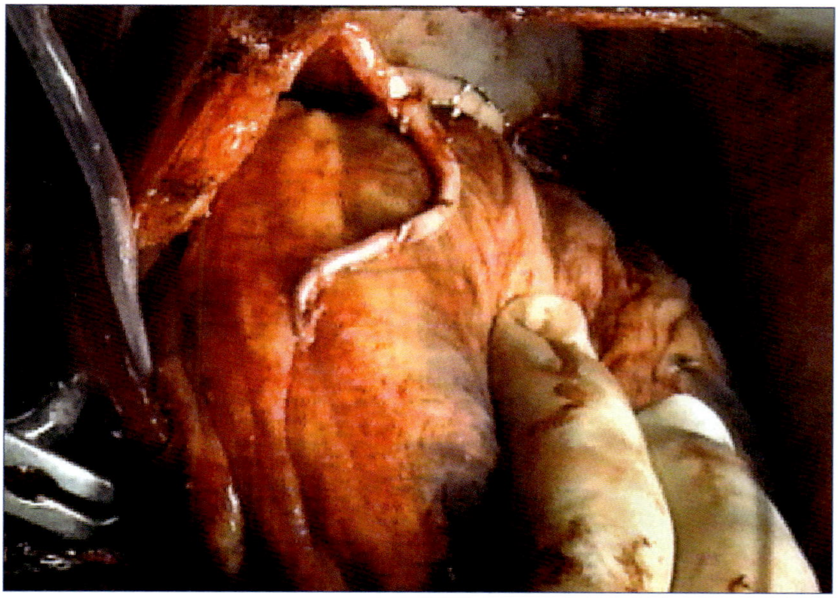

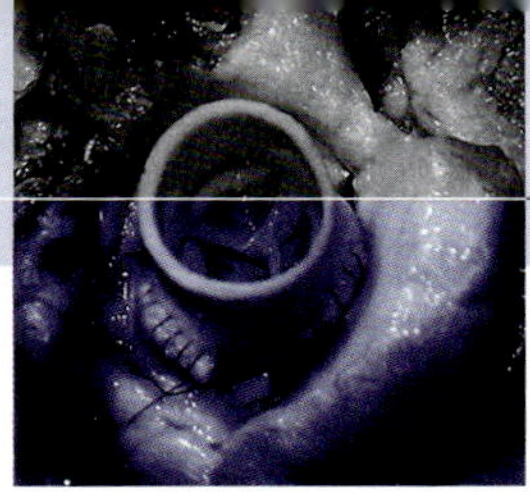

After complete revascularisation of the heart and with the "T"-graft already perfused via the left ITA, all anastomoses can be re-assessed on the decompressed heart, haemostasis and exact configuration can be secured. Once a satisfactory result is confirmed, the cross-clamp is removed and the ventilation can be restarted. While the lung is hyper-inflated by the anaesthetist, the length of the left ITA can be re-assessed and the ITA should be checked for tension. The patient can be weaned off cardiopulmonary bypass and it is important that the mean arterial blood pressure is maintained above 75 mmHg to prevent the grafts from vasospasm.

No general recommendation for a post operative and long-term medical prophylactic treatment against vasospasm can be made at present. Some groups use calcium antagonists, nitrates and phosphodiesterase inhibitors, however, others have achieved excellent results by avoiding systematic vasodilators intra-operatively because of the risk of hypotension. The authors always use the intra-luminal and topical medical treatment of the grafts as described. Whatever kind of medical vasodilation is used, it is important that the arterial perfusion pressure is kept high to guarantee adequate coronary perfusion. If the patient suffers from a hypoperfusion syndrome in the post-operative course, the placement of an intra aortic balloon pump is recommended.

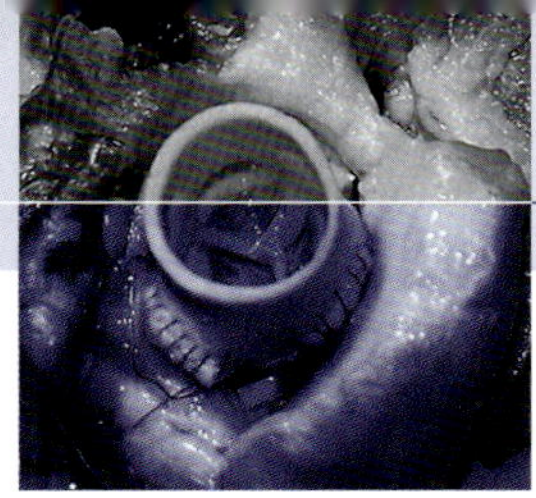

1 2 3 4 5 6 7 8 9 10 11 12 13 14 15

References

1. Hirose H, Amano A, Takahoshi A. Triple arterial coronary revascularization using the radial artery and bilateral internal mammary arteries versus the gastroepiploic artery and bilateral internal mammary arteries. Circ J 2002; 66: 544–8
2. Lytle BW. Prolonging patency-choosing coronary bypass grafts. N Engl J Med 2004; 351: 2262–64
3. Possati G, Gaudino M, Prati F, Alessandrini F, Trani C, Glieca F, Mazzari MA, Luciani N, Schiavoni G. Long-term results of the radial artery used for myocardial revascularization. Circulation 2003; 108: 1350–4
4. Suma H, Isomura T, Horij T, Sato T. Late angiographic results of using the right gastroepiploic artery as a graft. J Thorac Cardiovasc Surg 2000; 120: 496–8
5. Verma S, Szmitko PE, Weisel RD, Bonneau D, Latter D, Errett L, Leclerc Y, Fremes SE. Should radial arteries be used routinely for coronary artery bypass grafting? Circulation 2004; 110: E40–E46
6. Wendler O, Hennen B, Markwirth T, König J, Tscholl D, Huang Q, Shahangi E, Schäfers HJ. T-grafts with the right internal thoracic artery to left internal thoracic artery versus left internal thoracic artery and radial artery: Flow dynamics in the internal thoracic artery mainstem. J Thorac Cardiovasc Surg 1999; 118: 841–888
7. Wendler O, Hennen B, Demertzis S, Markwirth T, Tscholl D, Lausberg H, Huang Q, Dübener L, Langer F, Schäfers HJ. Complete arterial revascularization in multivessel coronary ar tery disease with 2 conduits (skeletonized grafts and T-grafts). Circulation 2000; 102 (suppl. 3): III 79–83
8. Zacharias A, Habib RH, Schwamm TA, Riordan CJ, Durham SJ, Shah A. Improved survival with radial artery versus vein conduits in coronary bypass surgery with left internal thoracic artery to left anterior descending artery grafting. Circulation 2004; 109: 1489–96

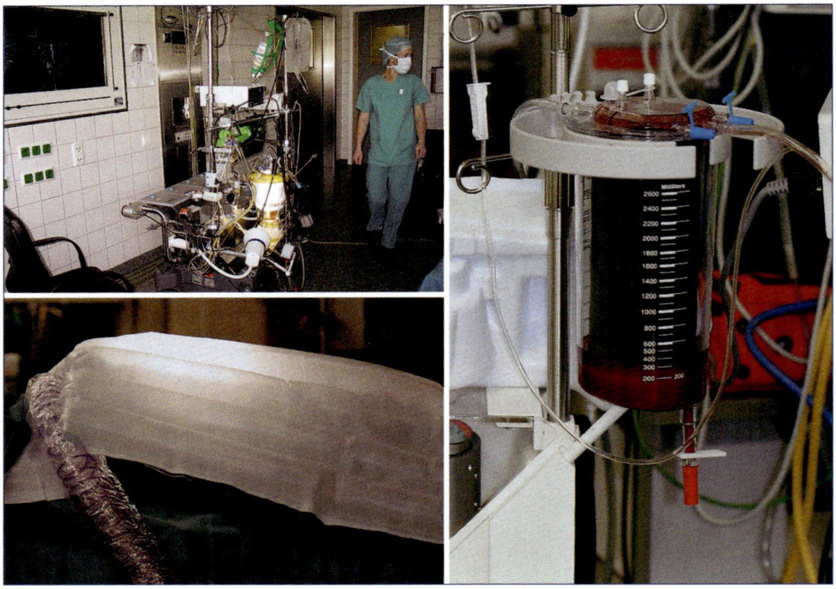

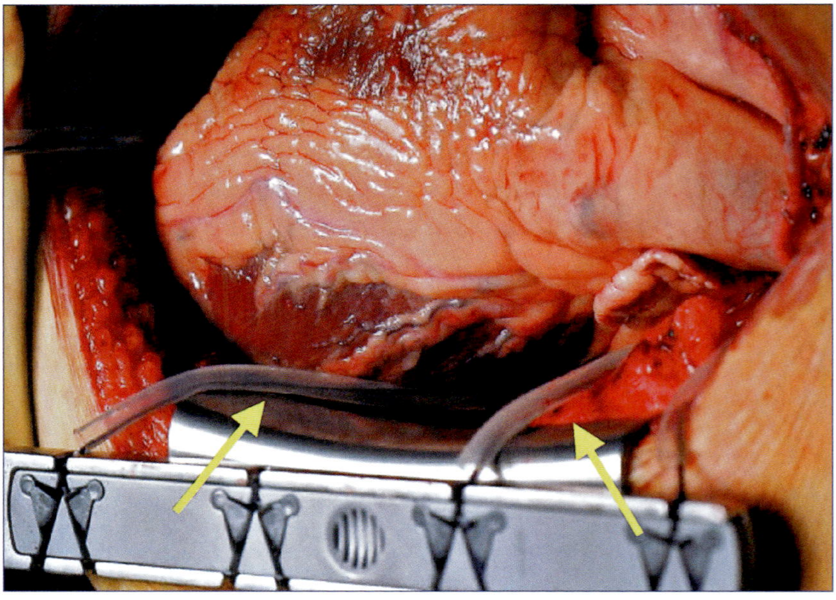

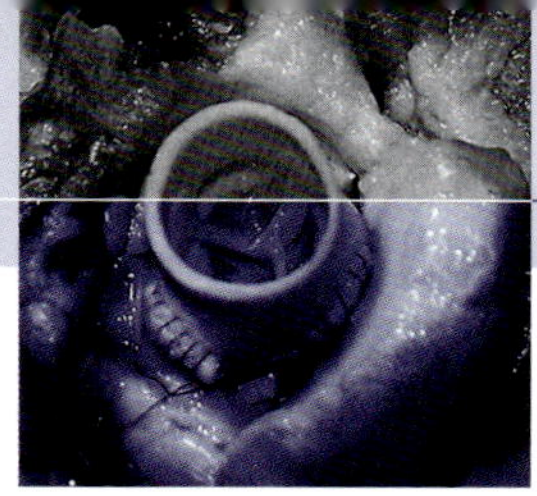

1 2 3 4 5 6 7 8 9 10 11 12 13 14 15

Perioperative management is important in OPCAB surgery. Cardiopulmonary bypass cannot be used for temperature management, therefore it is mandatory to prevent cooling of the patient to enable fast track extubation. Warm i.v. fluid replacement as well as disposable, heat-controlled blankets (figure1) have been proven useful.
The application of a cell saver is recommended. Intensity of anticoagulation is still controversial. My recommendation is to use 150 I.U/kg heparin to achieve an ACT above 300 sec. The heart lung machine must be readily available in the OR, however, with the tubing not yet in the sterile field. A pump technician must be available, especially during the distal anastomosis.

The heart can be exposed with two to three deep pericardial stitches on the left side. They are placed between the pulmonary veins and the phrenic nerve which should be visualised carefully. The descending aorta can be injured as well. To expose the right heart it might be necessary to use additional stitches on the right side. Depending on the anatomy it might be wise to cover the stitches with plastic tubes (figure 2) in order to avoid damage of the epicardial tissue.

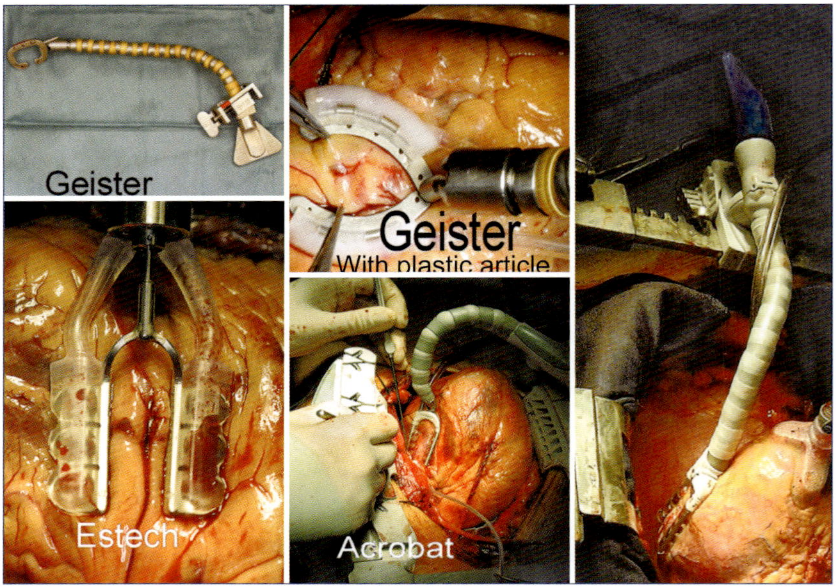
Geister
Geister
With plastic article
Estech
Acrobat

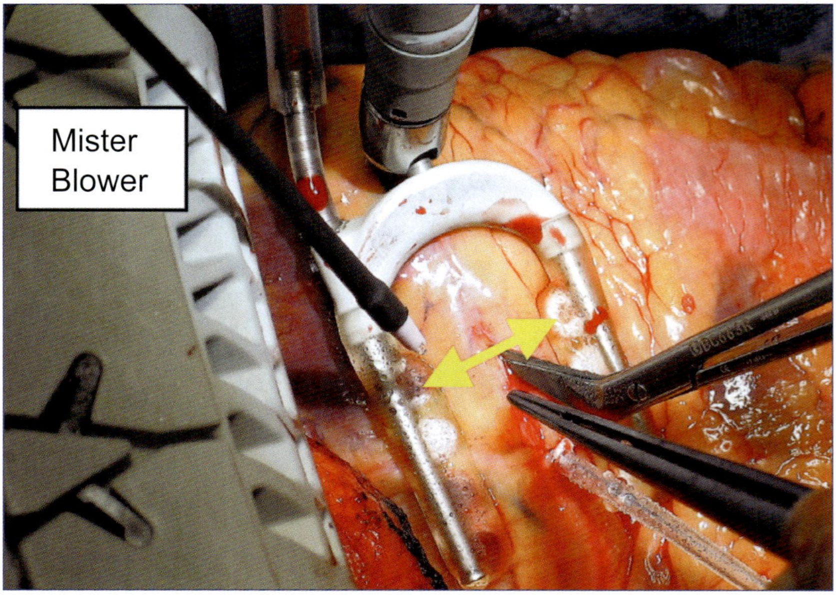
Mister
Blower

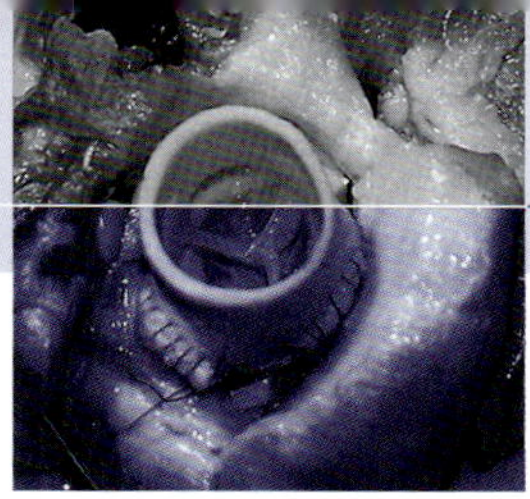

Since the first use of the octopus stabilizer many different stabilizers have been introduced to facilitate off pump cardiac surgery. Some companies have introduced the fifth generation of stabilizers. Some of those have not been a true improvement compared to previous generations. There are two principal types of stabilizers: (1) pressure stabilizers and (2) suction stabilizers (like the Octopus). Pressure stabilizers are usually made of metal and can be re-sterilised. They are mainly used for the anterior wall. Suction stabilizers are necessary if the target vessels are located on the lateral and posterior wall of the heart. Most of them are single use disposables, but in some countries they are re-sterilised many times depending on local laws. The different brands differ only in minor details. Some of those have a longer arm and may be beneficial in large patients.

Another criterion to select a suitable stabilizer is the distance between the two feet of the stabilizer (yellow arrow). If the distance is too large, the stabilizing effect is not sufficient, if the distance is too small it may be uncomfortable to suture the anastomosis. Distal anastomotic devices require more space. Most stabilizers are flexible in order to accommodate to those special needs. Stabilizers can be selected based on their capabilities to be attached to the sternal retractor. The mister blower is powered by CO_2 to minimise the risk of thrombembolic complications. Sodium in a physiologic concentration is used to keep the vessel wall wet and to minimise the risk of endothelial damage. One must be aware of the risk of dissection and the assistant should use the blower very carefully.

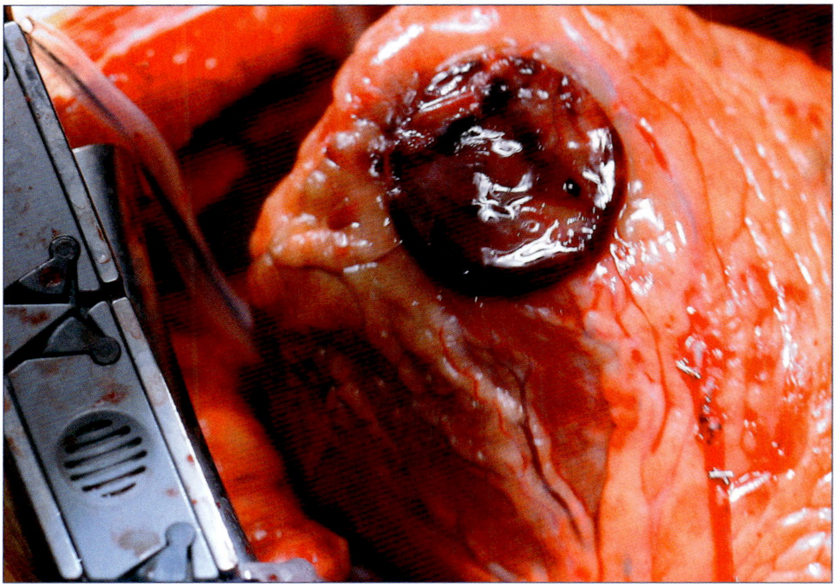

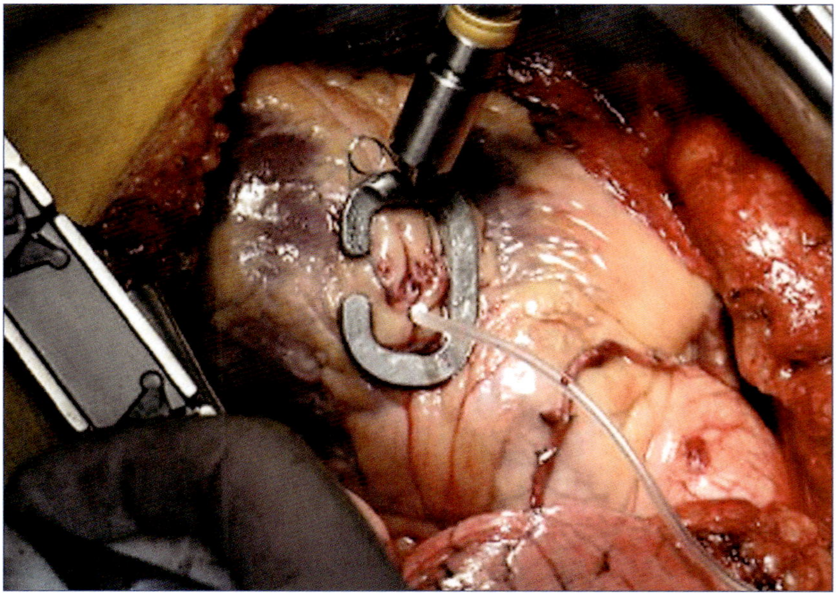

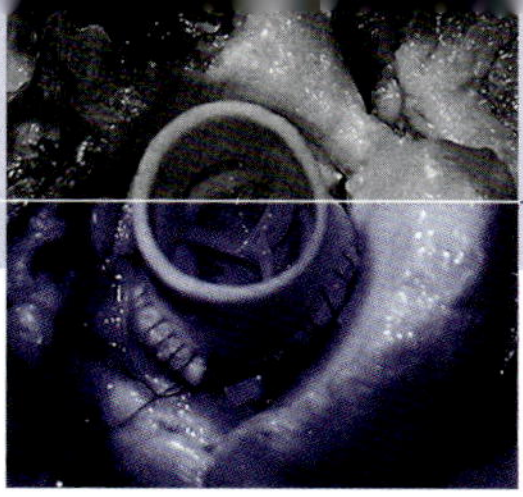

In general it is not necessary to use a heart positioner like the Xpose system or the star fish. Hemodynamic benefits have not been demonstrated conclusively. Under special anatomic circumstances a heart positioner can ease the handling of the heart and it is certainly more elegant. Based on the type of stabilizer a heart positioner can be even mandatory. Sometimes the stabilizer is not tight enough to control the position of the heart on its own. Other indications may be enlarged ventricles in patients with ischemic cardiomyopathy.
The resulting apex hematoma is harmless and clinically not relevant, it usually affects only the epicardial tissue. Studies have demonstrated no elevation of cardiac enzymes when using a heart positioner.

Intraluminal shunts, small vessel clamps or vessel loops (e.g. prolene 4-0) are used to control the bleeding during the anastomosis. To prevent endothelial damage vessel loops should not be used distally. Shunts are very useful and are used routinely in many centers. Depending on the center experience, however, they are certainly not mandatory.
Coronary retractors can be useful in exposing intramural coronaries, those retractors must be very atraumatic in order to prevent severe damage to the epicardial fat tissue.

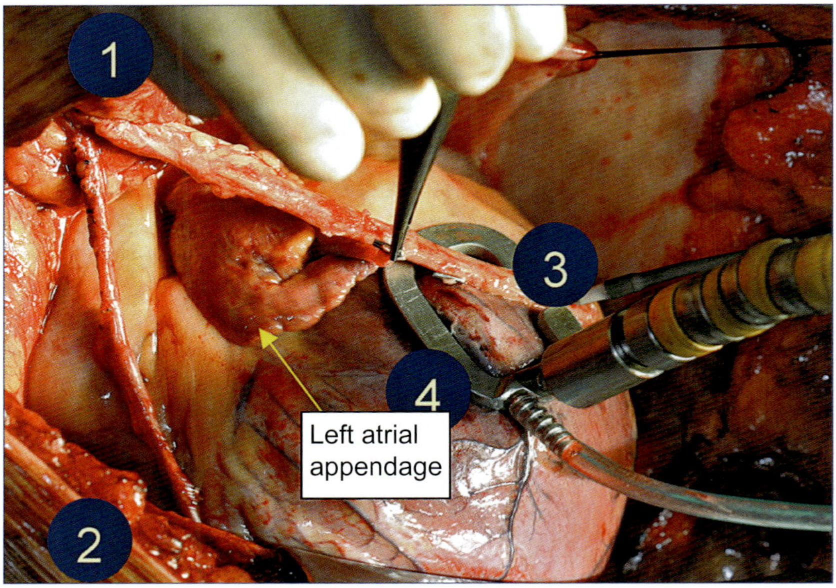
1
2
3
4
Left atrial appendage

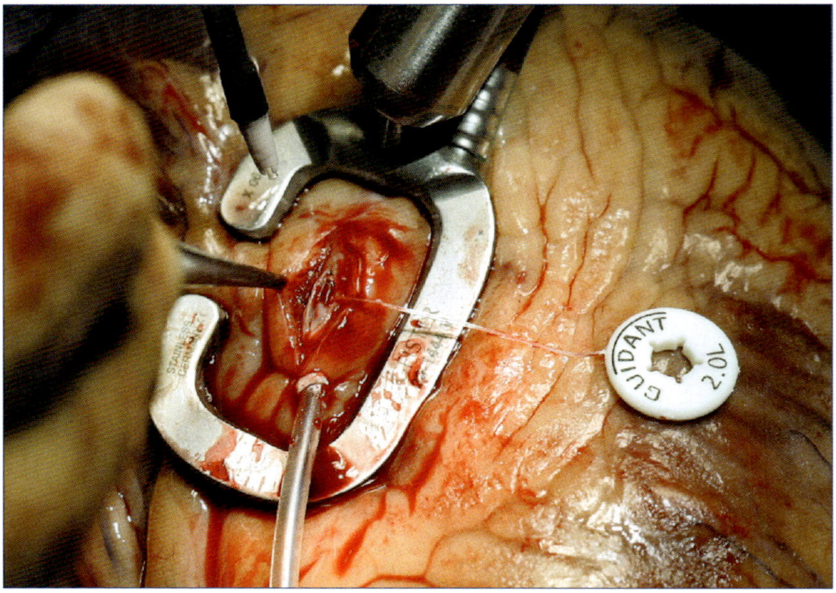
GUIDANT 2.0L

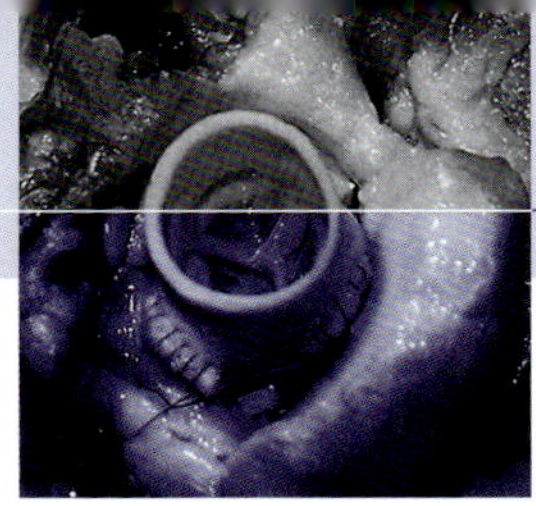

The sequence of grafting in OPCAB surgery is very important. There are issues regarding temporary ischemia and the position of the heart during anastomosis to be observed. In general the first anastomosis is the ITA – LAD anastomosis. The manipulation of the heart is not extensive and the patient benefits immediately from the blood flow to the left ventricular wall. The second anastomosis should be made to the vessel with the highest stenosis grade. It is very helpful to perform the proximal anastomosis first because that simplifies the de-airing of the graft and the heart has an immediate benefit after completion of the distal anastomosis. An example for a sequence in complete arterial grafting is shown on the figure. (1) T–graft anastomosis of the radial artery to the proximal ITA. (2) ITA to LAD anastomosis. (3) Sequential side-to-side anastomosis radial artery to distal circumflex artery and end-to-side anastomosis to the posterior descending artery (not visualised). (4) Finally the right ITA is guided through the transverse sulcus and anastomosed to the large OM 1. This specific sequence helps to avoid tension on the right ITA.

There is an ongoing debate about the necessity to use shunts in OPCAB surgery. I recommend to use shunts definitely in large vessels (> 2 mm). Temporary ischemia to the right heart can cause rhythm disturbance and a shunt should be used in all vessels with a stenosis grade less than 90%.

Dissection of LAD

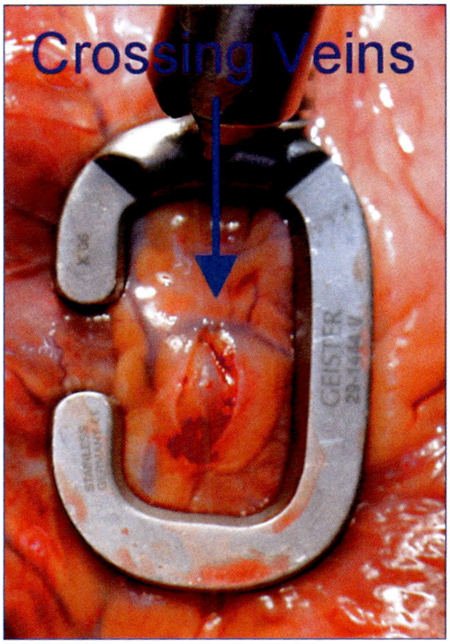

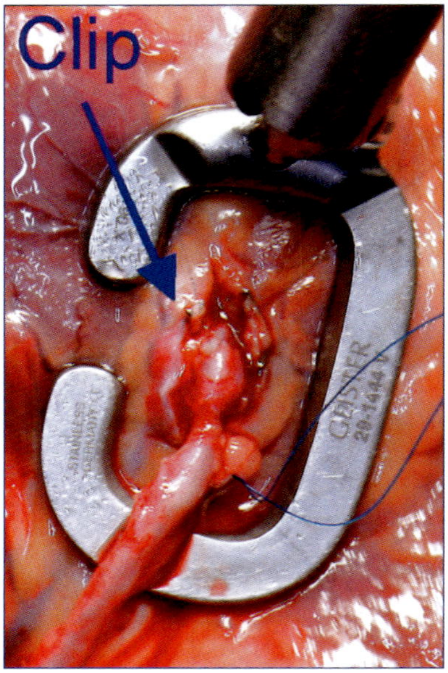

Course of LAD in epicardial fat

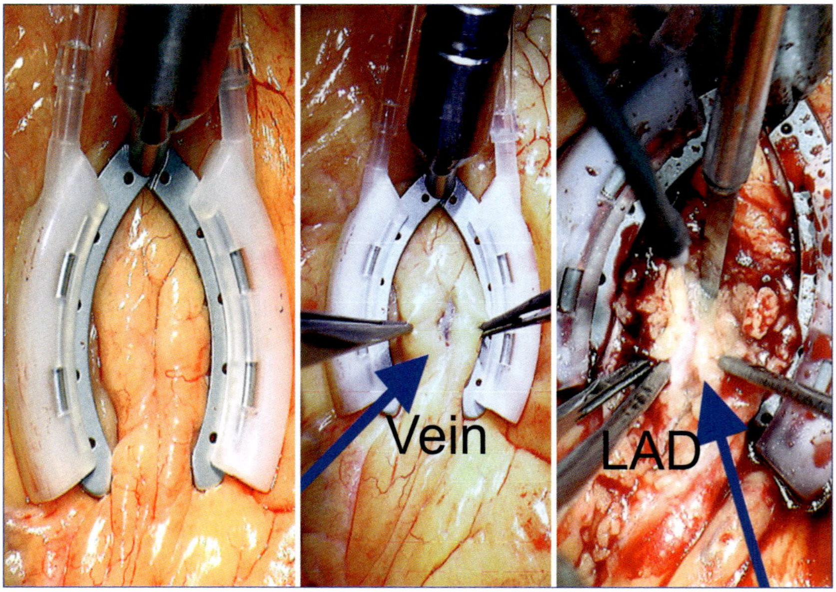

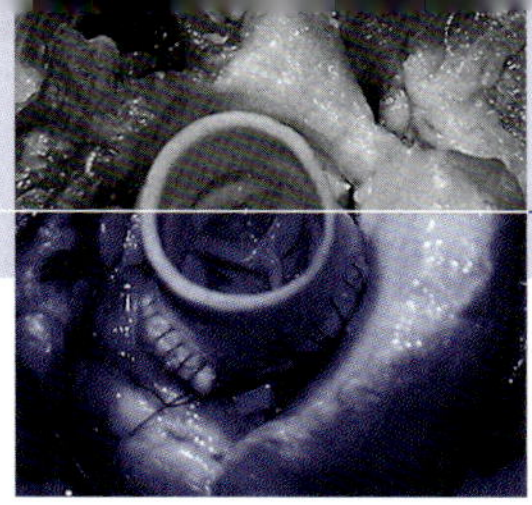

Exposition of the LAD can be challenging in case of a deep intramural situation. To deal with veins crossing the LAD can be tiring. Small veins can be coagulated, larger veins should be clipped to avoid bleeding complications.

Exposition of the LAD is even more difficult in OPCAB surgery compared to the arrested heart. The dissection is very time consuming. In some cases a conversion to on-pump surgery is necessary and one should not hesitate to do so to avoid catastrophic complications.
The strategies to identify the LAD and to dissect follow the same principles as in conventional surgery. If a high proximal anastomosis is necessary an intraluminal shunt is recommended. The risk of a hemodynamic relevant ischemia is very high and the threshold to convert should be very low.

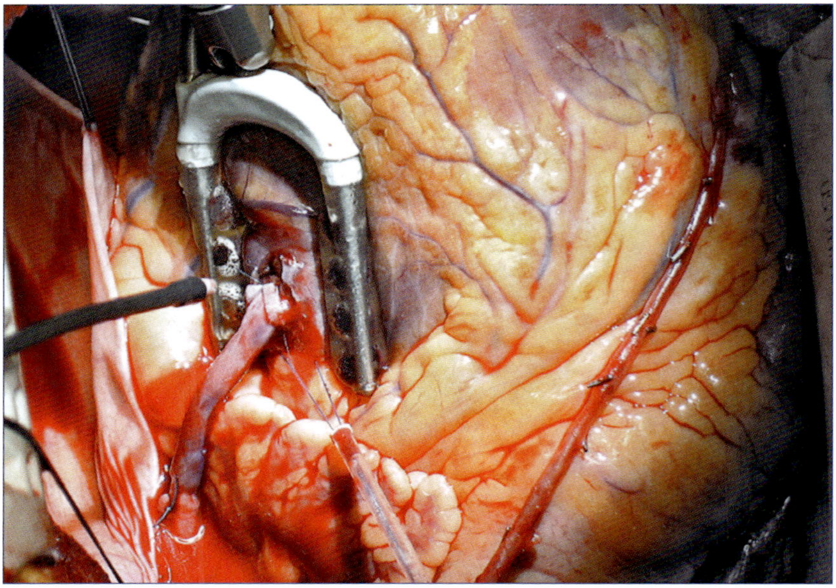

CAVE! Avoid tension on LIMA during exposition of the lateral wall!

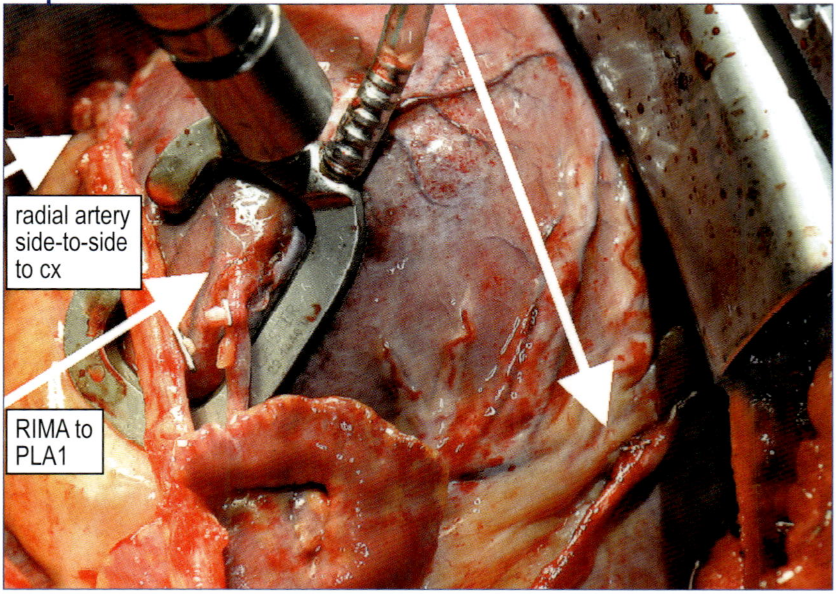

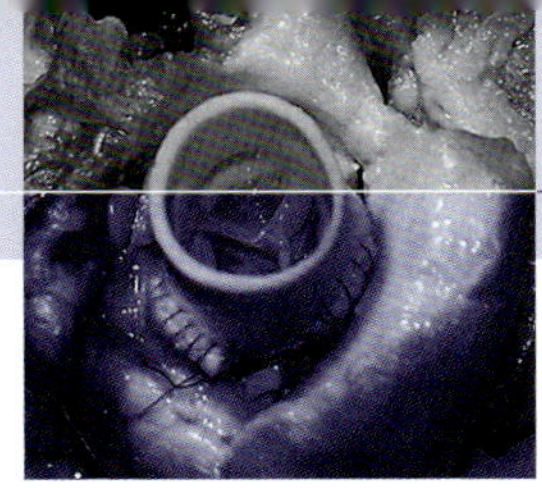

On this picture the heart is positioned for the anastomosis to a large OM branch. In this case the Cardica C-Port® system was used. This position is hemodynamically more challenging because the heart is compressed to the right pleura thus compromising adequate filling of the right ventricle.
In the beginning of the OPCAB surgery the right pleura was routinely opened. With increasing experience the same can be accomplished by gently positioning of the heart and an incision of the pericardium close to inferior vena cava without touching the pleura if possible. Pericardial stay sutures should not be placed on the right side. In critical cases of very large ventricles opening of the right pleural space can result in a hemodynamically more stable patient.

After finishing the left ITA to LAD anastomosis the exposition of the lateral wall can result in tension on the anastomosis. Special care must be taken to avoid this situation. In some cases the use of a heart positioner is very helpful.

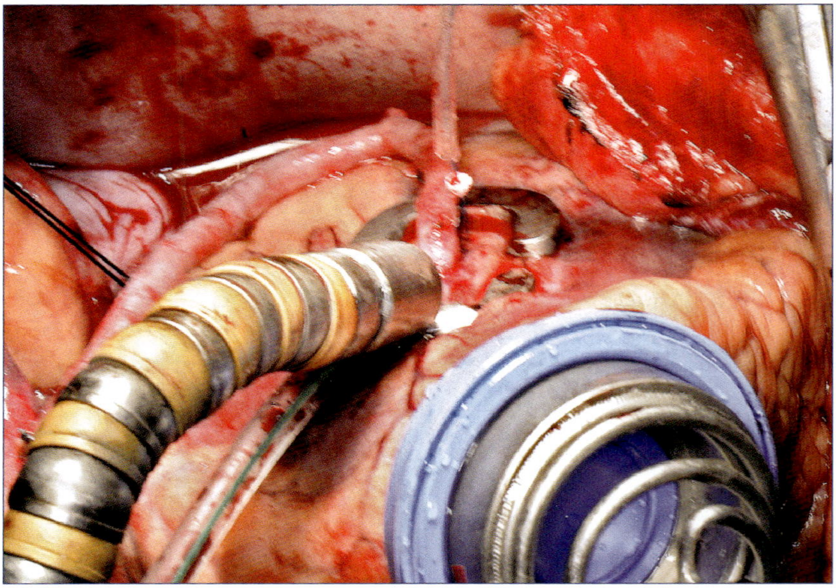

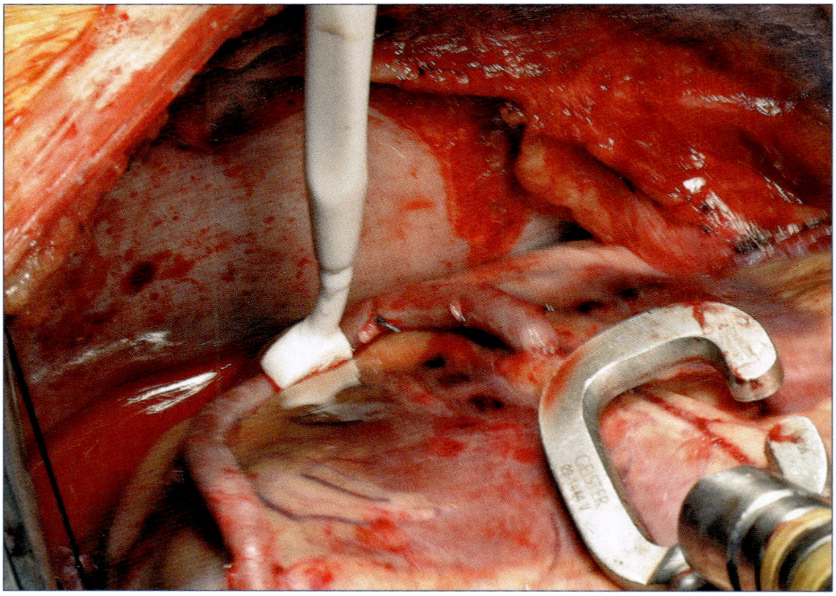

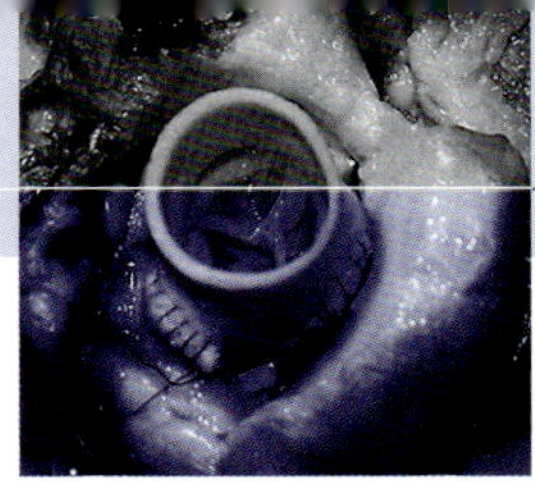

Sequential grafting is possible in OPCAB surgery without limitations. A meticulous planning of the procedures is necessary. Most often it is very easy to measure the exact length of the graft because the filling of the heart is unchanged. I recommend to perform the proximal anastomosis first in venous grafts. The de-airing process is simplified and the distal anastomoses of sequential grafts are performed from the most proximal to the very distal anastomosis. Again, de-airing is no problem in this situation. The position of the grafts can be secured with fibrin glue or stay sutures to the epicardial fat tissue to reliably avoid kinking of the graft.

Flow measurement is essential for quality control in OPCAB surgery and is highly recommended. Other techniques are not generally accepted. One should guarantee to measure all segments of a sequential graft

1 2 3 4 5 6 7 8 9 10 11 12 13 14 15

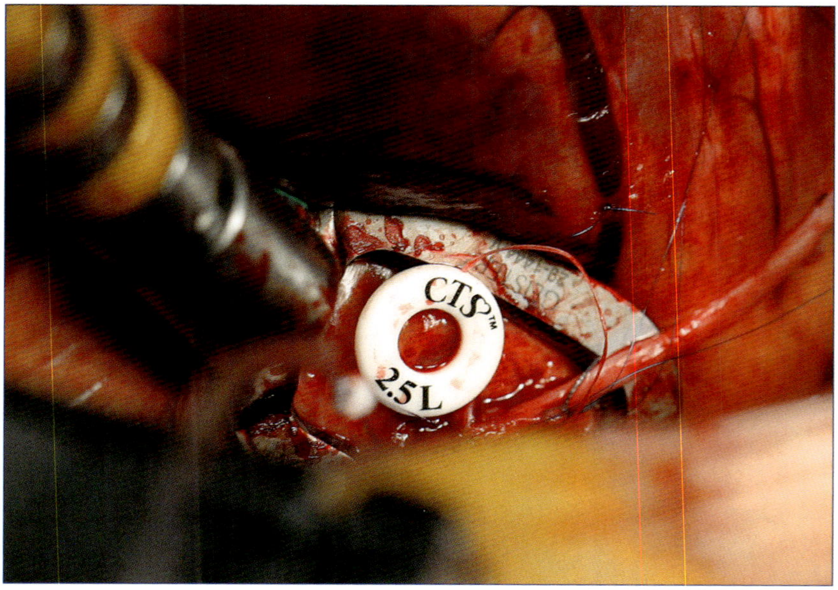
CTS™
2.5L

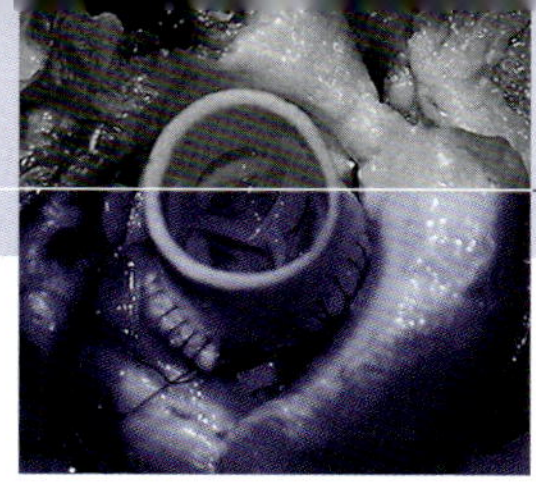

The anastomosis to the proximal right coronary artery can be complex, even brief episodes of ischemia can cause arrhythmias and right heart failure. It is generally recommended to use a shunt especially in the situation of large vessels and a stenosis grade lower than 90%. To avoid the potential problems of bradyarrhythmias temporary pacing wires are recommended.

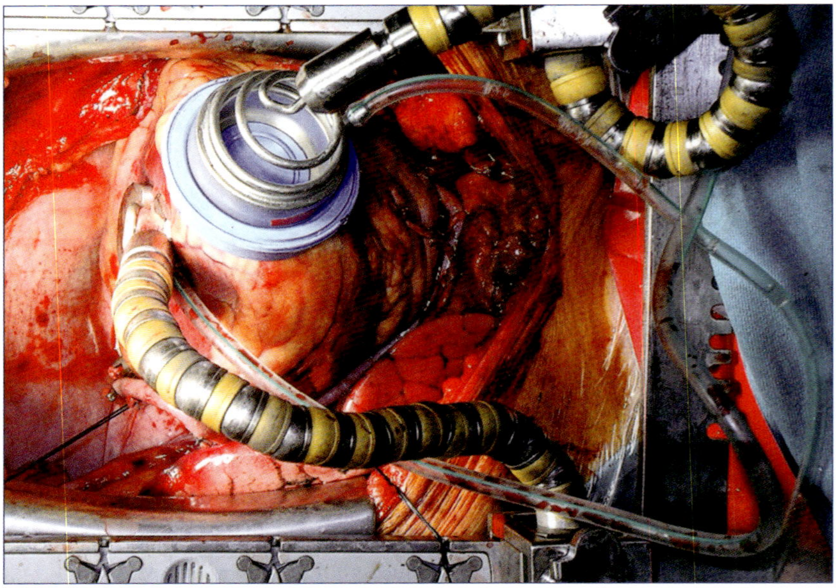

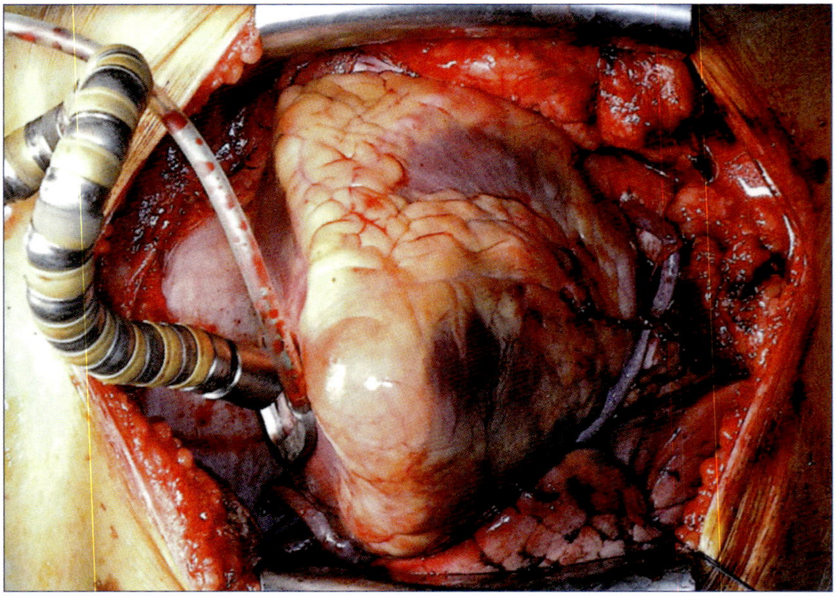

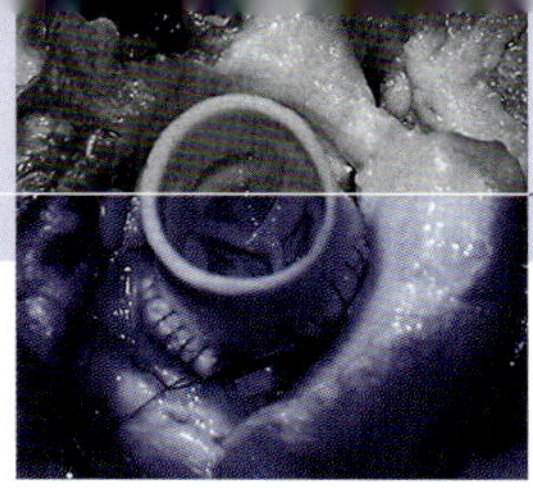

Anastomosis to branches of the inferior wall are in general technically not demanding because the necessary position is well tolerated in most patients. To gain more space the sternal retractor is replaced as shown in the figure. The use of a heart positioner can be considered.

Training in OPCAB surgery requires sufficient experience in conventional on pump coronary surgery. The different anastomotic techniques should be perfectly mastered.
In the future a more sophisticated training concept for young surgeons is mandatory because the so called "simple" cases will not be available any more. Beginners in OPCAB surgery should use shunts to allow tolerance of a prolonged ischemia time. The position technique and anastomosis can be trained on a beating heart with heart lung machine.

References

1. Bucerius J, Gummert JF, Borger MA, Walther T, Doll N, Falk V. et al. Predictors of delirium after cardiac surgery delirium: effect of beating-heart (off-pump) surgery. J Thorac Cardiovasc Surg 2004; 127(1): 57–64.
2. Bucerius J, Gummert JF, Walther T, Borger MA, Doll N, Falk V. et al. Impact of off-pump coronary bypass grafting on the prevalence of adverse perioperative outcome in women undergoing coronary artery bypass grafting surgery. Ann Thorac Surg 2005; 79(3): 807–812.
3. Puskas JD, Wright CE, Ronson RS, Brown WM, Gott JP, Guyton RA. Offpump multivessel coronary bypass via sternotomy is safe and effective. Ann Thorac Surg 1998; 66(3): 1068–1072.
4. Puskas JD, Wright CE, Ronson RS, Brown WM, III, Gott JP, Guyton RA. Clinical outcomes and angiographic patency in 125 consecutive off-pump coronary bypass patients. 1999.
5. Leacche M, Carrier M, Bouchard D, Pellerin M, Perrault LP, Paga P. et al. Improving neurologic outcome in off-pump surgery: the "no touch" technique. Heart Surg Forum 2003; 6(3): 169–175.
6. Lund C, Hol PK, Lundblad R, Fosse E, Sundet K, Tennoe B. et al. Comparison of cerebral embolization during off-pump and on-pump coronary artery bypass surgery. Ann Thorac Surg 2003; 76(3): 765–770.
7. Mazzone A, Gianetti J, Picano E, Bevilacqua S, Zucchelli G, Biagini A. et al. Correlation between inflammatory response and markers of neuronal damage in coronary revascularization with and without cardiopulmonary bypass. Perfusion 2003; 18(1): 3–8.
8. Nathoe HM, van Dijk D, Jansen EW, Suyker WJ, Diephuis JC, van Boven WJ. et al. A comparison of on-pump and off-pump coronary bypass surgery in low-risk patients. N Engl J Med 2003; 348(5): 394–402.
9. Athanasiou T, Aziz O, Mangoush O, Weerasinghe A, Al Ruzzeh S, Purkayastha S. et al. Do off-pump techniques reduce the incidence of postoperative atrial fibrillation in elderly patients undergoing coronary artery bypass grafting? Ann Thorac Surg 2004; 77(5): 1567–1574.

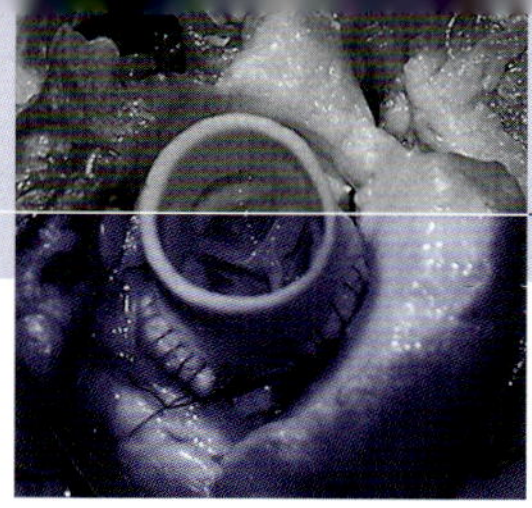

10. Mack MJ, Brown P, Houser F, Katz M, Kugelmass A, Simon A. et al. Onpump versus off-pump coronary artery bypass surgery in a matched sample of women: a comparison of outcomes. Circulation 2004; 110(11 Suppl 1): II1–II6.
11. Mack MJ, Pfister A, Bachand D, Emery R, Magee MJ, Connolly M. et al. Comparison of coronary bypass surgery with and without cardiopulmonary bypass in patients with multivessel disease. J Thorac Cardiovasc Surg 2004; 127(1): 167–173.
12. Mack MJ. Off-pump surgery and alternatives to standard operation in redo coronary surgery. J Card Surg 2004; 19(4): 313–319.
13. Sergeant P, Wouters P, Meyns B, Bert C, Van Hemelrijck J, Bogaerts C. et al. OPCAB versus early mortality and morbidity: an issue between clinical relevance and statistical significance. Eur J Cardiothorac Surg 2004; 25(5): 779–785.
14. Thanikachalam M, Lombardi P, Tehrani HY, Katariya K, Salerno TA. The history and development of direct coronary surgery without cardiopulmonary bypass. J Card Surg 2004; 19(6): 516–519.
15. Herz I, Moshkovitz Y, Hendler A, Adam SZ, Uretzky G, Ben Gal Y. et al. Revascularization of left anterior descending artery with drug-eluting stents: comparison with off-pump surgery. Ann Thorac Surg 2005; 79(1): 88–92.
16. Pandey R, Grayson AD, Pullan DM, Fabri BM, Dihmis WC. Total arterial revascularisation: effect of avoiding cardiopulmonary bypass on in-hospital mortality and morbidity in a propensity-matched cohort. Eur J Cardiothorac Surg 2005; 27(1): 94–98.

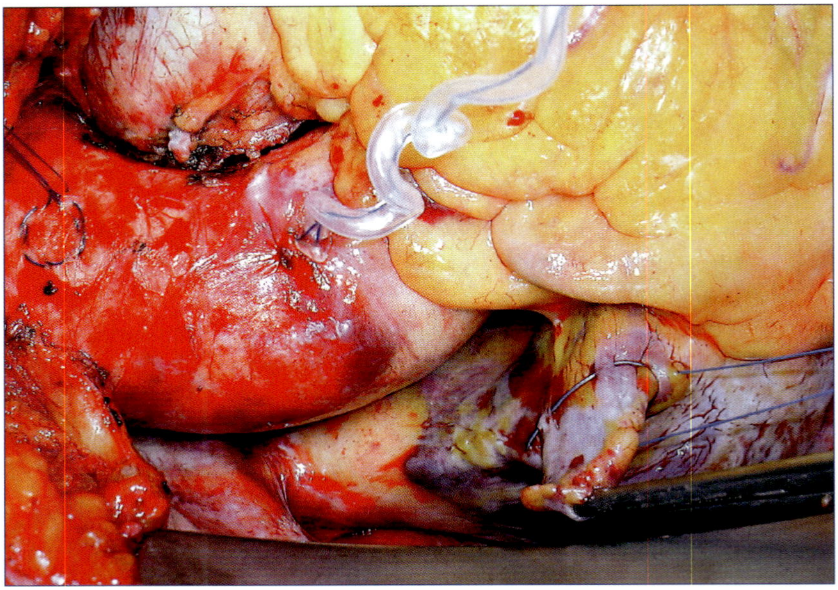

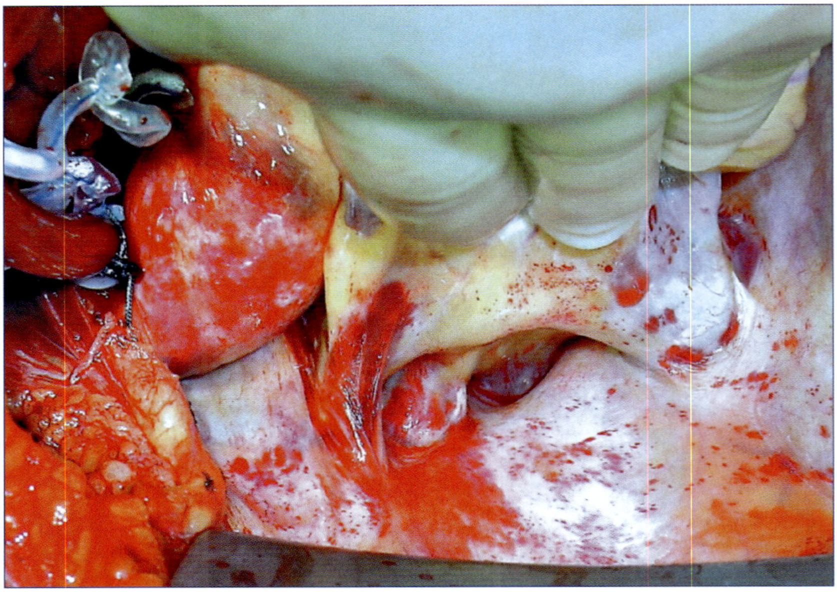

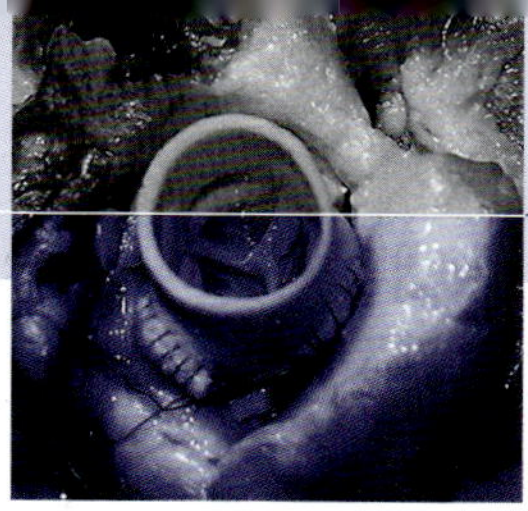

Aortic valve replacement (AVR):
Implantation of mechanical or stented biological cardiac valve prosthesis. Surgical site before cannulation. The purse-string sutures have been placed on the distal ascending aorta as well as around the tip of the right atrium for single venous two-stage cannulation. Aortic wall calcification most frequently accompanies aortic valve stenosis. Be cautious of any calcification at any aortic site, especially near the origin of the brachiocephalic trunk. If the ascending aorta is ectatic and requires reduction plasty, the proximal aortic arch will be cannulated. It is possible to employ bicaval venous cannulation, however it is not necessary as neither cavae need to be snared. In cases of isolated aortic valve stenosis, a cannulation stitch for cardioplegia is used.

Illustration of the interatrial groove:
Immediately after arterial and venous cannulation, the interatrial groove is exposed once the heart is unloaded.

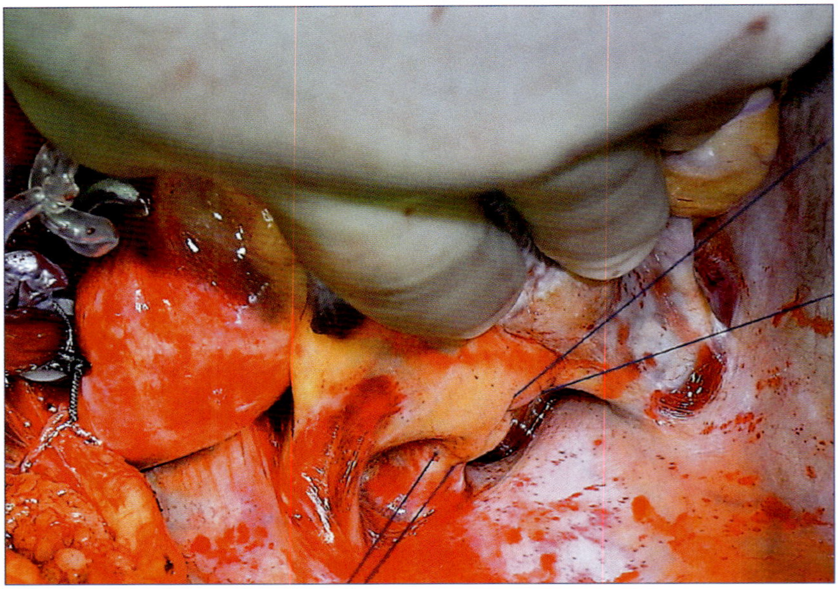

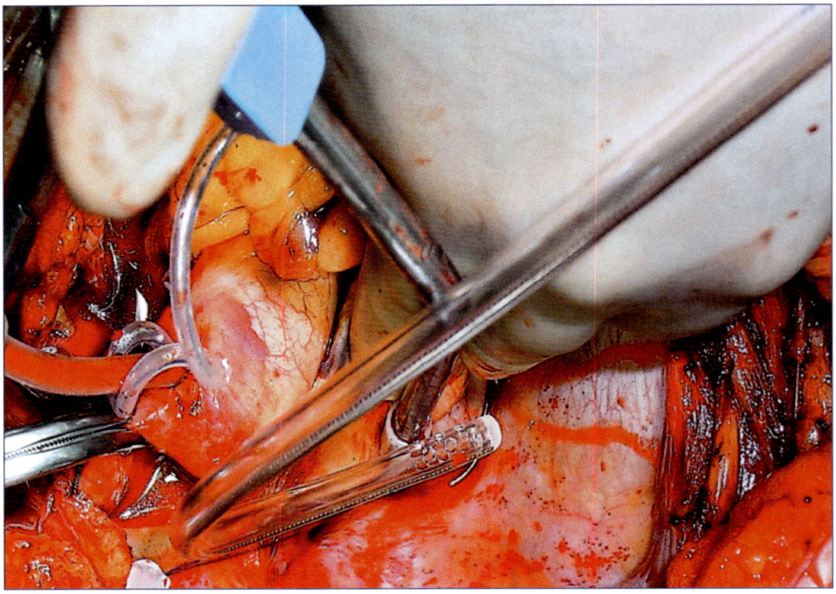

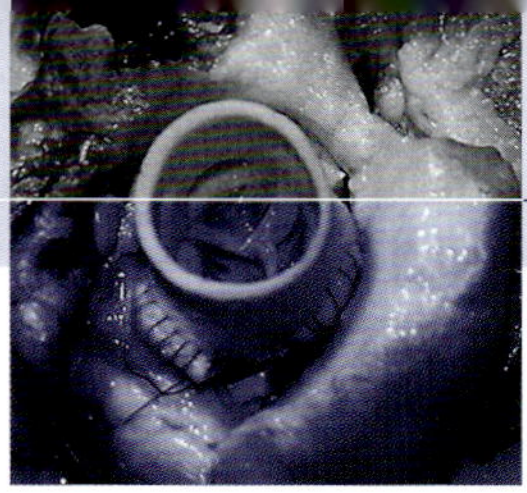

Placing the vent suture:

The vent suture is placed as a backhand U stitch from the right atrial wall of the interatrial groove in the direction of the right upper pulmonary veins (not necessarily entering the pulmonary veins). The thick tissue layers of the interatrial groove allow for a primary tightness of the suture. Lacerations of the pulmonary veins are avoided.

Placing of the left ventricular vent catheter:

In cases of aortic valve regurgitation, the left ventricular vent catheter is inserted immediately after aortic cross clamping, whereas in cases of aortic valve stenosis, the left ventricular vent catheter is inserted immediately after cardioplegia. The picture shows a malleable vent catheter. By palpating from outside the heart, the catheter is guided trans-atrially and trans-mitrally into the left ventricle. Care must be taken not to perforate the left ventricle in cases of end-stage disease with dilated ventricles or in combination surgery for post-infarct coronary disease.

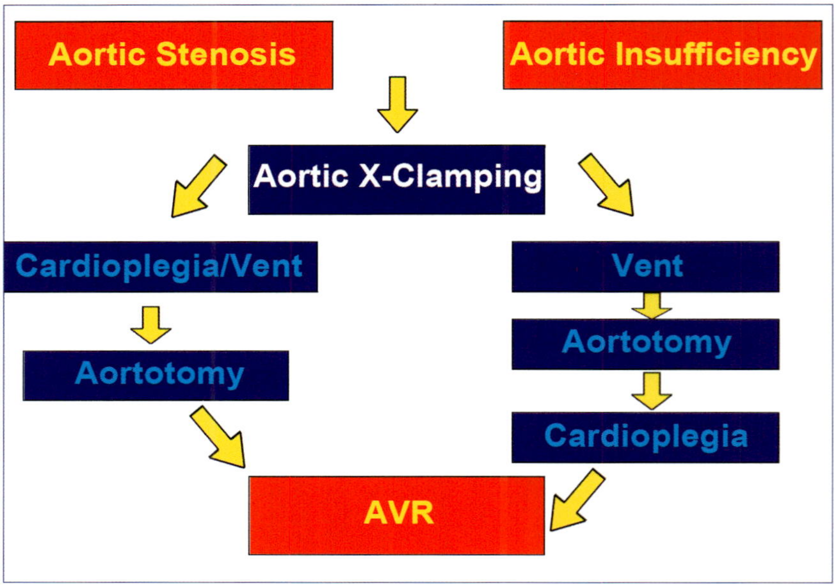
Aortic Stenosis
Aortic Insufficiency
Aortic X-Clamping
Cardioplegia/Vent
Aortotomy
Vent
Aortotomy
Cardioplegia
AVR

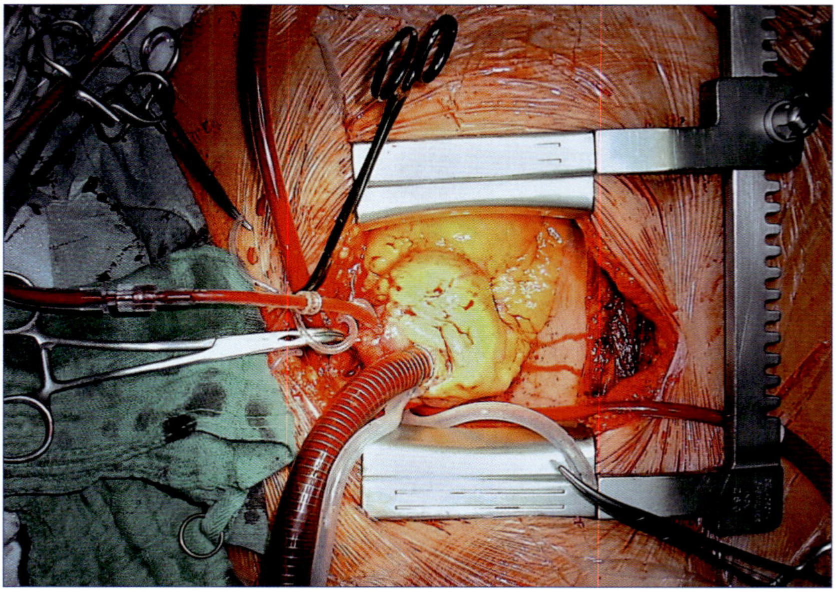

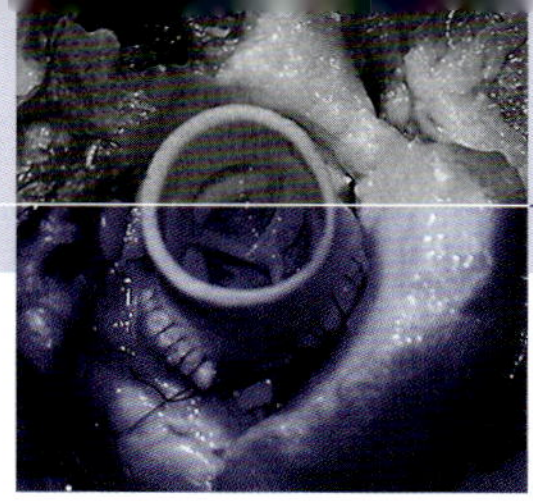

Schematic sequence from aortic cross clamping to aortic valve replacement:
In isolated aortic valve stenosis, cardioplegia infusion and insertion of the left ventricular vent are initiated simultaneously, immediately after aortic cross clamping. In cases of aortic valve regurgitation, the sequence is different. Immediately after aortic cross clamping, the vent is inserted into the left ventricle followed by the aortotomy when the left ventricle is decompressed. Cardioplegia is then given directly into the coronary ostia.

Surgical site during extracorporeal circulation:
This is the cannulation site for an aortic stenosis case. The heart is completely drained and empty and cardioplegia is being infused. There is a single venous two-stage cannula in the right atrium. The vent catheter tubing enters the field from below, running underneath the sternal retractor. The aortic cannula can be secured at the upper edge of the skin incision either with a suture or, as in this case, a Backhaus clamp (towel clip). The cardioplegia line enters the surgical site straight from above and is secured together with a 120° angled aortic clamp at the surgical drapes (Backhaus clamp sharp or blunt).

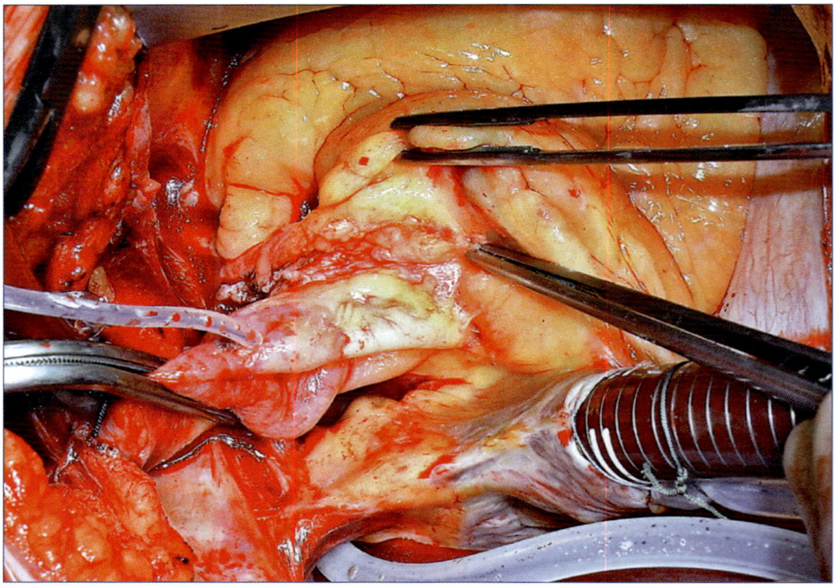

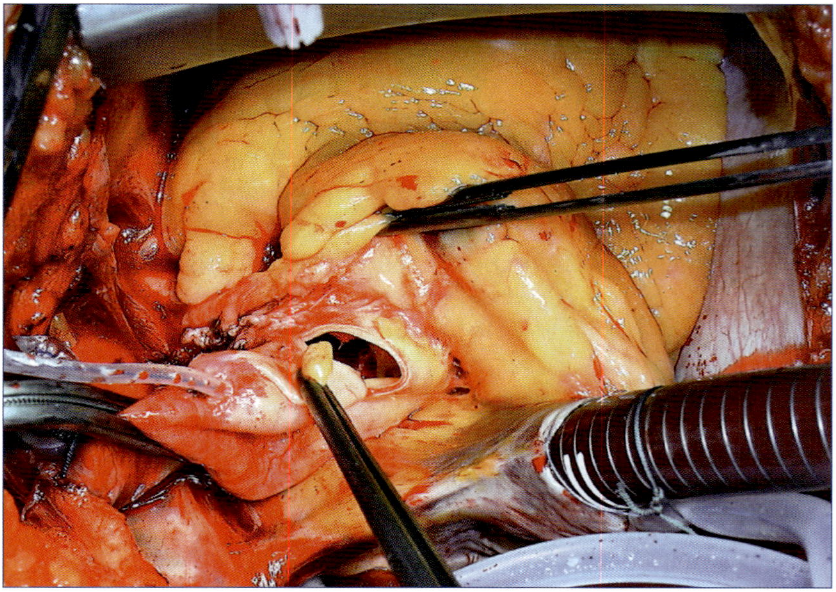

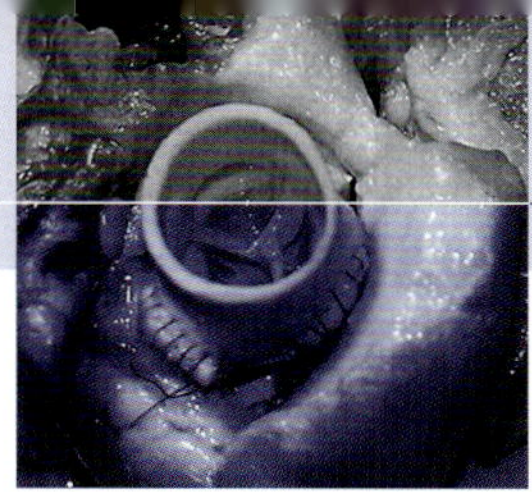

Where is the right coronary artery?
With inspection of the flaccid aortic root (in cases of aortic regurgitation before, and in cases of aortic stenosis, after infusion of cardioplegia) make sure to visualize the take-off of the right coronary artery at the outer aspect of the aortic root. Therefore the slight dissection of the aortic adventitia down to the heart is necessary.

Aortotomy:
Start with a small aortotomy incision and verify the intraaortic anatomy: distance to the right coronary artery ostium, distance to the commissures or to the sino-tubular junction. Then open the aorta completely, either oblique or in a hockey-stick shape, ending medially in the acoronary sinus; for the latter incision stop 0.5 to 1 cm above the annulus, otherwise the aortotomy closure is complicated.

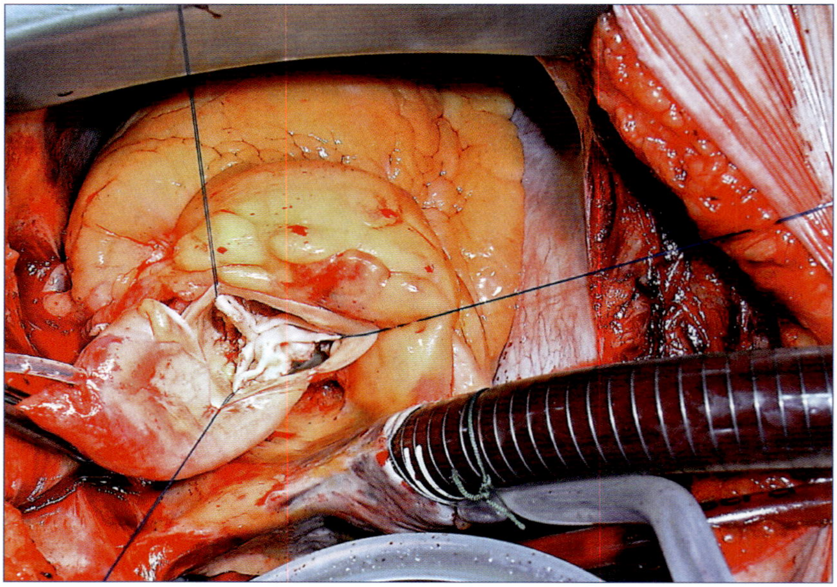

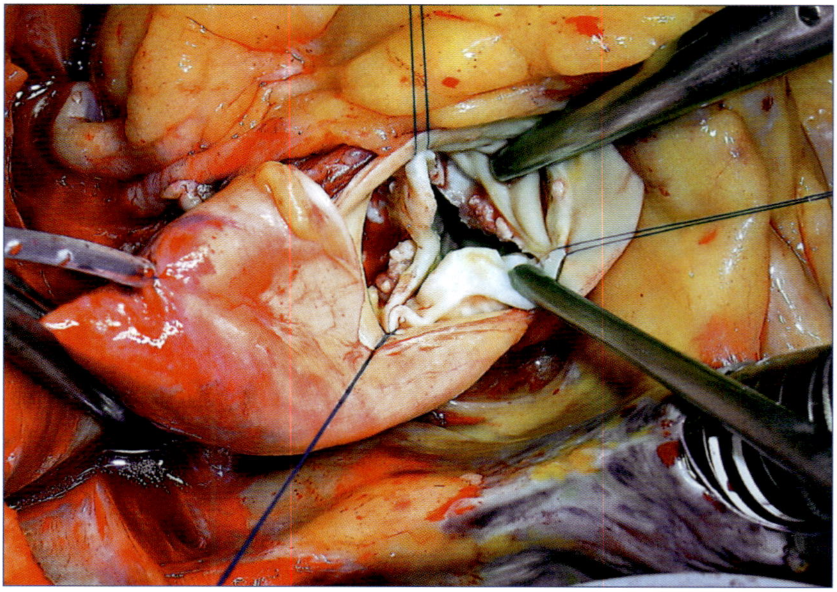

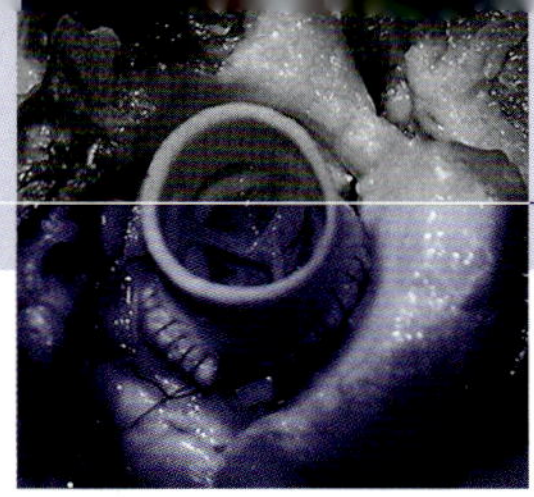

Exposure of the aortic valve:
After the standard aortotomy is completed, here oblique to the left and in a right angle direction into the acoronary sinus to the right ("hockey stick"), three staged sutures are placed into the commissures at their distal end. Even bicuspid aortic valves almost always have a third commissure which tends to be quite rudimentary.

Aortic valve excision I:
Especially in cases of heavily calcified valves, it is suggested to excise each cusp separately in a stepwise fashion. Before the next cusp is excised, the previous sinus section of the annulus is completely decalcified and cleaned. This stepwise approach allows for ideal management of calcium debris loss which increases the risk of embolism.

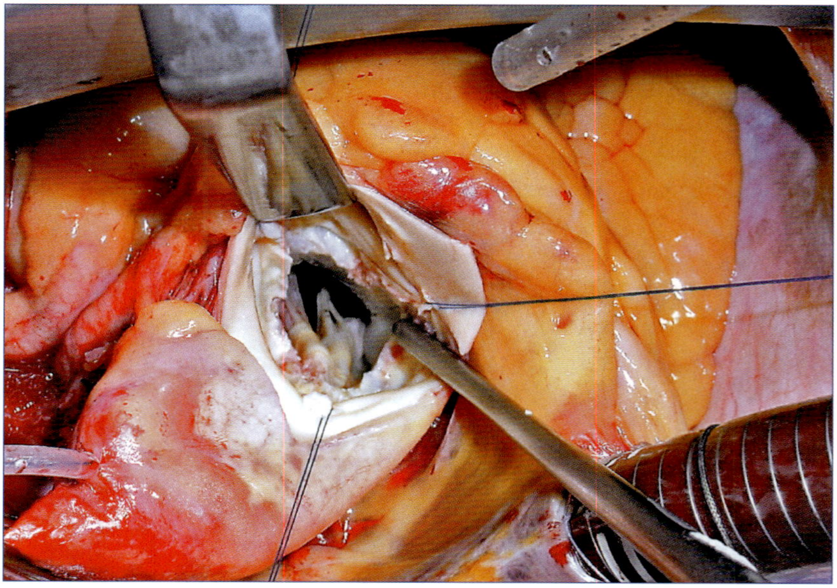

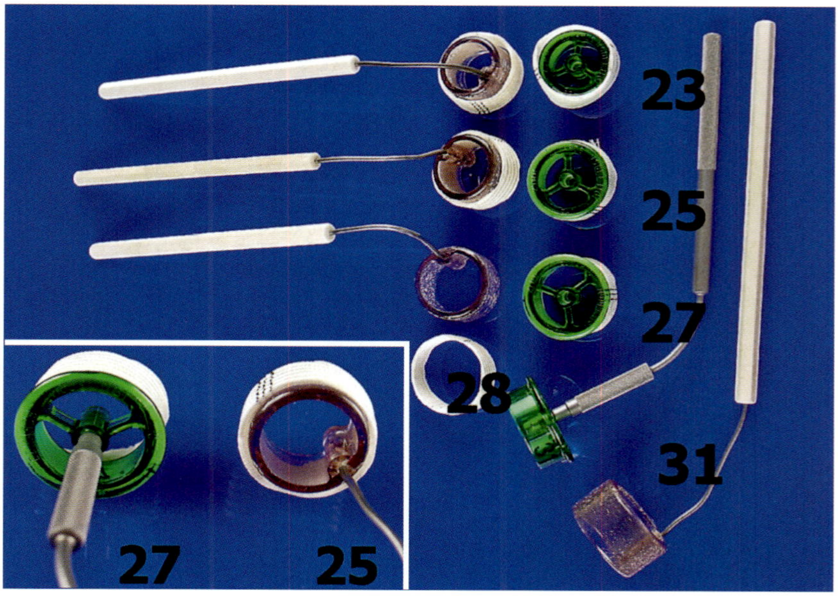
23
25
27
28
31
27
25

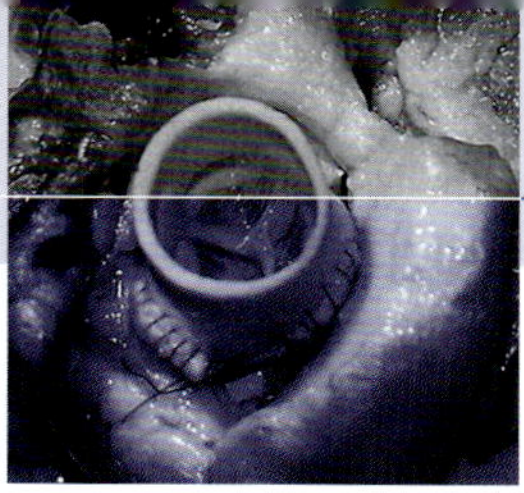

Aortic valve excision II:

After complete excision of the aortic valve and decalcification of the annulus, the interior of the left ventricle and the left ventricular aspect of the anterior mitral valve leaflet (aorto-mitral continuity) may be easily inspected. The stepwise excision procedure of the valve, as outlined before, omits the need for an intra left ventricular gauze to catch possible calcium fragments since each step has managed and eliminated all evidence of calcium fragments. Postoperatively these left ventricular gauzes, if not caught in the mechanical aortic valve prosthesis, have been found in various regions of the aorto-arterial tree!

Valve sizers:

This picture shows in detail the size labelling by manufacturers of cardiac valves. On the left side only the sizers 23 and 25 fit into a 28 mm Dacron tube, while on the right side even sizer 27 can also be introduced. In the small picture (bottom, left), a #27 sizer is compared to a #25 sizer. This difference does not depend on the implantation technique, supra- or intraannularly.

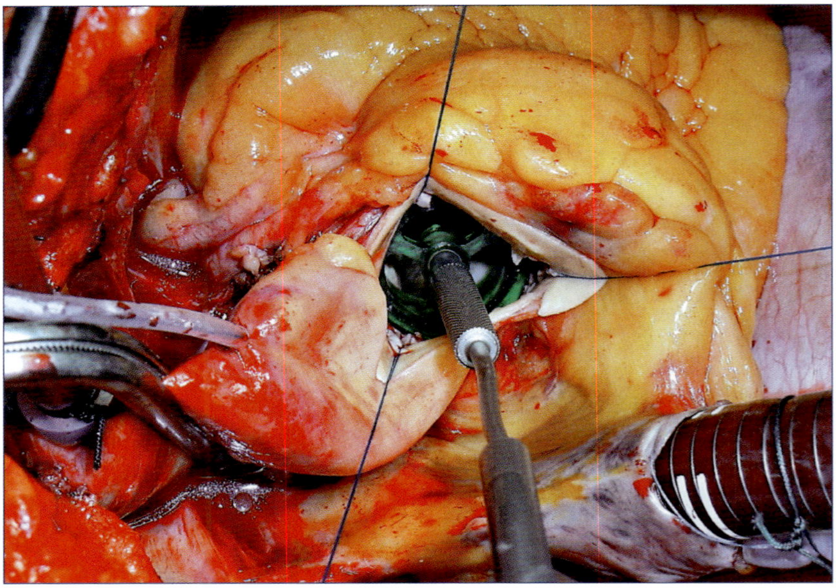

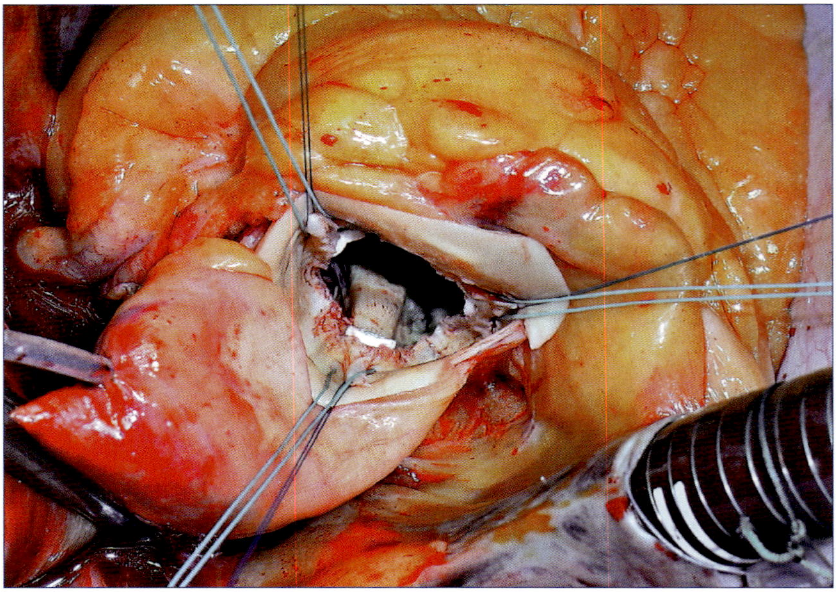

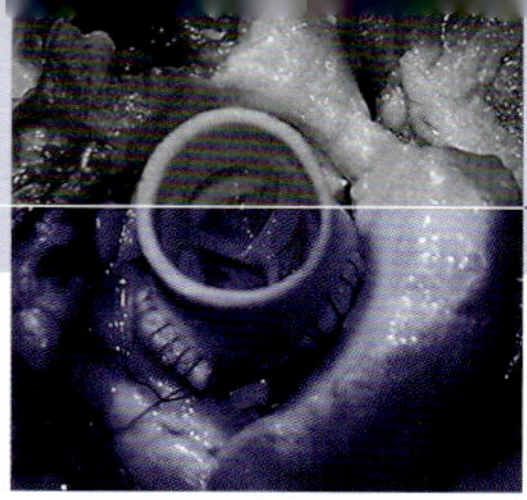

Sizing the annulus for supra-(epi-)annular implantation:
To measure the annulus for implantation of a valve in supraannular position, the rim of the sizer fits onto the annulus while the rest of the sizer is introduced into the orifice. It is important to assess the unrestricted coronary ostia and also the lower end of the aortotomy within the acoronary sinus. A smaller valve should be chosen if at least one coronary ostium is compromised and then should be implanted with everting sutures in intraannular position.

Commissural sutures:
To facilitate and secure symmetrical placement of all valve sutures, three commissural sutures should be positioned so that their location within the circumference has a certain distance below the sinotubular junction. Mechanical valves are implanted in a tangental plane to the deepest points of the aortic sinuses so the commissural sutures are therefore stitched at a relatively deep level. Biological valve prostheses, however, come with a scalopped suture-ring, mimicking the normal course of the ventricular aortic junction. Therefore commissure sutures for implantation of a biological valve are somewhat higher. We always use double armed multifilament polyester sutures ("1x0") with Teflon felt. Others employ "2x0" with or without felt.

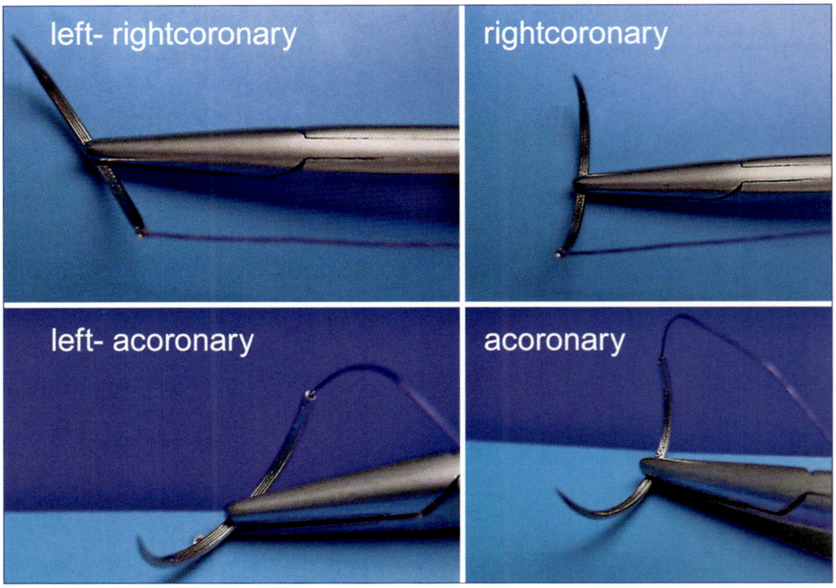
left- rightcoronary
rightcoronary
left- acoronary
acoronary

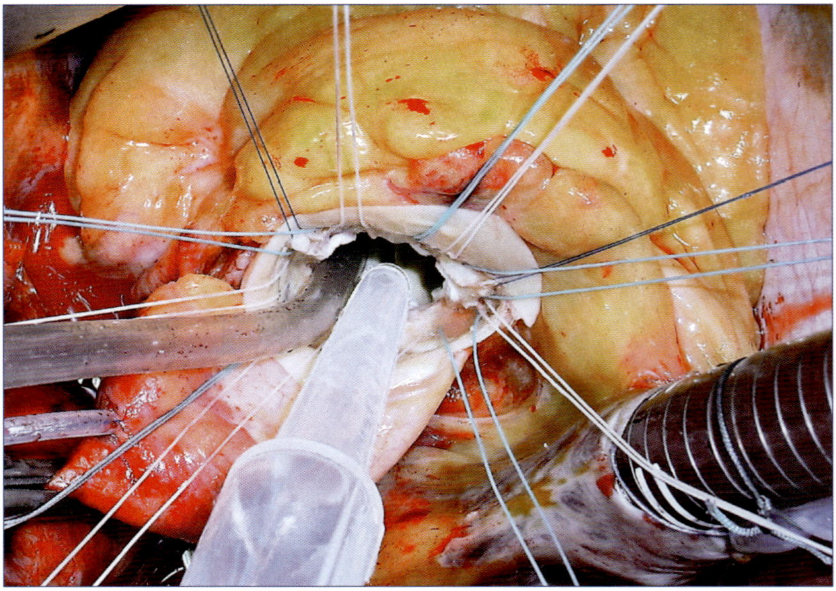

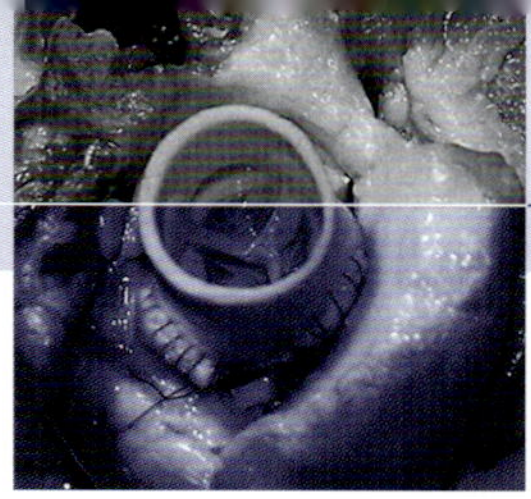

Needle orientation for supraannular aortic valve implantation: For supraannular implantation, the stitches come from the left ventricular outflow tract, through the annulus and into the aorta. The Teflon-felt pledget ("U"-stitch) ends up on the ventricular aspect of the annulus. In principle, any sequence for the stitches are possible. Frequently used is the sequence: left coronary, right coronary, acoronary. "While artists sew towards themselves, idiots sew away from themselves" (An elderly staff surgeon's advice to residents in training). In a smooth sequence with a balanced rhythm and adequate discipline, this results in three commissural sutures, and three U-stitches for each sinus (exceptions may support this rule). By planning the next stitch, the needles can be placed on the needle holder in such a way as to allow suturing without any distorsion of hand, arm or shoulder joints.

The last flush:
After all sutures are in place, the left ventricular cavity may be rinsed again with saline, even though it had been rinsed after decalcification of the annulus. The sutures should be layed out in the field in a star fashion to facilitate a rapid order in stitching the suture-ring of the valve prosthesis. For laying out the sutures in the operative field, an additional drape is necessary only when a skin drape is not in place. On the hand, additional drapes may support the outlayed order of sutures. Direct sequential stitching of patient and prosthetic annulus should be done only by the experienced surgeon. In real life it adds only to a hectic atmosphere than to saving time.

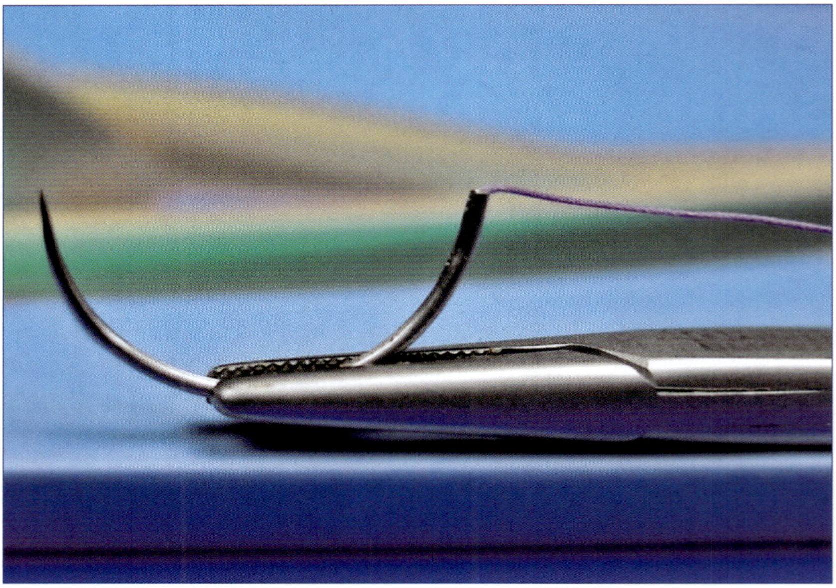

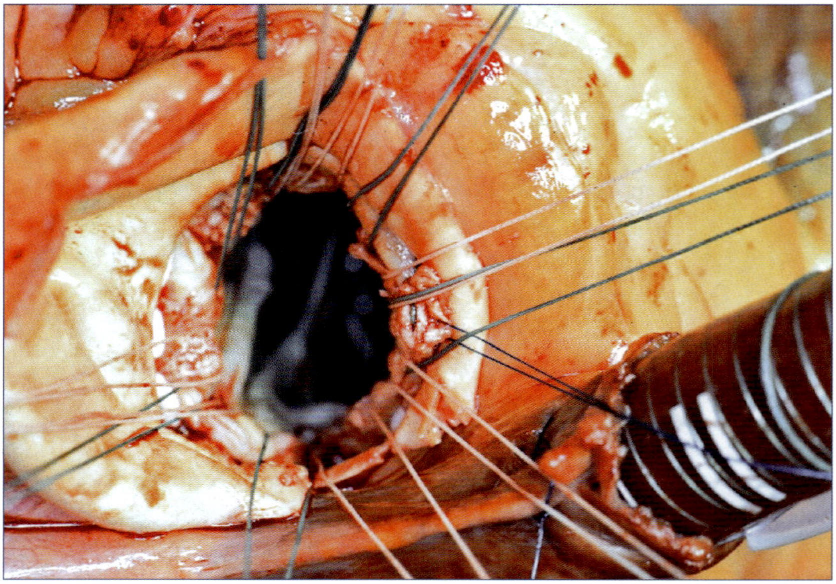

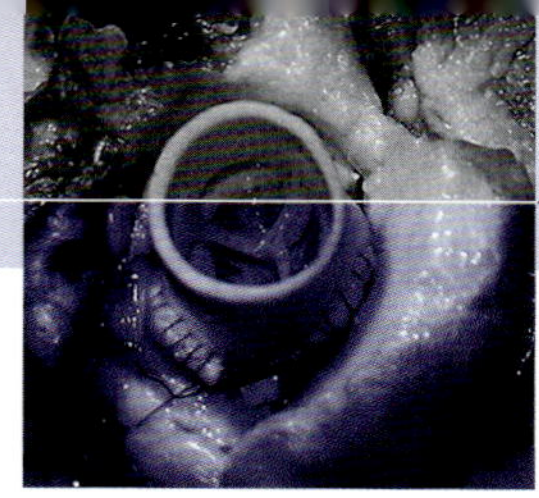

Needle placement for intraannular implantation of an aortic valve prosthesis:

For intraannular implantation, the stitches are run from the aorta, through the annulus into the left ventricular outflow tract and come back through the aortic valve orifice, into the aorta. For this technique we employ only one identical needle position in the needle holder as depicted on the photograph: The curved needle is mounted in tangent to the needle holder. The only change in stitching, while placing the different sutures, is a change between forehand and backhand and appropriate side movements.

Once the prosthesis is tied into the annulus, an eversion of the annulus results. For sequence of the stitches and tension of the sutures, the same procedure applies as described for the supraannular position. For a valve size of 23 mm and larger, regardless of the manufacturer, we prefer the intraannular technique of implantation.

The intraannular implantation technique is safer in avoiding coronary ostia obstruction.

Sutures in place for intraannular implantation of the valvular prosthesis. Three sutures for the commissures and three sutures each for the sinuses.

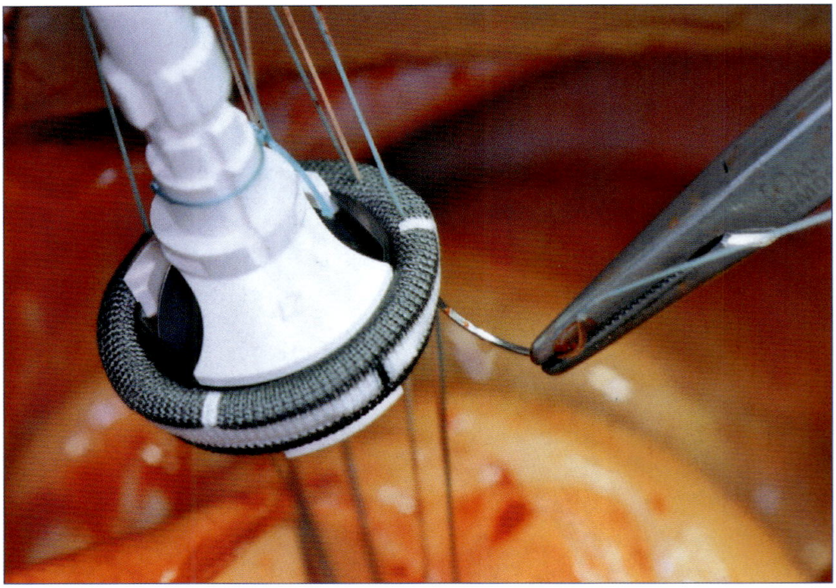

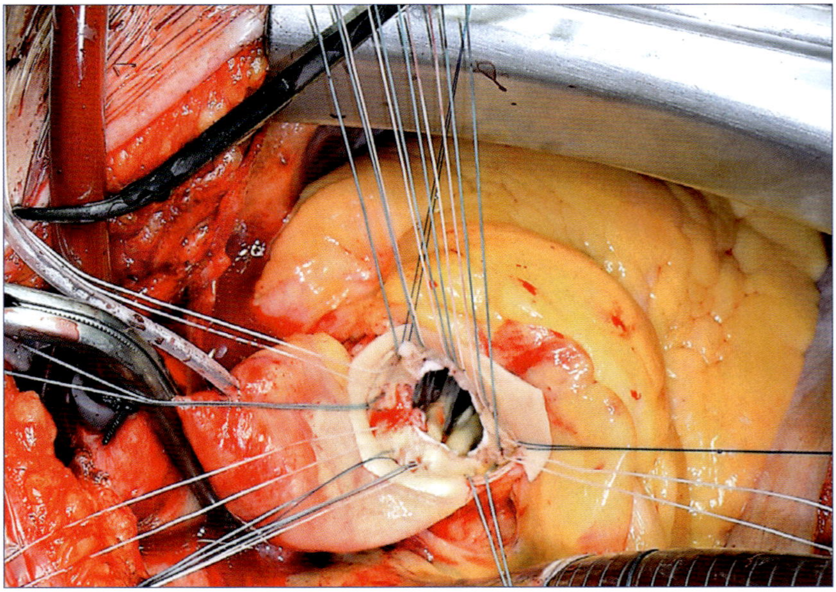

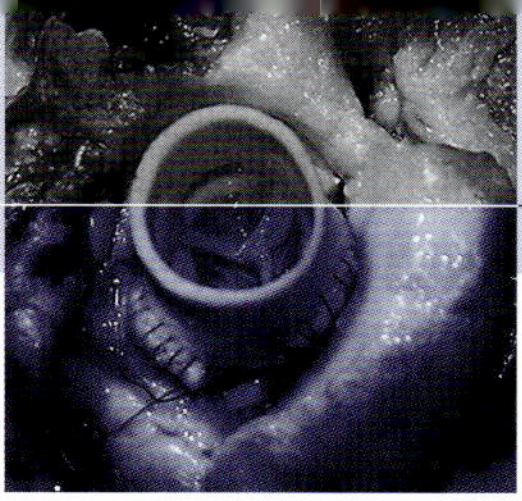

Hold the valve!

Placing the stitches in the suture-ring of the prosthesis can be done either in a backhand or forehand technique. The sequence is the same for suture placement in the annulus. The first assistant who really likes to help a surgeon, turns the valve according to the suture sequence. To ask a German resident to hold the valve ("Klappe halten") translates from German to English also as "shut up!"

Seating the valve:

After careful positioning of the prosthesis, with the sutures aligned, the valve is run down along the sutures into the annulus. In a very tight fit situation, a small dissector may have the same helping effect as a shoehorn for large feet that must fit into delicate Italian shoes.

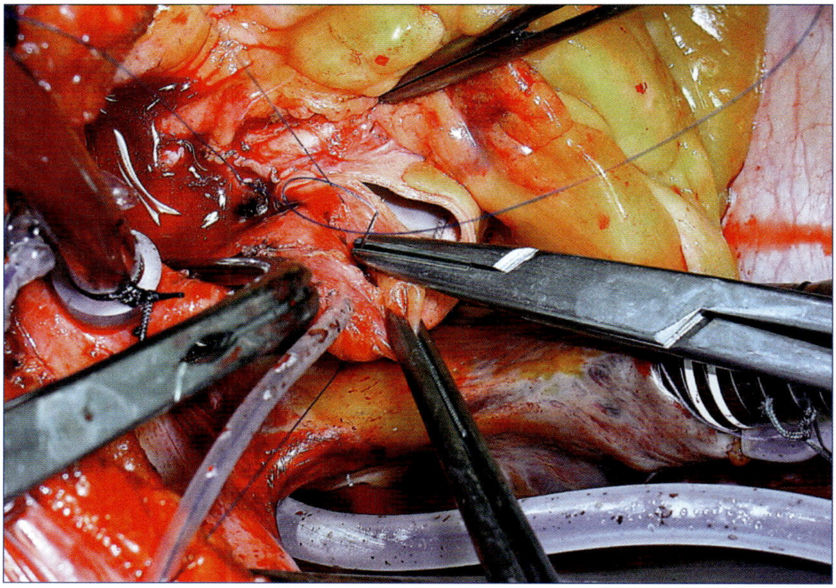

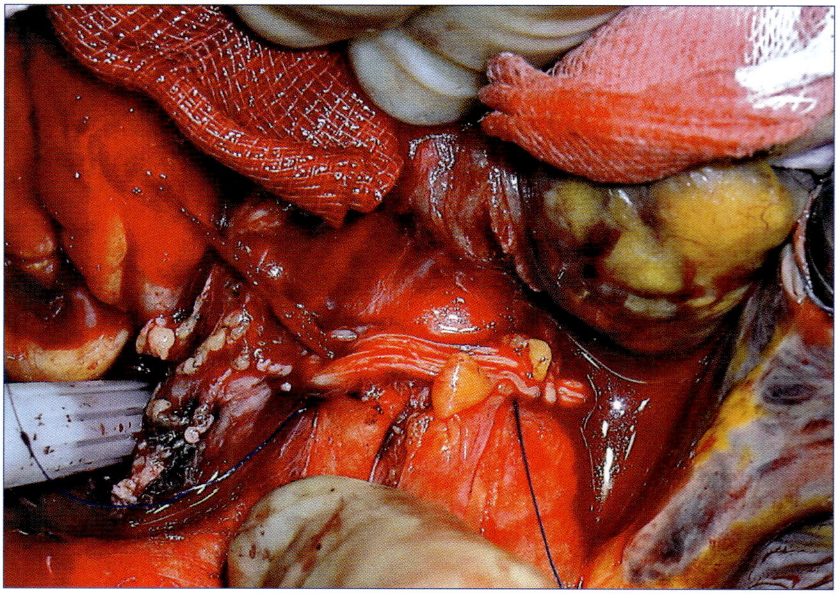

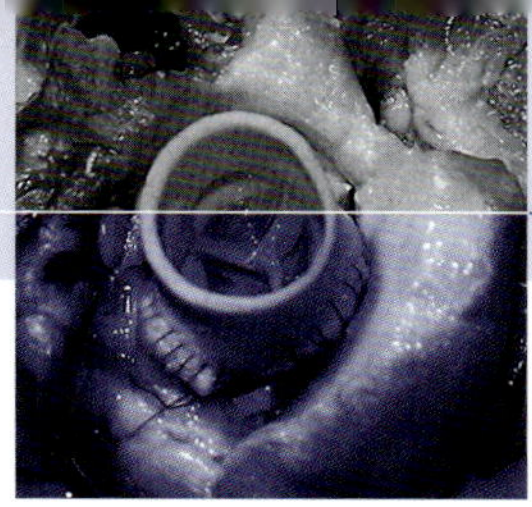

Aortotomy closure I:
While in young patients without aortic wall calcifications a single suture line may be sufficient, in elderly patients we always employ a double layer aortotomy closure. The first suture layer is done using a mattress technique and should result in an everting rim of both aortotomy cut edges. When the first layer of the aortotomy is almost closed, the patient may be rewarmed, if he had been moderately cooled before

Aortotomy closure II:
The rim of the first suture line is tested for leakage. Leakage, however, in this state is not a sign of poor suturing as a sufficient tightness cannot be achieved alone with the mattress suture.

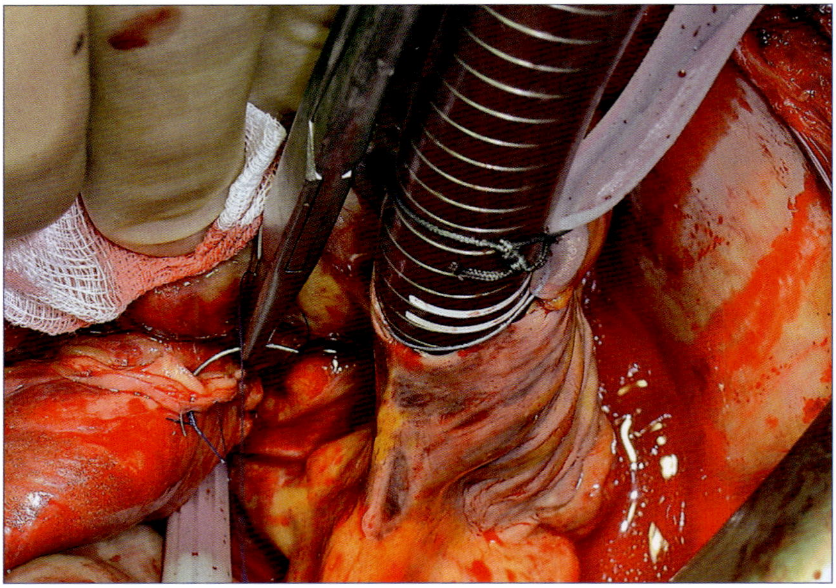

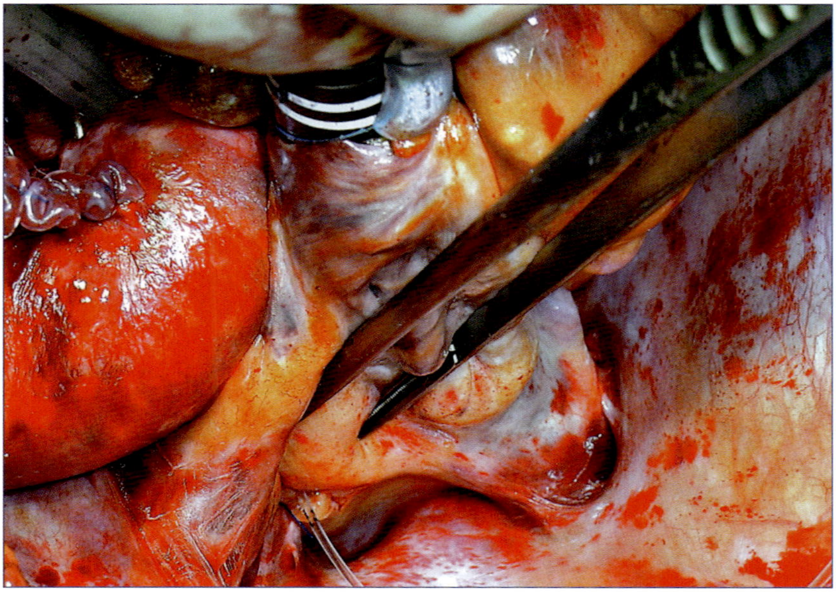

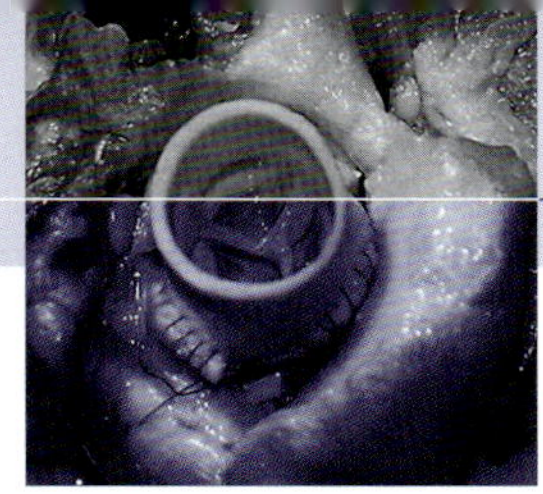

1 2 3 4 5 6 7 8 9 10 11 12 13 14 15

Aortotomy closure III:
The second layer of a double layer aortotomy closure is a simple over and over continuous suture. Ideally only the rim above the first mattress suture line is stitched. If this is accomplished there is no new intraluminal contact with more stitches and therefore no generation of new bleeding sites.

Left atrial catheter:
The last step before coming off bypass is the placement of a left atrial catheter for continuous monitoring of the left atrial pressure. If the catheter is introduced into the left atrium through the fat of the inter-atrial groove, no additional suture is necessary and this aids in reducing the bleeding after the catheter is taken out. The de-airing manoeuvres before and during weaning of extracorporeal circulation are the same as outlined in the chapter for mitral valve replacement.

1
2
3
4
5
6
7
8
9
10
11
12
13
14
15

References

1. Baskett R-J, Buth K-J, Legare J-F, Hassan A, Friesen CH, Hirsch G-M, Ross D-B, Sullivan J-A. Is it safe to train residents to perform cardiac surgery? Ann Thorac Surgery 2002 Oct; 74(4): 1043–8; DISCUSSION 1048–9
2. Brose S, Autschbach R, Rauch T, Engel M, Mohr F-W. Patienten-adaptierte Klappenselektion: biologischer vs. mechanischer Herzklappenersatz bei Aortenklappenvitien. [Patient-adapted valve selection: biological vs. mechanical heart valve replacement in aortic valve diseases] Z-Kardiol. 2001; 90 Suppl 6: 48–57
3. Collart F, Feier H, Kerbaul F, Mouly-Bandini A, Riberi A, Mesana T-G, Metras D. Valvular surgery in octogenarians: operative risks factors, evaluation of Euroscore and long term results. Eur J Cardiothorac-Surgery 2005 Feb; 27(2): 276–80
4. Corbineau H, De-La-Tour B, Verhoye J-P, Langanay T, Lelong B, Leguerrier A. Carpentier-Edwards supraannular porcine bioprosthesis in aortic position: 16-year experience. Ann Thorac Surgery 2001 May; 71(5 Suppl): 228–31
5. Gao G, Wu Y, Grunkemeier G-L, Furnary A-P, Starr A. Durability of pericardial versus porcine aortic valves. J Am Coll-Cardiol. 2004 Jul 21; 44(2): 384–8
6. Kolh P, Kerzmann A, Lahaye L, Gerard P, Limet R. Cardiac surgery in octogenarians; peri-operative outcome and long-term results. Eur Heart J. 2001 Jul; 22(14): 1235–43
7. Kolh P, Lahaye L, Gerard P. Limet R Aortic valve replacement in the octogenarians: perioperative outcome and clinical follow-up. Eur J Cardiothorac-Surgery 1999 Jul; 16(1): 68–73
8. Milano A-D, De-Carlo M, Mecozzi G, D'Alfonso A, Scioti G, Nardi C, Bortolotti U. Clinical outcome in patients with 19-mm and 21-mm St. Jude aortic prostheses: comparison at long-term follow-up. Ann Thorac Surgery 2002 Jan; 73(1): 37–43
9. Mistiaen W, Van-Cauwelaert P, Sys S-U, Muylaert P, Harrisson F, Bortier H. Role of age, gender and association of CABG on long-term results after aortic valve replacement with a Carpentier-Edwards bioprosthesis in the elderly. J Cardiovasc Surgery (Torino). 2003 Dec; 44(6): 701–6

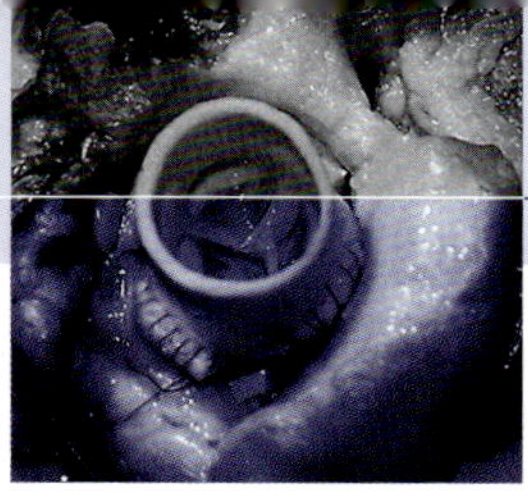

10. Mortasawi A, Gehle S, Yaghmaie M, Schroder T, Ennker IC, Rosendahl U, Albert A, Ennker J. Kurz- und Langzeitergebnisse des Aortenklappenersatzes bei 80- und über 80-Jährigen. [Short and long term results of aortic valve replacement in patients 80 years of age and older] Herz. 2001 Mar; 26(2): 140–8
11. Russo C-F, Mazzetti S, Garatti A, Ribera E, Milazzo A, Bruschi G, Lanfranconi M, Colombo T, Vitali E. Aortic complications after bicuspid aortic valve replacement: long-term results. Ann Thorac Surgery 2002 Nov; 74(5): 1773-6; discussion S1792–9
12. Seitelberger R, Bialy J, Gottardi R, Seebacher G, Moidl R, Mittel bock M, Simon P, Wolner E. Relation between size of prosthesis and valve gradient: comparison of two aortic bioprosthesis. Eur J Cardiothorac Surgery 2004 Mar; 25(3): 358–63
13. Sethi G-K, Hammermeister K-E, Oprian C, Henderson W. Impact of resident training on postoperative morbidity in patients undergoing single valve replacement. Department of Veterans Affairs Cooperative Study on Valvular Heart Disease. J Thorac Cardiovasc Surgery 1991 Jun; 101(6): 1053–9
14. Sethi G, Oprian C, Miller D-C, Khuri S, Cantor A, Henderson W-G, Hammermeister K-E. Operative mortality in patients undergoing single valve replacement in teaching institutions–early mortality as a function of resident versus staff surgeon. Surgery 1988 Aug; 104(2): 301–10
15. Sioris T, David T-E, Ivanov J, Armstrong S, Feindel C-M. Clinical outcomes after separate and composite replacement of the aortic valve and ascending aorta. J Thorac Cardiovasc Surgery 2004 Aug; 128(2): 260–5
16. Ura M, Sakata R, Nakayama Y, Fukui H. Bileaflet mechanical valve (St. Jude Medical valve) replacement in long-term dialysis patients. Ann Thorac Surgery 1999 Sep; 68(3): 870–3
17. Yamasaki M, Sasaguri S, Hosoda Y, Takazawa K, Yamamoto T, Hariya A Long-term results for aortic valve replacement with small aortic annulus. Artif-Organs. 2002 May; 26(5): 474–8

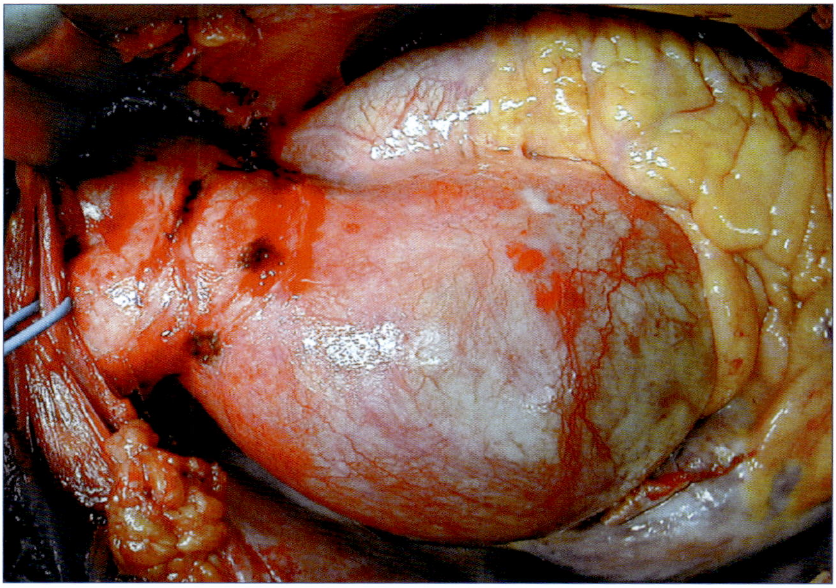

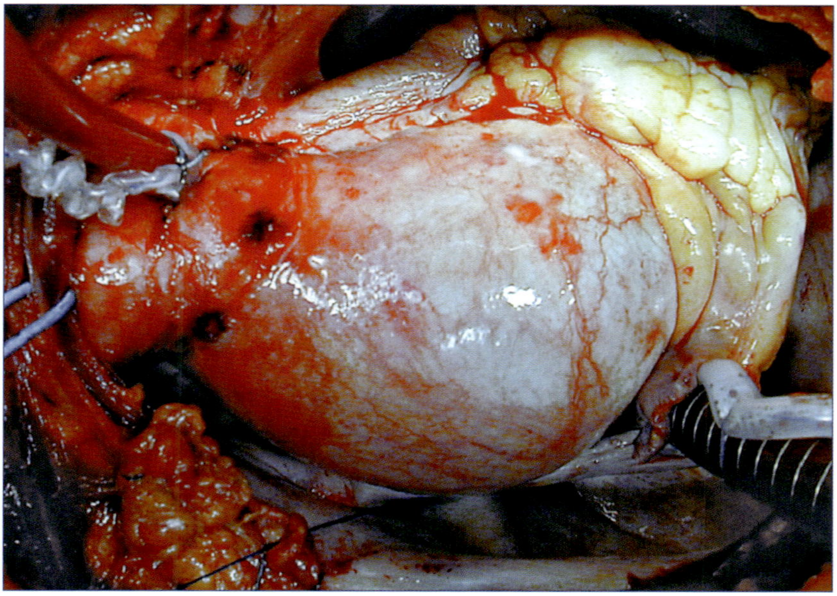

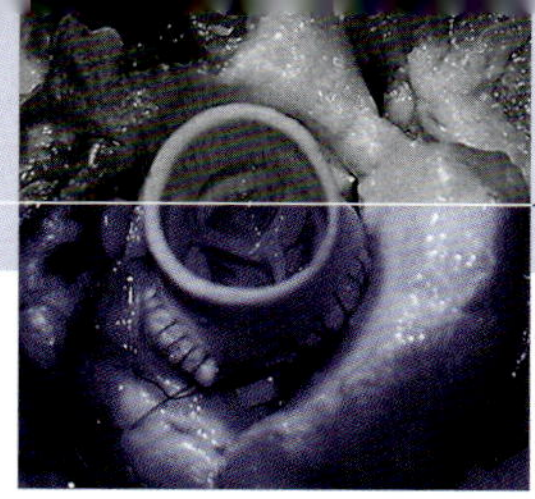

Replacement of the Ascending Aorta

J. M. Albes

Aneurysms of the ascending aorta with or without concomitant aortic valve disease can reach considerable extents. The risk of dissection or rupture increases rapidly from a diameter of 5 cm. In these instances, the benefit of a replacement markedly outweighs the operative risks. A concomitant aortic valve disease can prevailingly influence the prognosis. In case of a moderate aneurysm and concomitant hemodynamically relevant aortic stenosis or insufficiency additional replacement of the aorta is recommended already at a diameter of 4.5 cm because progression of the aneurysm can be expected. Early mortality of ascending aortic surgery, however, lies around 10% and must therefore be kept in mind. In contrast, early mortality of isolated aortic valve replacement is only 6%. For the purpose of risk reduction in elderly patients with valve disease and concomitant moderate aortic ectasia simplified measures such as aortic valve replacement and tailoring of the ascending aorta or prosthetic wrapping can be considered as an alternative.

Cannulation for the heart-lung-machine follows standard recommendations. The aortic cannula is placed in the proximal arch, if the procedure can be confined to the ascending aorta in order to generate space for x-clamping or to ensure an open anastomosis at the junction to the arch in short deep-hypothermic arrest. If the arch is involved cannulation of the ascending aorta is recommended. The anastomosis between prosthesis and aorta is then performed in deep-hypothermic arrest and the cannula is thereafter repositioned into the prosthesis. Venous drainage can be performed with a two-stage cannula. The U-suture for the left-atrial venting catheter can be readily performed once extracorporeal circulation is commenced and the heart is unloaded. A retrograde cardioplegic cannula facilitates the procedure because cardioplegic solution can be intermittently applied without jeopardizing exposition. Positioning of the catheter, however, can be arduous at times in case of a large aneurysm displacing the right atrium. If the aortic valve is unaltered cardioplegia may be applied directly via the aortic root.

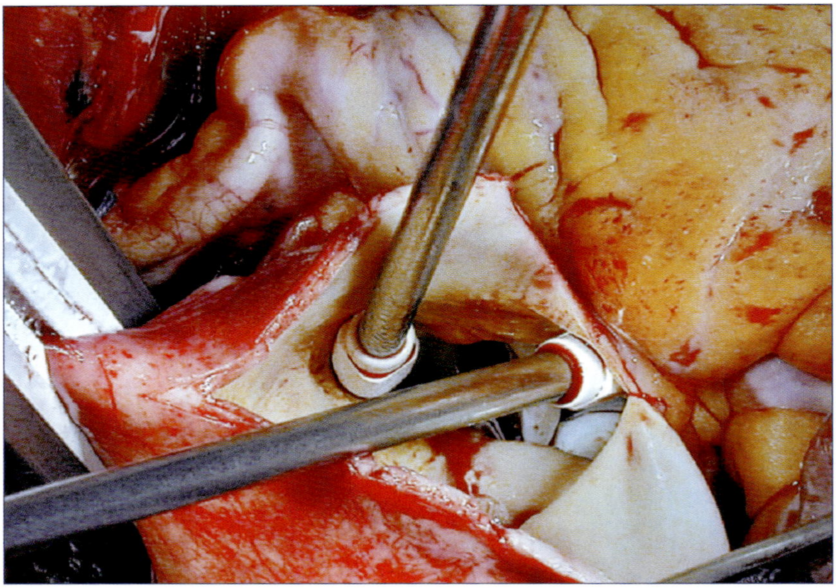

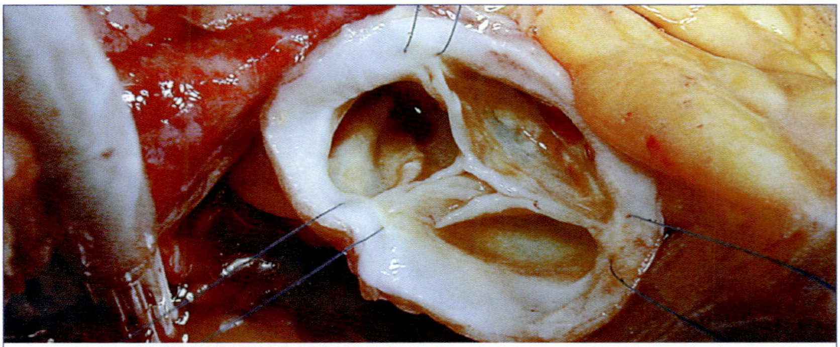

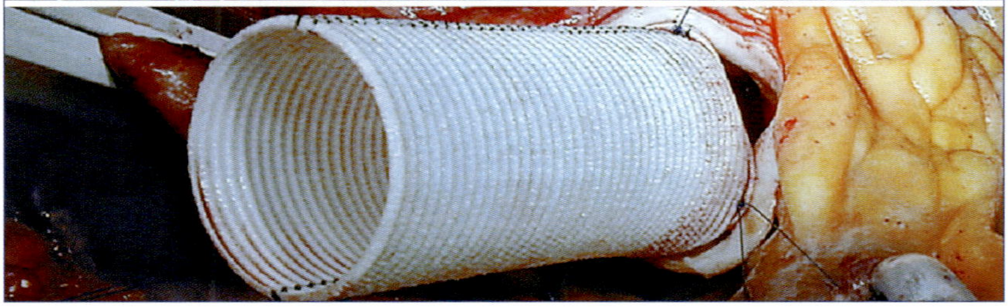

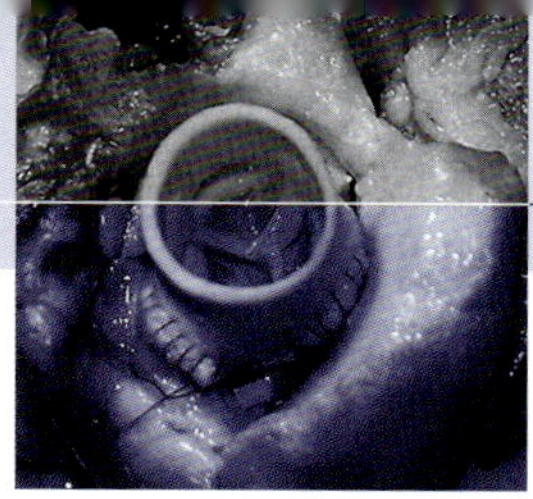

After start of extracorporeal circulation and consecutive cooling to 32° C (no arrest) or 20° C (deep-hypothermic arrest) non-traumatic X-clamping of the aorta with a rubber-armed clamp is performed. The aneurysm is opened in a longitudinal fashion. Cardioplegia is applied via both ostia.

Isolated aortic aneurysm: The ascending aorta is circumferentially transsected directly above the commissures. Fixation of the commissures with polypropylene 4/0 U-sutures is performed. A collagen-coated prosthesis is chosen. A valve sizer is recommended to verify proper diameter (typical sizes: 26 or 28mm; at times 30 mm). The prosthesis is cut in halves. The commissural sutures are placed i n the edge of the prosthesis in a isosceles triangular fashion. The sutures are knot down. Completion of the anastomois with these sutures in a running fashion. Final knots are thus located between the commissures.

1
2
3
4
5
6
7
8
9
10
11
12
13
14
15

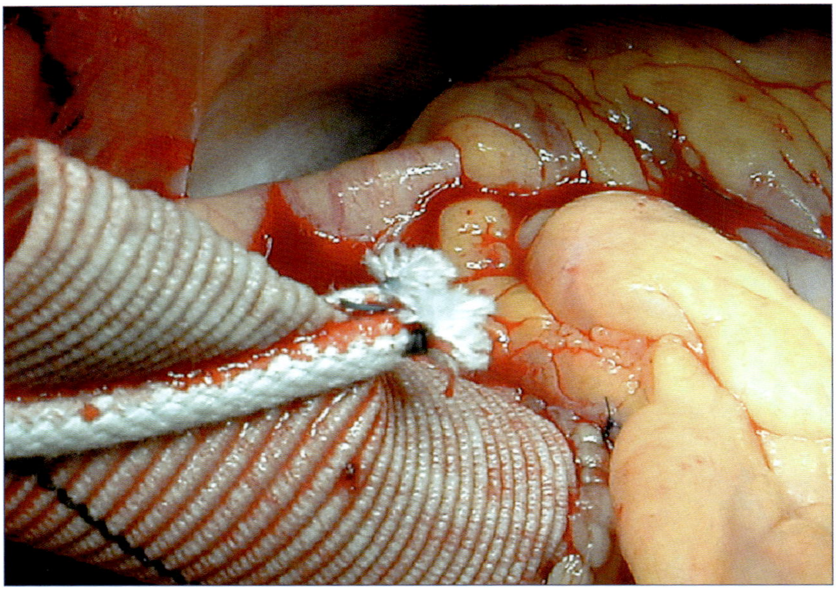

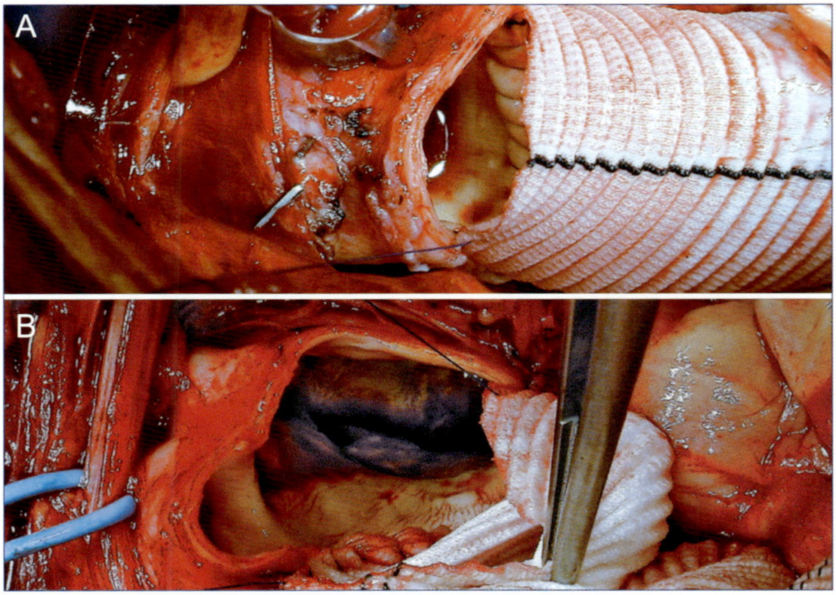

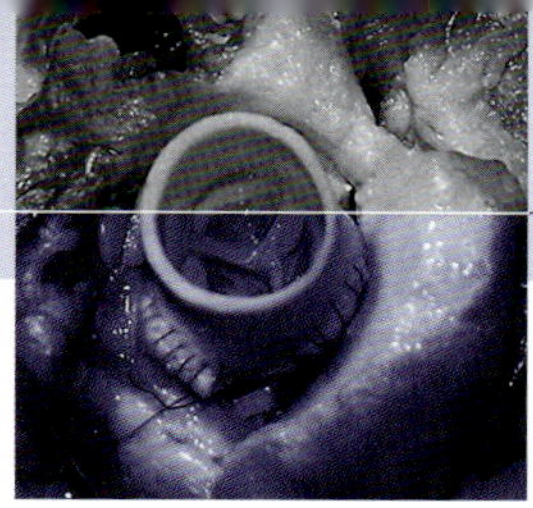

Application of cardioplegia via the aortic root (pressure 100–150mm Hg). Thus, sufficient coaptation of the valve cusps as well as tightness of the anastomosis can be tested simultaneously. Important: a fabric-covered non-traumatic, curved clamp should be used for the prosthesis in order to avoid microfractures. A small mosquito-clamp (arrow) placed between cardioplegic cannula and curved clamp improves tightness during application of cardioplegia.

The prosthesis is nearly always shortened in an oblique fashion in order to match the larger diameter of the native proximal arch. Attention: The prosthesis requires almost always considerable shortening in order to avoid kinking of the posterior wall. Quite often is the posterior length of the prosthesis only 2 cm (figure A).
In case of clamped aorta (isolated ascending aortic replacement) the clamp is gently lowered towards the heart by the first assistant in order to verify proper length ("too short" does not occur, "too long", however, often): This position is maintained during the proximal anastomosis with polypropylene 4/0 or 3/0 running suture.
In case of an open anastomosis or proximal arch replacement (deep hypothermic arrest) the heart-lung-machine is stopped once 20° C is reached. The aneurysm is liberally resected including the aortic cannulation site, if necessary, and the prosthesio-aortic anastomosis is accomplished. At times, it may be useful to perform this anastomosis with he second half of the initially cut prosthesis in order to facilitate the anastomosis to the arch (figure B).

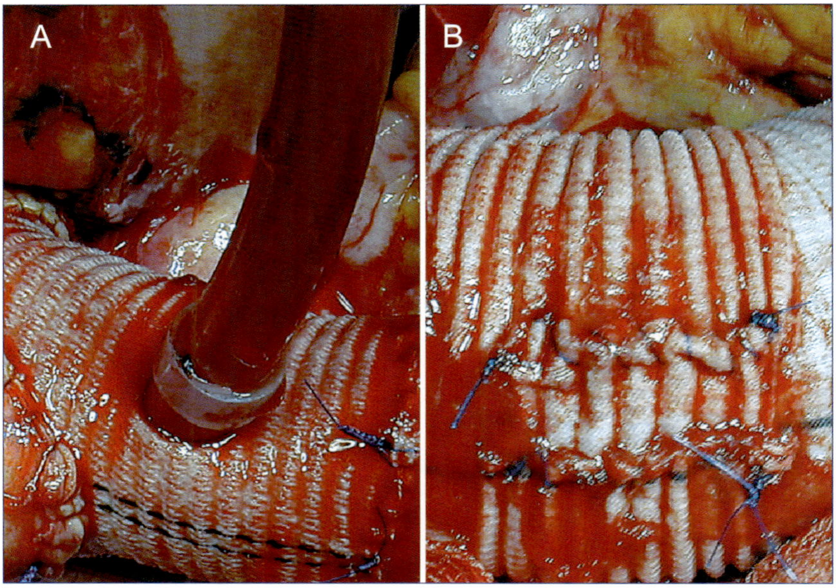
A
B

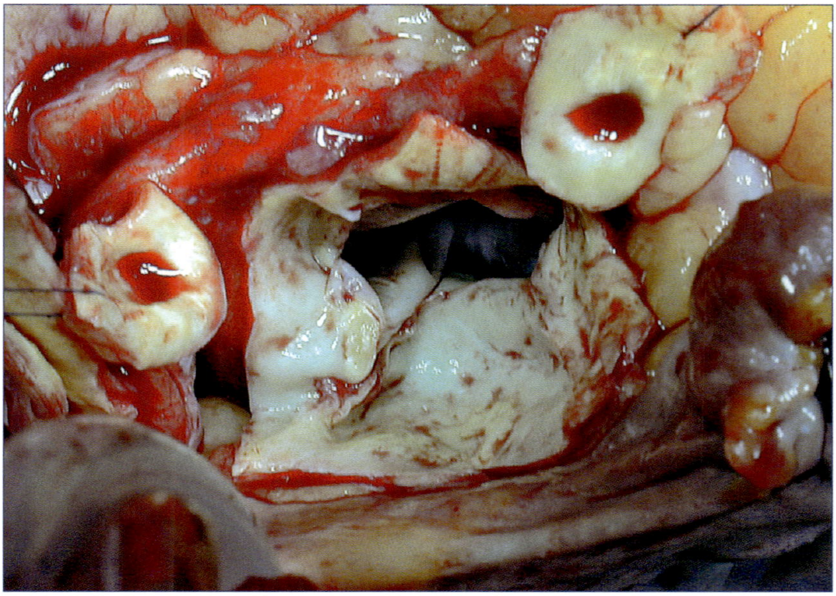

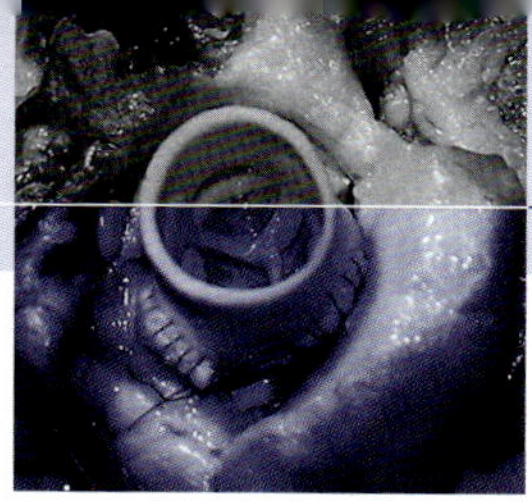

Repositioning of the aortic cannulation into the prosthesis. A rather small, horizontal incision is recommended. Placement of 2 pledget-reinforced polypropylene 4/0 U-sutures facilitates tight closure after decannulation (not seen). It is noteworthy to maintain adequate space for clamping of the prosthesis proximal to the cannulation site for proper de-airing of the heart after resuming extracorporeal circulation (A). Anastomosis of the two prosthetic parts is performed with 4/0 polypropylene running sutures. Tightness of this always oozing anastomosis can be improved by covering the region with a sleeve constructed from two stripes of surplus prosthesis material (B).
After weaning from extracorporeal circulation and decannulation the prosthesis may be rinsed with non-absorbable antibiotic solution (Neomycine/Bacitracine) and covered with fibrin-glue in order to achieve a bacteriostatic milieu.

Aortic valve and ascending aortic replacement with a conduit: Button-technique: In a first step, the aneurysm is transsected circumferentially. Thereafter, both ostia are excised resembling a funnel and suspended with polypropylene 4/0-sutures. The cusps are resected and the valve is sized (typically 23 or 25 mm). The appropriate composite graft is chosen (23/26mm or 25/28mm). Tight approximation of the tissue of the annulus in case of a rigid, fibrotic rim, however, can be difficult. Therefore, "defensive" sizing (i.e. choice of the next smaller size) is recommended.

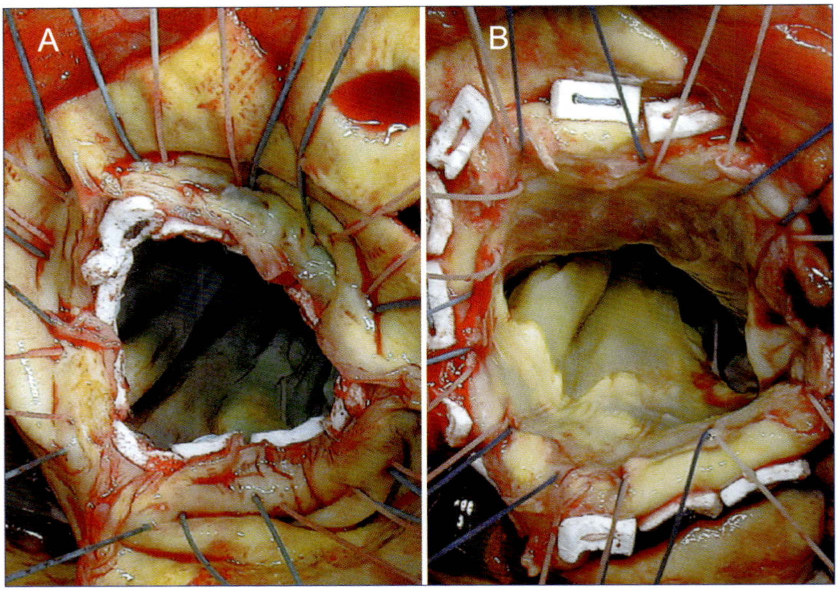
A
B

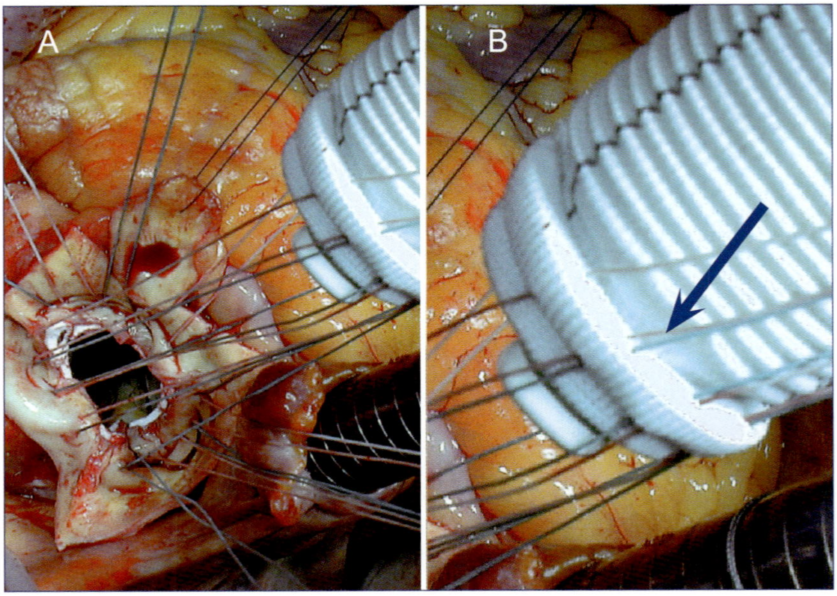
A
B

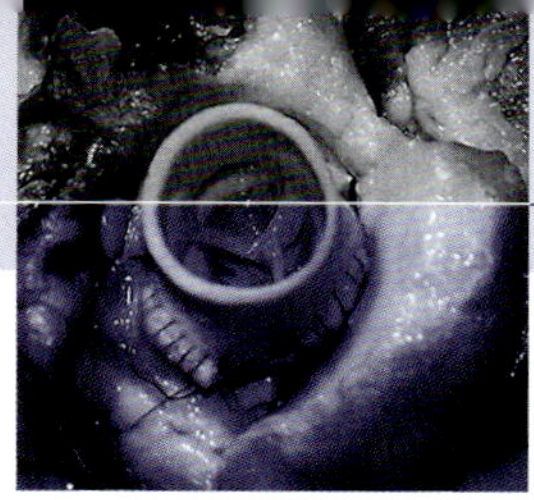

Epiannular placement of approximately 12–14 pledget-reinforced non-absorbable, braided 2/0-sutures in case of a small annulus (A). Consequently, the valve is positioned above the annulus. Intraannular placement in case of a large annulus. Thereby a reduction of the annulus size can be achieved. Consequently, the prosthesis is positioned inside the native annulus (B).

Placement of the sutures in the valve rim of the prosthesis (A). The adjacent U-sutures are stiched in tight proximity in order to avoid leakage of this entirely uncovered area (B). Attention: Do not pass the next needle through the already placed braided suture.

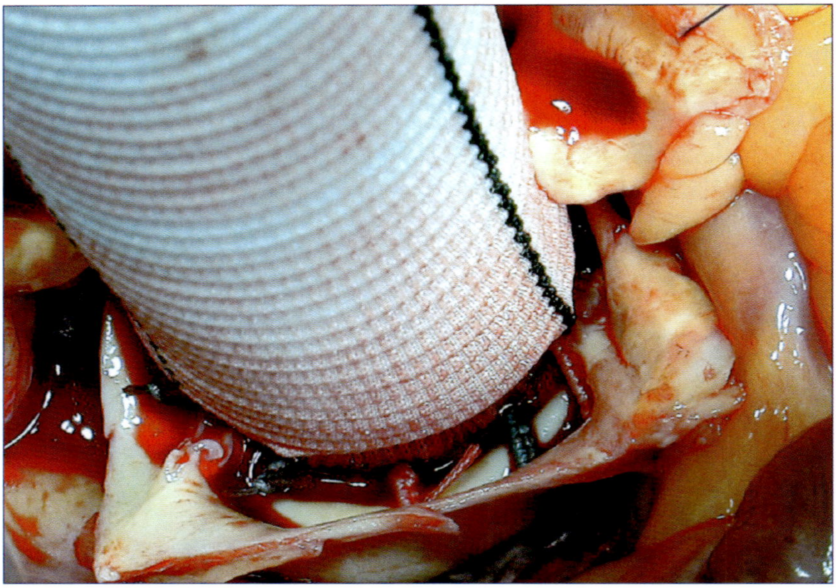

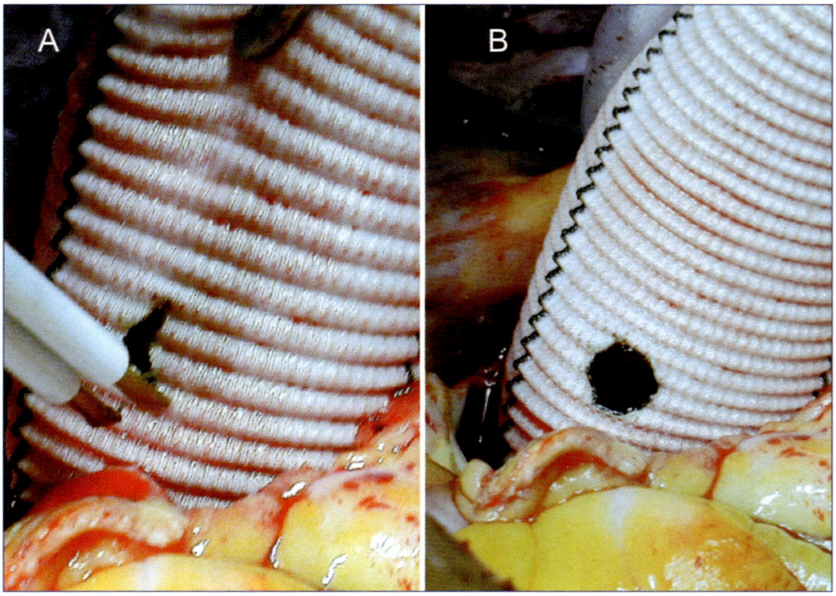
A
B

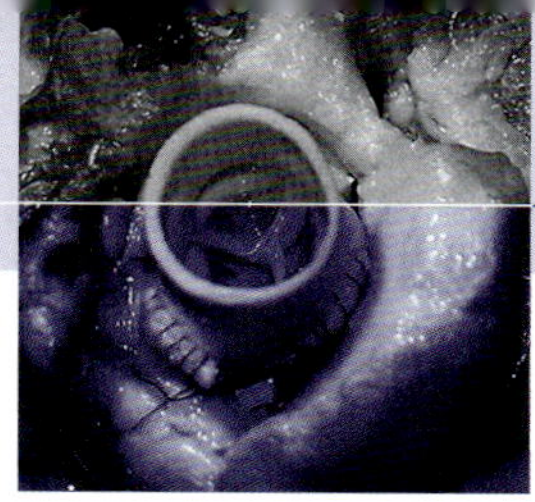

Approximation of the prosthesis and knotting

Positioning of the holes in the prosthesis for the anastomosis to the native ostia require utmost care. The correct position can be evaluated by means of tense-free approximation of the respective ostium with a forceps. A little blood remaining in the ostium marks the exact position. A battery driven electro-coagulator provided by the manufacturer is used. During burning utmost care is taken to avoid any contact of the hot wire with the surrounding prosthesis. The hole can be made rather large (6–8mm).

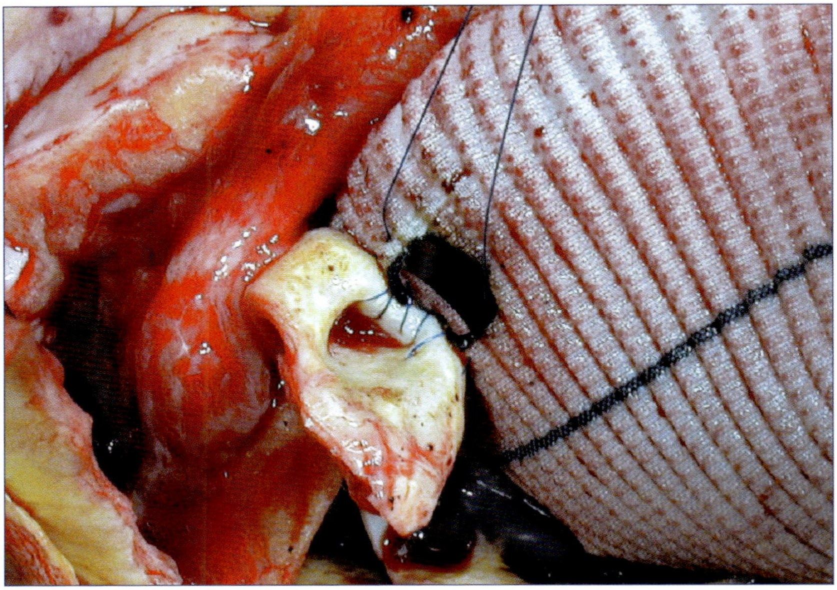

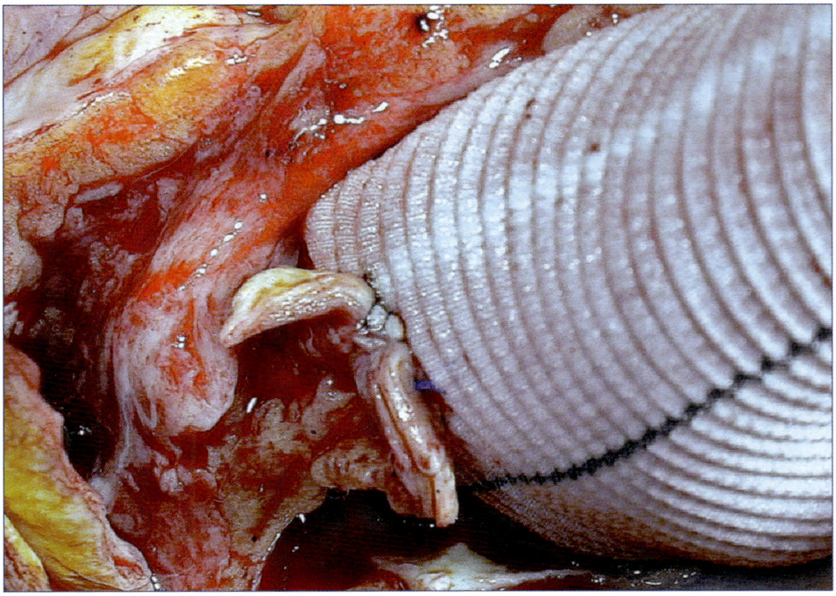

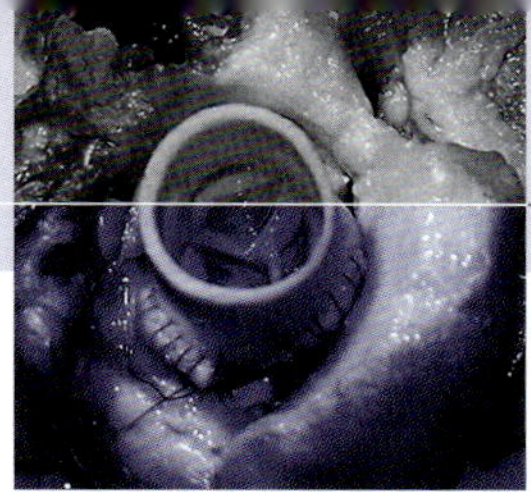

Anastomosis of the ostium onto the prosthesis is performed with polypropylene 4/0 or 5-0 suture in a running fashion. 4–5 stitches are carried out at distance on the posterior wall with narrow intervals.

Completion of the suture

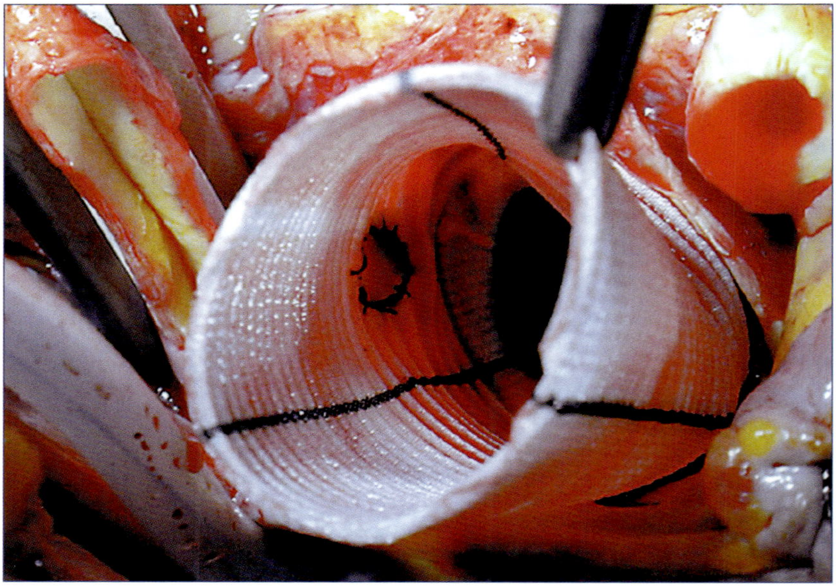

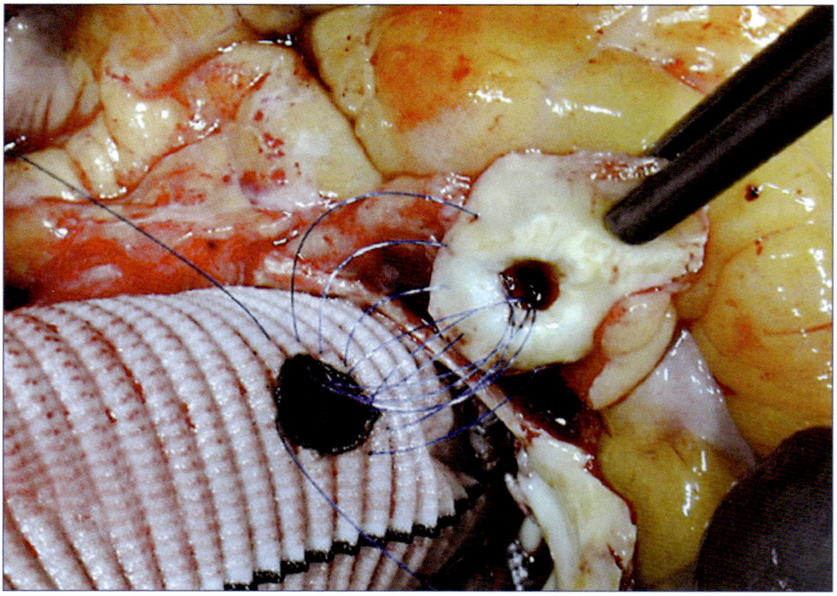

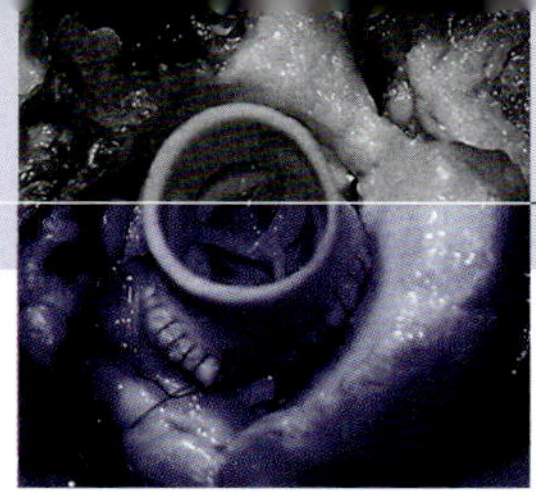

Patency of the anastomosis can be tested visually and with a curved clamp. Attention: Do not probe with too much force.

The right coronary ostium is accomplished in an identical fashion. Passing the needle through the funnel can be performed as an everting suture (in- and out on the intimal aspect). Leakage and folds can thereby be minimized. As an option, both ostia as well as the valve basis can be sealed with fibrin glue.

1
2
3
4
5
6
7
8
9
10
11
12
13
14
15

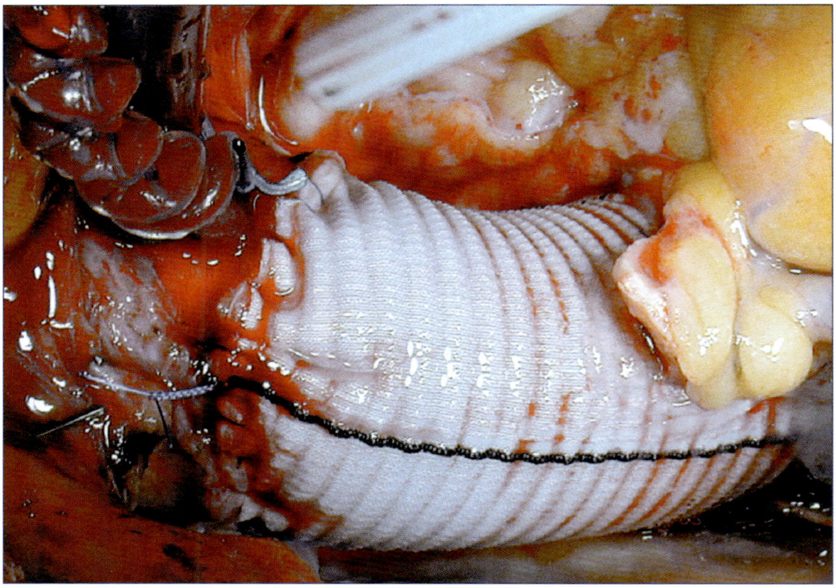

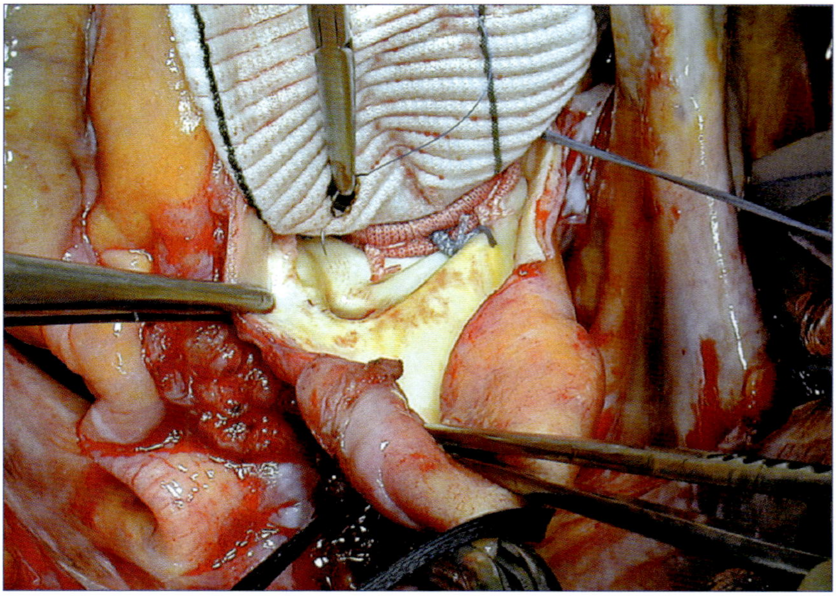

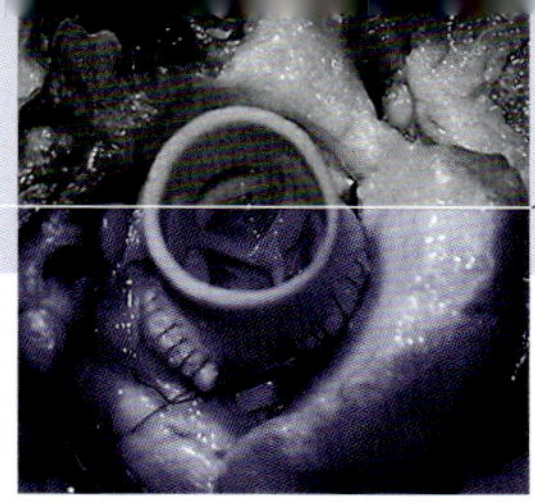

Completion of the anastomosis at the proximal arch according to the given situation with aorta X-clamped or in deep hypothermic arrest with one or two prostheses (see above).

As an alternative to the Button-technique the original Bentall-technique can be chosen. The aneurysmatic aortic wall is preserved. The procedure is thus virtually carried out inside the aneurysm. The dilated wall is used as a coat at the end of the procedure. Fixation of the valve as well as cutting of the ostia-holes are performed equivalent to the open technique.

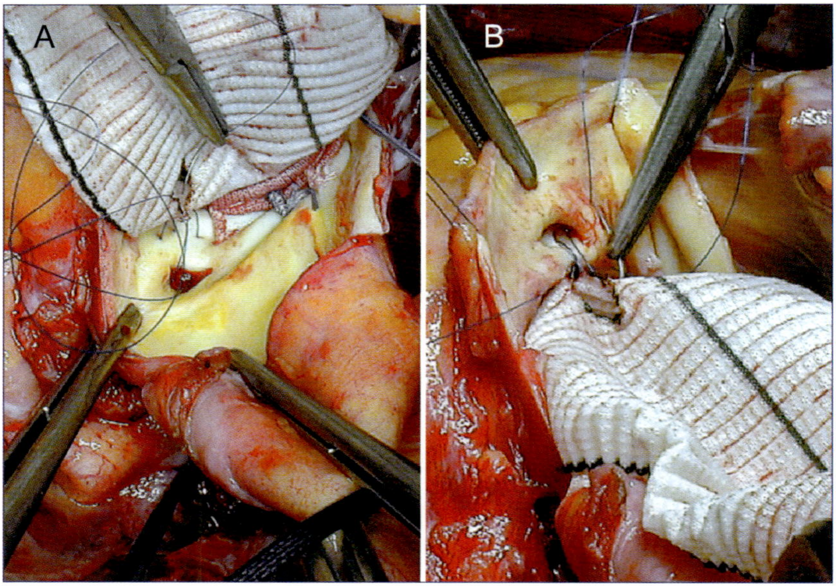
A
B

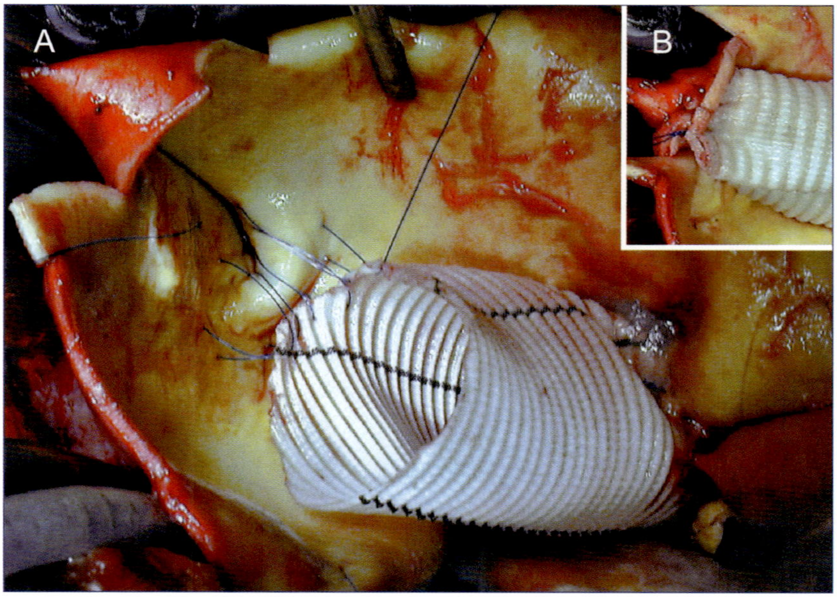
A
B

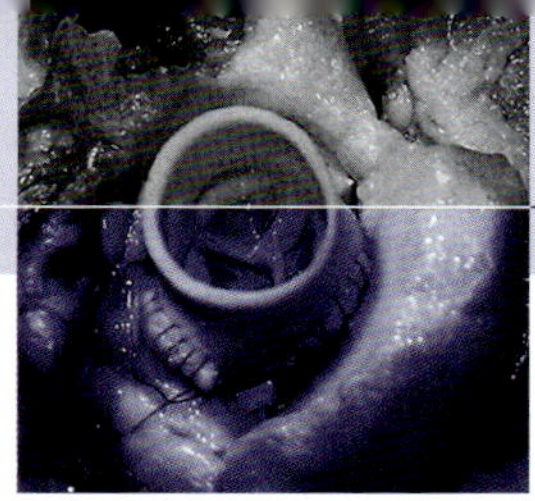

Five stitches are placed at distance with polypropylene 4/0-sutures at the unprepared, native ostium (A). Thereafter, the ostium is approximated to the prosthesis and the anastomosis is completed. The right ostium is treated in an identical manner (B). Fibrin glue may help to seal ostia and basis.

The prosthesio-aortic anastomosis is accomplished from the inside with polypropylene 4/0 or 3/0 in a running fashion as well (A). Attention: Approximation of the prosthesis (B) may result in distortion of the anastomosis with consecutive leakage. Pulling the suture loops of the posterior wall with a nerve-hook or a needle prior to knotting can help to overcome this obstacle.

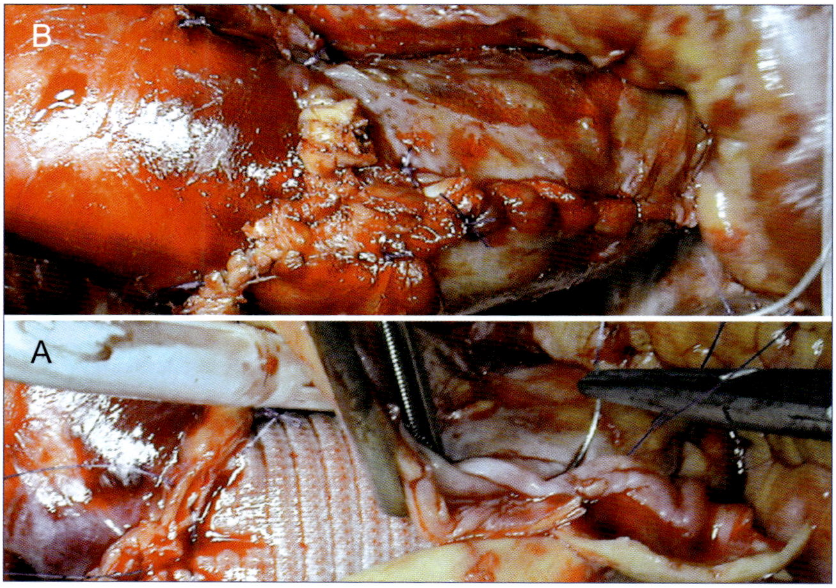
B
A

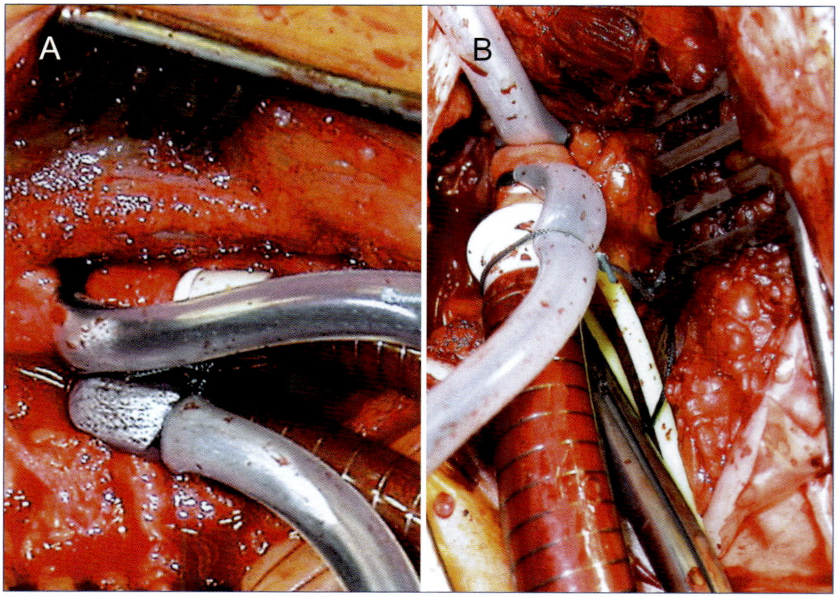
A
B

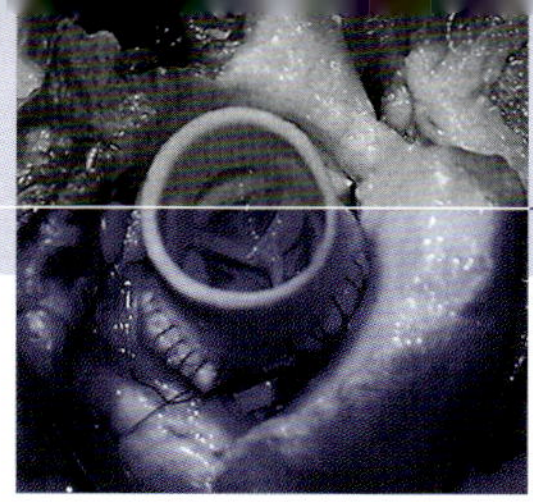

The aneurysmatic wall will be wrapped around the entire construction at the end of the procedure. This "graft-inclusion" will be sutured with a polypropylene 3/0 running suture in a tight fashion (A). Thereafter, fibrin glue can be injected into the cavity between prosthesis and graft-inclusion. Attention: Careless tightening of the coat can distort the anastomoses. At the end, the prosthesis is entirely covered and thus invisible and may therefore be protected in case of a deep sternal wound infection (B). Evidence indicating less infections in the Bentall-technique with graft- inclusion as compared to the Button-technique, however, does not exist. In contrast, evidence does exist regarding less postoperative complications in the open "Button" technique such as development of "perigraft" perfusion and aneurysm.

As an alternative to a cannulation of the ascending aorta or the aortic arch cannulation of the femoral vessels (A) or the axillary artery may be chosen instead (B). Cannulation of the axillary artery can be performed directly without any prosthetic sock. A transverse incision allows introduction of a standard femoral cannula. Closure at the end of the procedure is carried out with several polypropylene 6/0 single sutures. The invaluable advantage of an axillary cannulation lies in the possibility of antegrade cerebral perfusion during operative maneuvers at the arch without having perfusion catheters blocking the operative field.

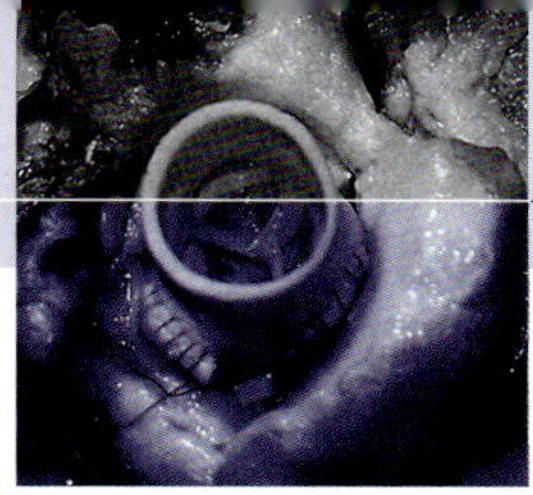

References

1. Bentall H. et al. A technique for complete replacement of the ascending aorta. Thorax 1968; 23: 338
2. Cabrol C. et al. Complete replacement of the ascending aorta with reimplantation of the coronary arteries: New surgical approach. J Thorac Cardiovasc Surg 1981; 81: 309
3. Borst HG. et al. Replacement of ascending aorta and aortic valve: How to do it. Ann Thorac Surg 1981, 32: 613
4. Vogt PR. et al. Modification of surgical aortoatrial shunts for inaccessible bleeding in aortic surgery – modification of the Ca brolshunt technique. Thorac Cardiovasc Surg 1001; 49: 240
5. Jacobs MJ. et al. Aortic arch and proximal supraaortic arterial repair under continuous antegrade cerebral perfusion and moderate hypothermia. Cardiovasc Surg 2001; 9: 396
6. Hagl C. et al. Is aortic surgery using hypothermic circulatory arrest in octogenarians justifiable? Eur J Cardiothorac Surg 2001; 19: 417
7. Yagdi T. et al. Determinants of early mortality and neurological morbidity in aortic operations performed under circulatory arrest. J Card Surg 2000; 15: 186–93
8. Ehrlich MP. et al. Predictors of adverse outcome and transient neurological dysfunction after ascending aorta/hemiarch replacement. Ann Thorac Surg 2000; 69: 1755
9. Niederhauser U. et al. Surgery for acute type A aortic dissection: comparison of techniques. Eur J Cardiothorac Surg 2000; 18: 307
10. Vogt PR. et al. Modification of surgical aortoatrial shunts for inaccessible bleeding in aortic surgery – modification of the Ca brolshunt technique. Thorac Cardiovasc Surg 2001; 49: 240
11. Whitlark JD. et al. Axillary cannulation in acute ascending aortic dissections. Ann Thorac Surg 2000; 69: 1127
12. Mathes DW. et al. Successful treatment of an infected ascen ding aortic graft. Ann Thorac Surg 2000; 70: 1410
13. Davies RR. et al. Yearly rupture and dissection rates for thoracic aortic aneurysms: simple prediction based on size. Ann Thorac Surg 2002; 73: 17–28

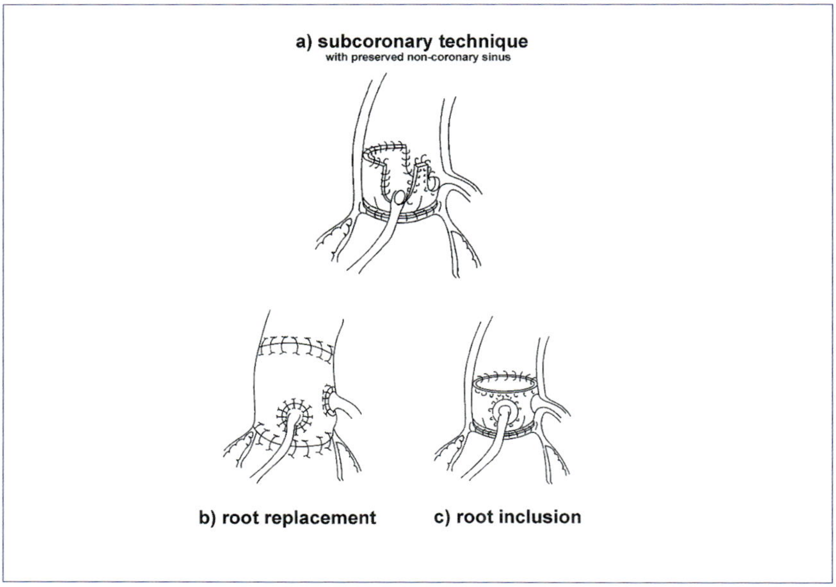
a) subcoronary technique
with preserved non-coronary sinus
b) root replacement
c) root inclusion

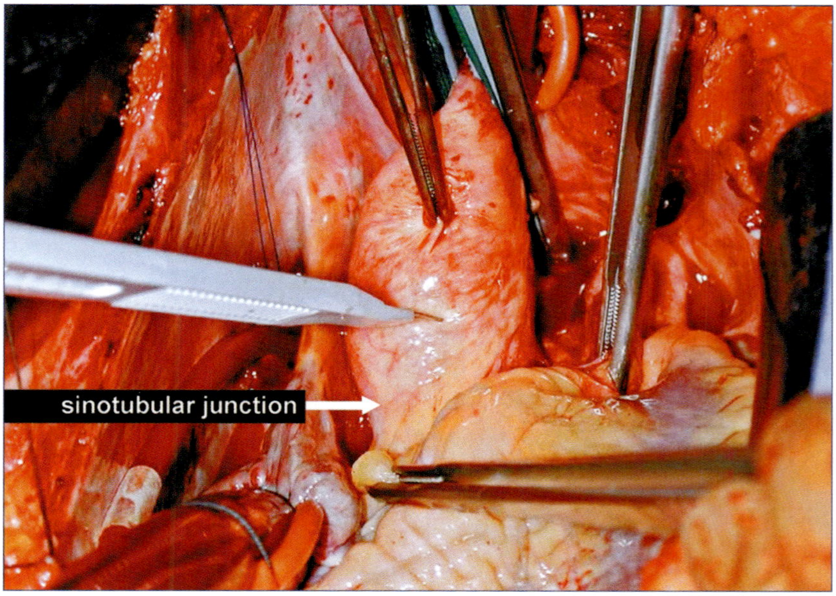
sinotubular junction

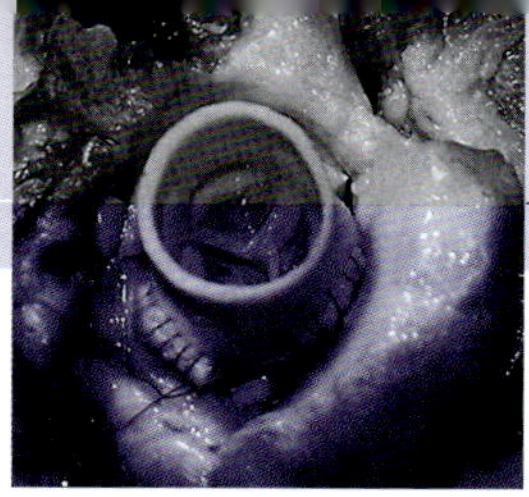

a) **subcoronary technique:** the stentless prosthesis is inserted completely **into** the aortic root of the patient. This can be challenging in small or very large aortic roots and may involve root enlargement or root reduction techniques. The subcoronary technique is the prefered method of implantation at our department because aortic root motion is closest to normal with this technique; and because the conserved wall of the patient's aortic root is a reinforcement for the stentless prosthesis and facilitates reoperations.
b) **full root replacement technique:** the aortic root of the patient is completely resected except for small buttons around the coronary ostiae. Then, the stentless prosthesis is inserted as a neo-aortic root. Advantage: it is relatively easy to implant the stentless prosthesis without distortion of its anatomy/symmetry. Disadvantages: mandatory Reimplantation of the coronary arteries into the prosthesis; no external reinforcement; many suture lines that can bleed.
c) **root-inclusion technique:** technically very demanding, combines the advantages of a) and b). The coronary arteries are left in place; instead, two ostiae are cut into the prosthesis. Then, the stentless prosthesis is implanted **as a root into the autologous aortic root** with additional sutures lines around the coronary ostiae.

The aortotomy is made into the ascending aorta approximately 1 cm above the sinotubular junction. This way, one does not have to fear that the incision is too close to the right coronary artery (which often originates quite high from the right coronary sinus).

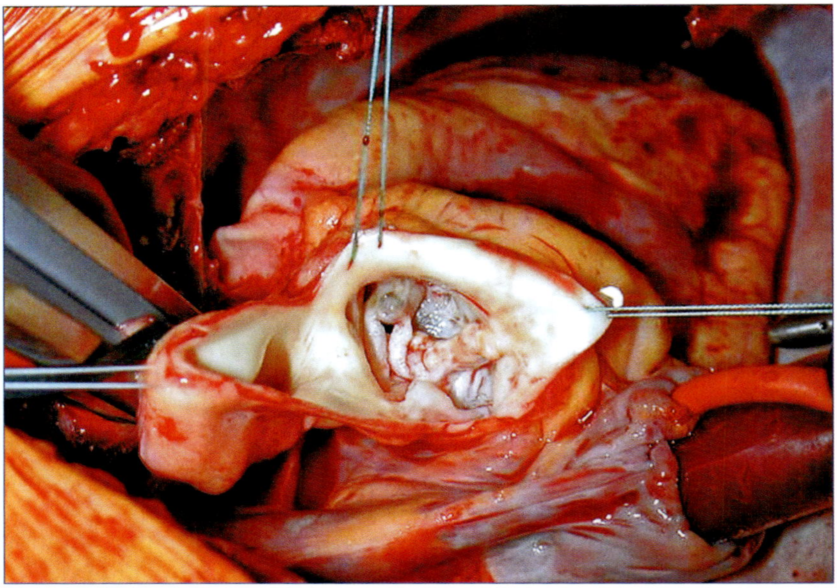

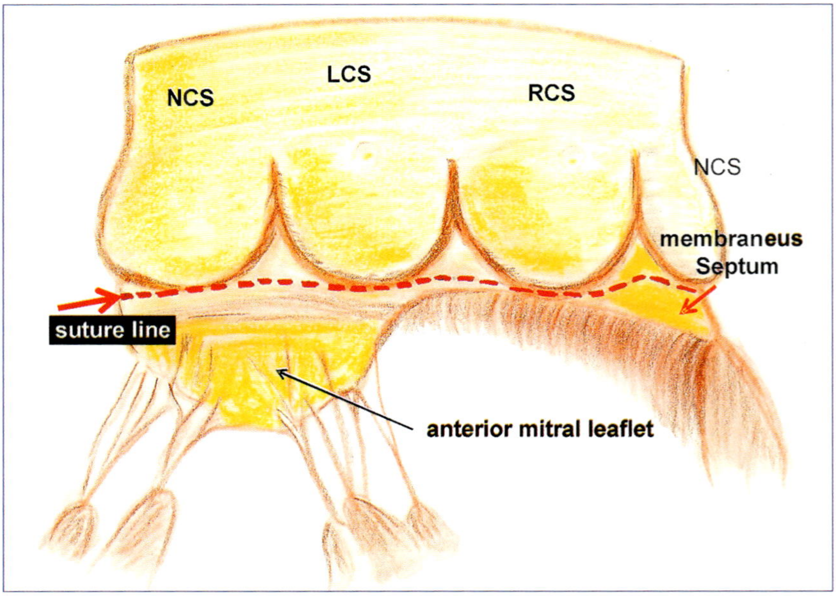
NCS
LCS
RCS
NCS
membraneus
Septum
suture line
anterior mitral leaflet

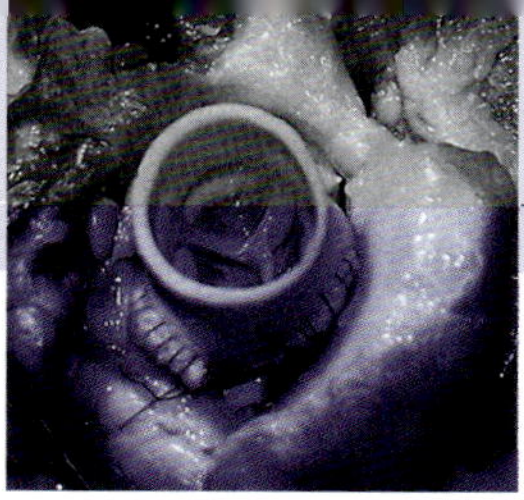

The aortotomy is extended S-shaped deep into the non-coronary aortic sinus close to the left/non-coronary commissure. If needed, the incision can be further extended into the aorto-mitral curtain for aortic root enlargement. If root enlargement is definitely not needed, it may be more easy to make a transverse incision that stays above the sinutubular junction. Closure of the aorta is more simple with such an incision, and the geometry of the aortic root is not changed. Optimal exposition of the aortic valve is then achieved by ≥ 3 sutures placed at the edges of the incision and pulling the aorta open. Afterwards, the semilunar valves are resected and all calcified parts that may interfere with implantation of the prosthesis are carefully removed from the aortic root. Be cautious that no loose debris is left in the aortic root or in the left ventricle: embolization-hazard!

At the base of the aortic root, the stentless prosthesis must be implanted on level with the deepest point of the aortic sinus (also see figure 13). In the intervalvular trigones, this level is maintained. The suture-line must not follow the hinge line of the semilunar valves! Exception: the bundle of HIS lies between the right [RCS] and non-coronary sinus [NCS]. The suture-line must be elevated slightly here to avoid an AV-block.

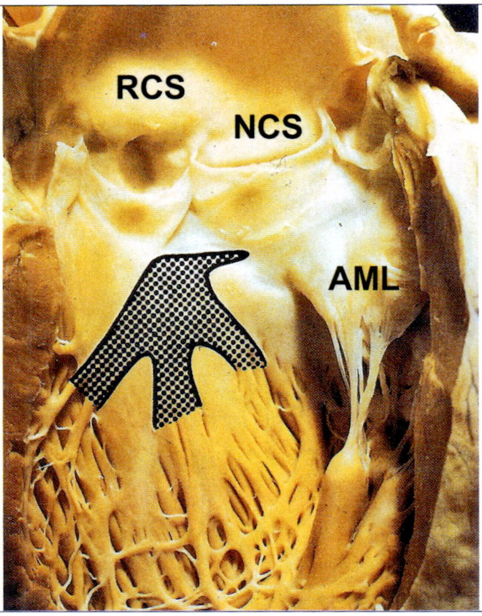
RCS
NCS
AML

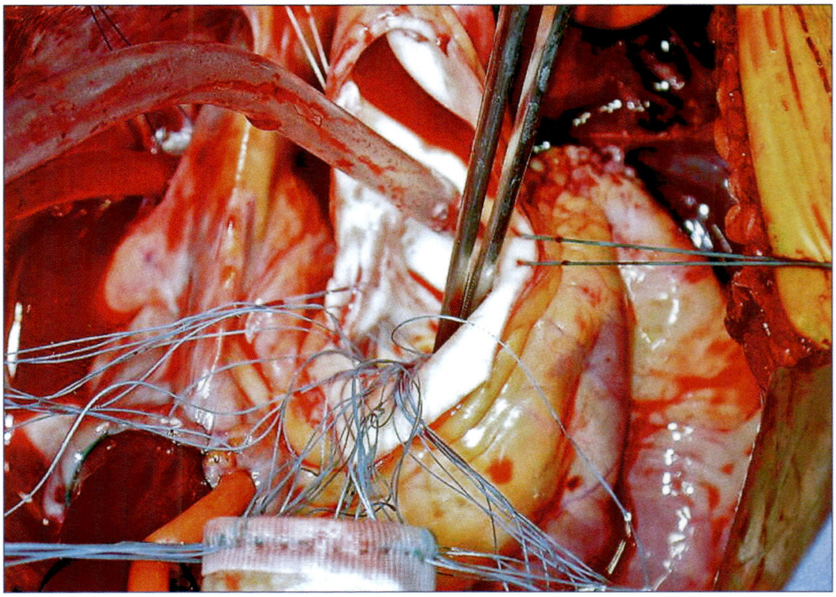

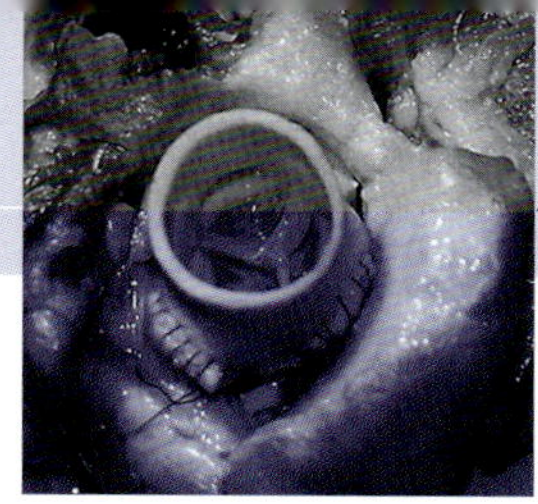

Relation of the conduction system and the aortic root. In this photo, the left-coronary sinus is divided, and the aortic root and the left ventricle are opened. The bundle of HIS penetrates the intervalvular trigone between right [RCS] and non-coronary sinus [NCS] and branches on the septum as indicated by the dotted area. AML: anterior mitral leaflet.

Basal implantation of the stentless prosthesis is performed by 4-0 sutures through the prosthesis and the aortic root. The sutures are passed one-on-one with a distance of approximately 1.5 mm from each other. All stiches are done with the prosthesis held on distance. It is mandatory that the basal ring of the prosthesis and of the aortic annulus match each other exactly! Otherwise the prosthesis will be distorted which may cause regurgitation or stenosis. To achieve perfect symmetry, one may choose to pass three sutures every 120° initally.

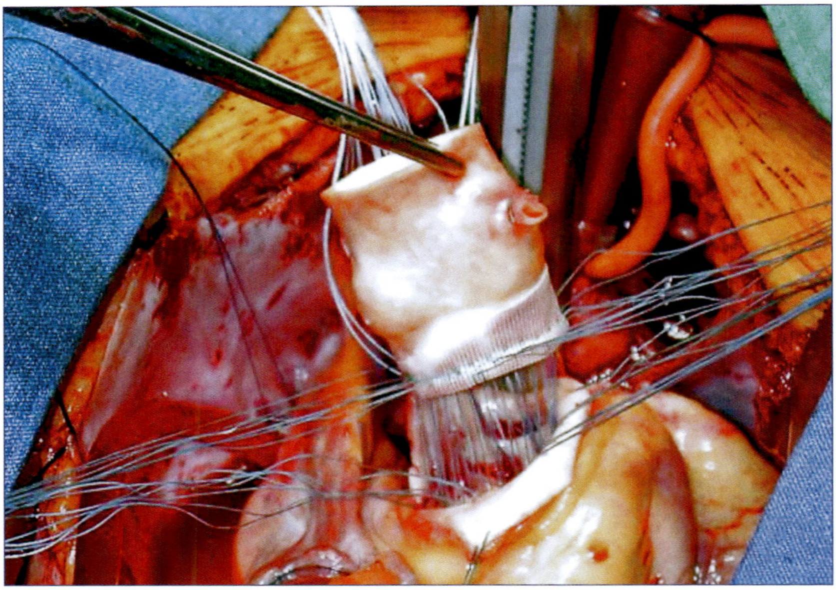

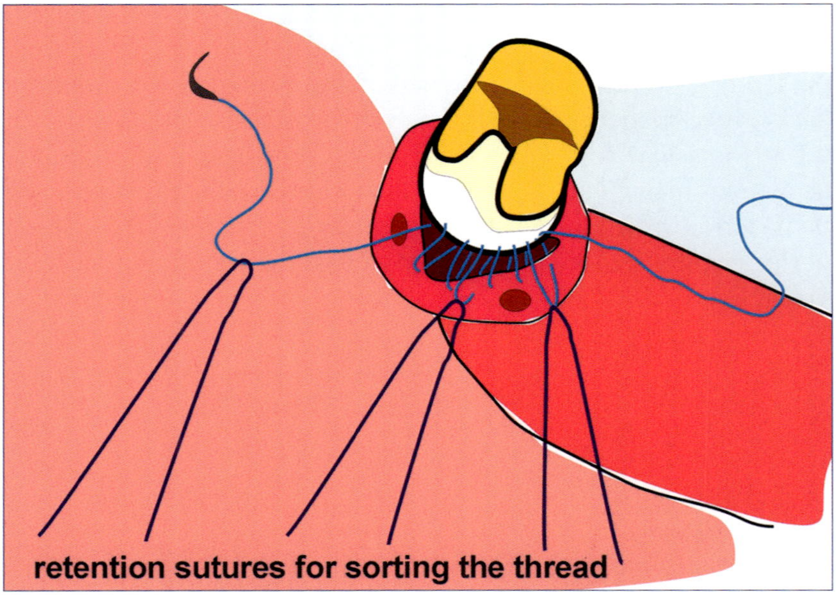
retention sutures for sorting the thread

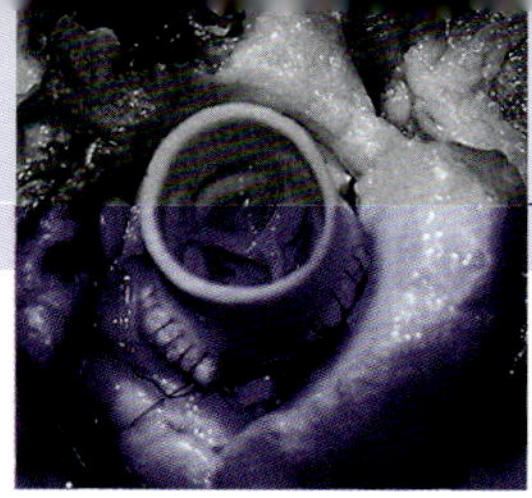

Only after the last suture has been made, the prosthesis is lowered into its destinated position. Be careful that the threads are always under tension and that no loops develop while lowering the prosthesis! Actively look for loops and correct them!

The basal suture can also be done as a continuous running suture. However, exact matching of prosthesis and aortic annulus is more difficult to achieve. It is also more difficult to be sure that the thread is adequately tightened at its complete length after the stentless prosthesis has been lowered into its destinated position and that no loops develop. It may be helpful to use retention sutures every 3-5 stitches to keep the continuous running suture ordered and to use a nerve hook for tightening it while lowering the stentless prosthesis.

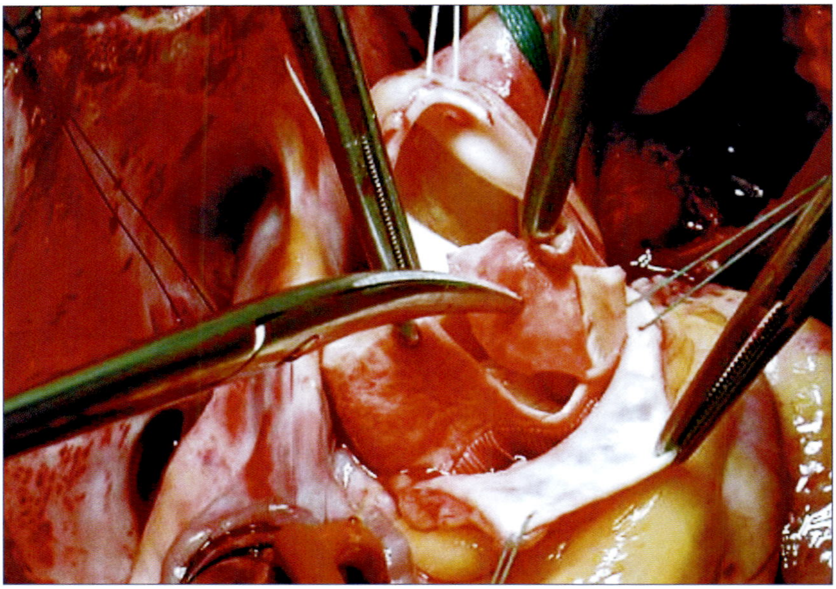

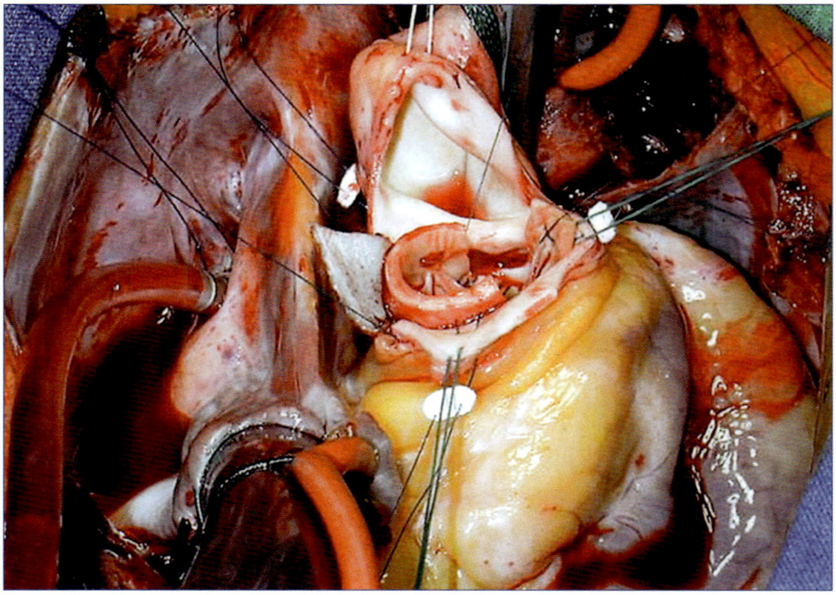

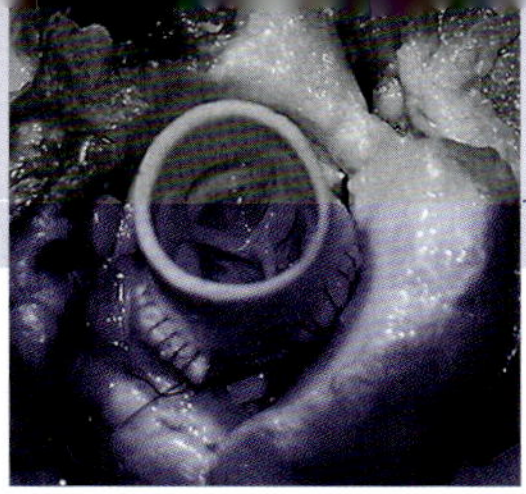

Subcoronary technique:
After the basal sutures have been knotted, the left- and right-coronary sinus of the prosthesis must be resected. 2mm of tissue above the aortic cusps should be left to facilitate the subcoronary sutures. The non-coronary sinus does not need to be resected.

It is crucial that the commissures of the stentless prosthesis are sutured to the right position on the autologous aortic wall. They need to be high enough and must be 120° apart from each other. We use U-stitches with 4-0 prolene (with PTFE-pledgets at the outside of the aorta) to bring the commissures into their destinated position. However, these sutures are not knotted, but kept loose. This way, making the subcoronary sutures is easier because the stentless prosthesis can be slightly moved while stitching.

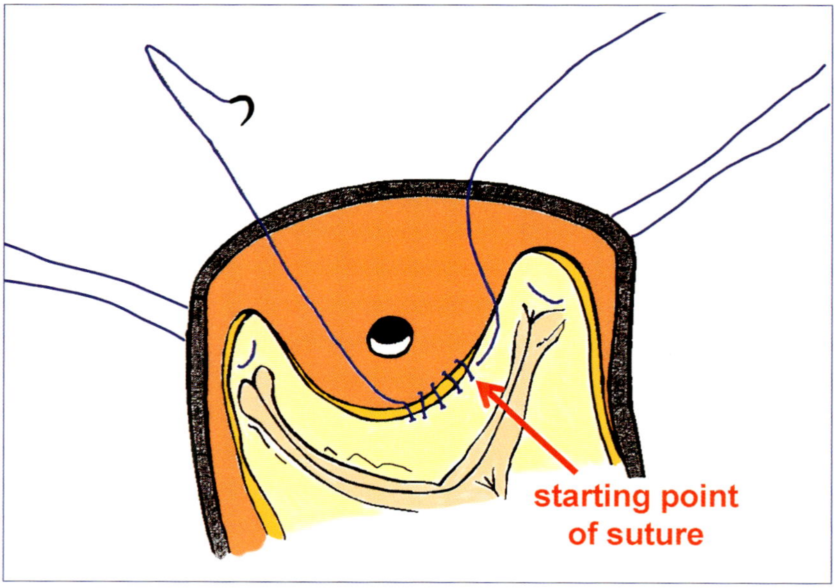
starting point
of suture

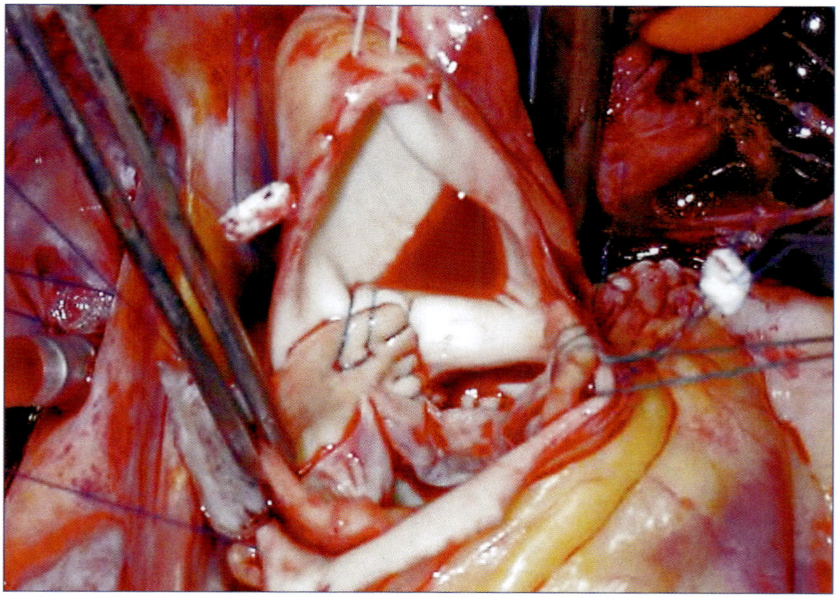

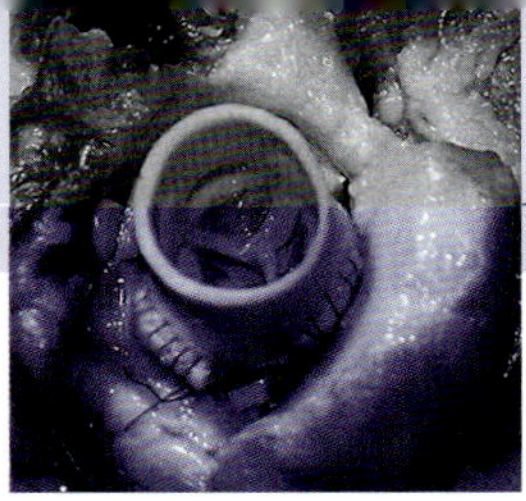

After having fixed (but not knotted) the commissures to their correct positions, the subcoronary suture is done (5-0 prolene). As shown, the suture starts at the left side of the base of the left/right commissure and is continued in a running fashion to the left/non-coronary commissure. Here, the thread is stitched to the outside and through the pledget of the suture that fixes this commissure. Then – with the other side of the 5-0 thread – the suture in the left coronary sinus is finished by continuing it up to the left/right commissure. Large parts of this suture can be done this way: stitch from inside through the sinus wall to the outside, then from the outside through the wall of the stentless prosthesis to the inside, and so on. This is easier than doing the complete suture from the inside. Finally, the needle is passed to the outside and through the pledget of the suture that fixes this commissure.
Then, the subcoronary suture to the right coronary sinus is done analogous. This suture starts at the right side of the base of the left/right commissure and is continued in a running fashion to the right/non-coronary commissure.
Before the upper rim of the non-coronary sinus (not resected from the prosthesis!) of the stentless prosthesis is sutured to the aortic wall, the S-shaped aortic incision needs to be partly closed.

Intraoperative view. The left subcoronary suture is finished, both ends of the thread are passed through the pledgets of the sutures that fix this commissures.

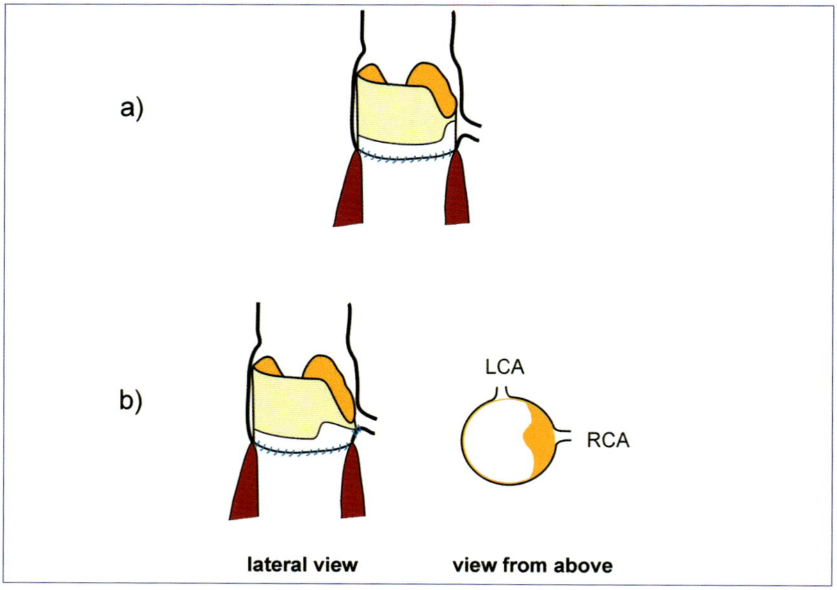
a)
b)
LCA
RCA
lateral view
view from above

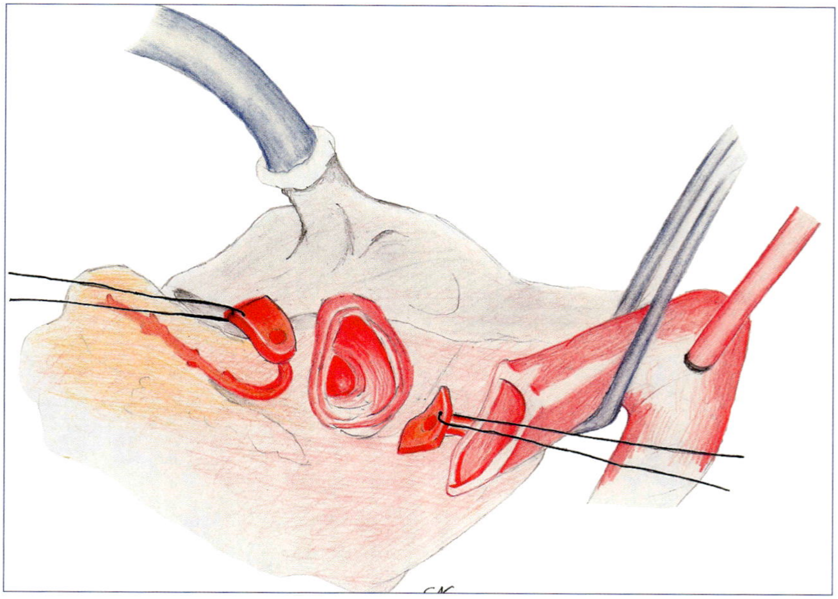

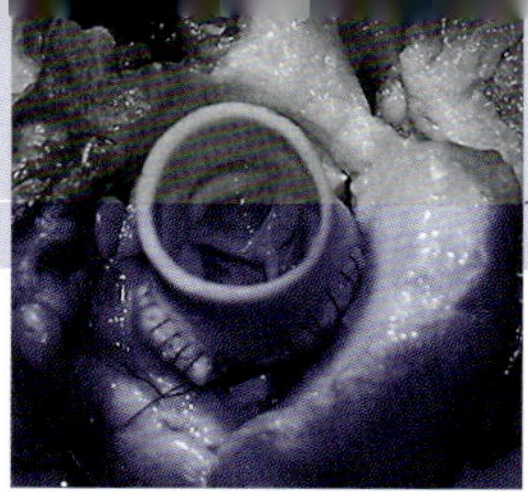

It is important that the stentless prosthesis is sutured deep enough into the aortic root. The remaining parts of the sinuses of the prosthesis must not obstruct the coronary ostiae (as it had happened in a)). Otherwise, the subcoronary suture will cause bulging of the stentless prosthesis which may cause partial obstruction of the valve orifice (b).

If the right coronary ostium is located rather low in the aortic root, it may be necessary to rotate the prosthesis anti-anatomically (i.e. the prosthetic non-coronary sinus to the right coronary sinus) in order to be able to resect enough sinus tissue without cutting into the basal Dacron-grommet of the prosthesis or risking the problem described above. Cave: this must be considered in advance before placing the basal sutures!

Full root replacement technique:
The aortic valve and its root is completely resected, except for small buttons of tissue around the coronary ostiae. For better exposition of the aortic basis, these buttons can be gently pulled away by 5-0 sutures.

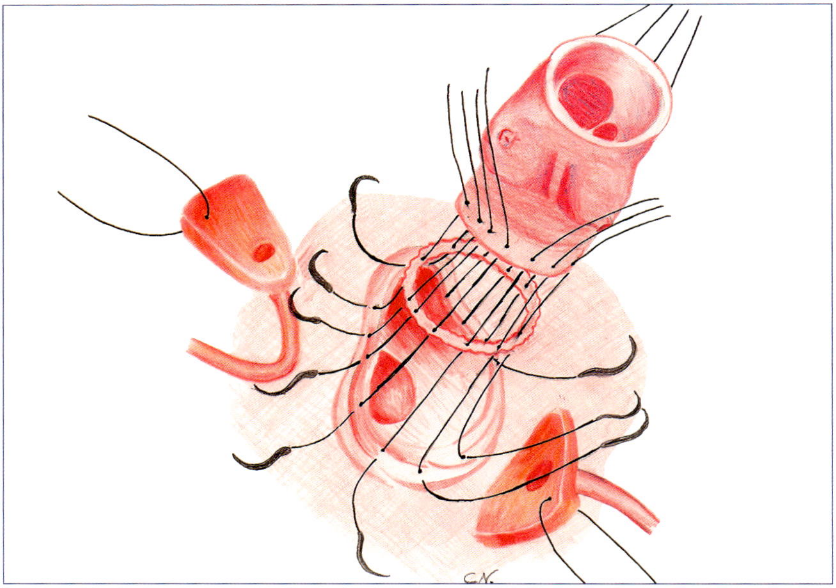
C.N.

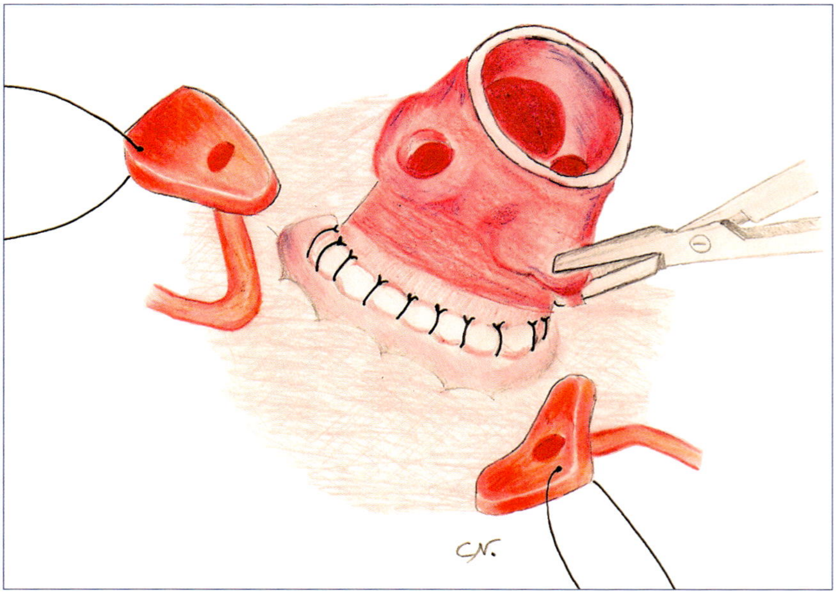
C.N.

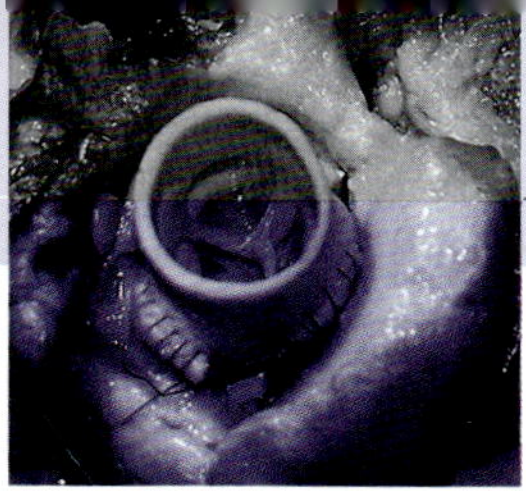

The basal sutures are done as previously explained and shown. However, with the full root replacement technique we recommend that the sutures are also passed through a teflon or pericardial strap that is placed around the stentless prosthesis on the outside. Doing so improves hemostasis.

After the basal sutures have been knotted, holes are cut into the stentless prosthesis for Reimplantation of the coronary arteries. Usually, the coronary arteries can be inserted where the coronary arteries of the prosthetic root originate, but occasionally these places will not fit anatomically. In such cases, holes have to be cut into the prosthesis where it fits the patient's anatomy. (If the origins of the prosthetic coronary arteries cannot be used for reinsertion of the patient's coronary arteries, we recommend that proper occlusion the origins of the prosthetic coronary arteries is assured by additional sutures.)

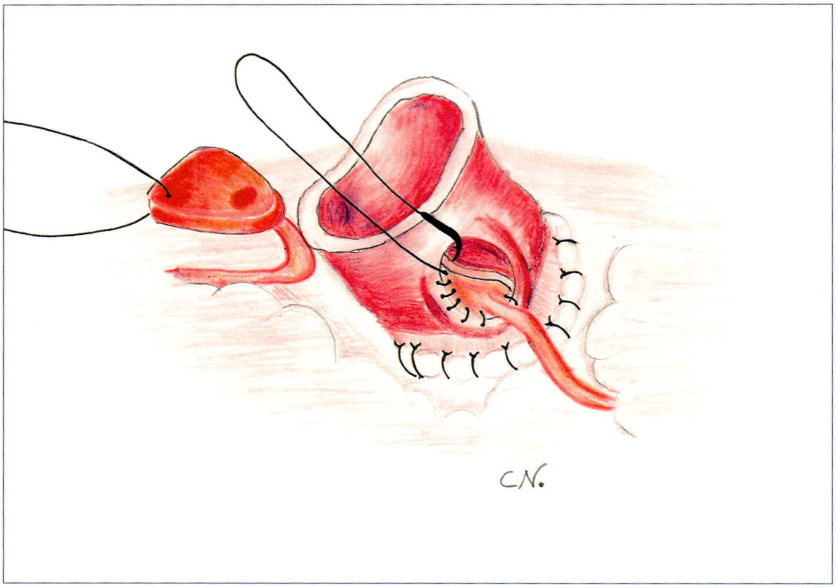
CN.

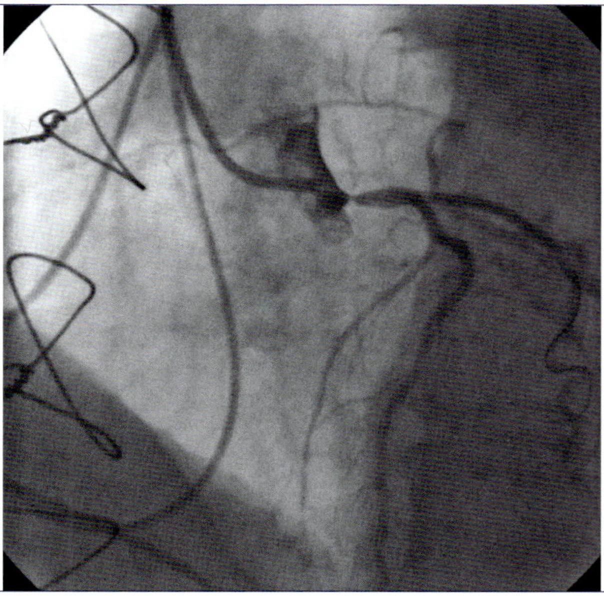

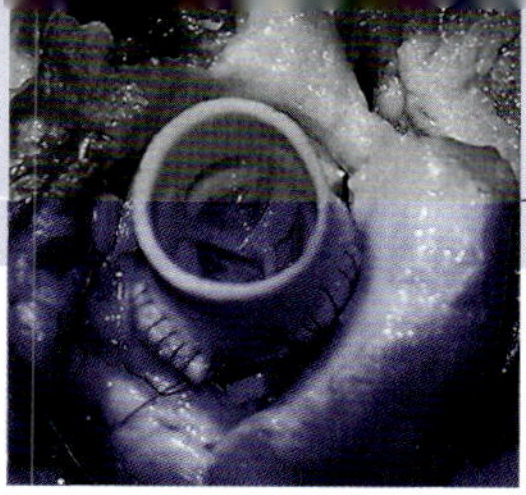

A 5-0 prolene running suture is used for reimplantation of the coronary arteries. First, the left coronary artery is reimplanted. It is important that the stitches are close to the coronary ostiae in order to prevent aneurysm formation. However, be careful not to narrow the coronary ostiae (or to distort them)!

This angiogram shows that reimplantation of the coronary arteries needs to be performed with maximum meticulousness to prevent complications.

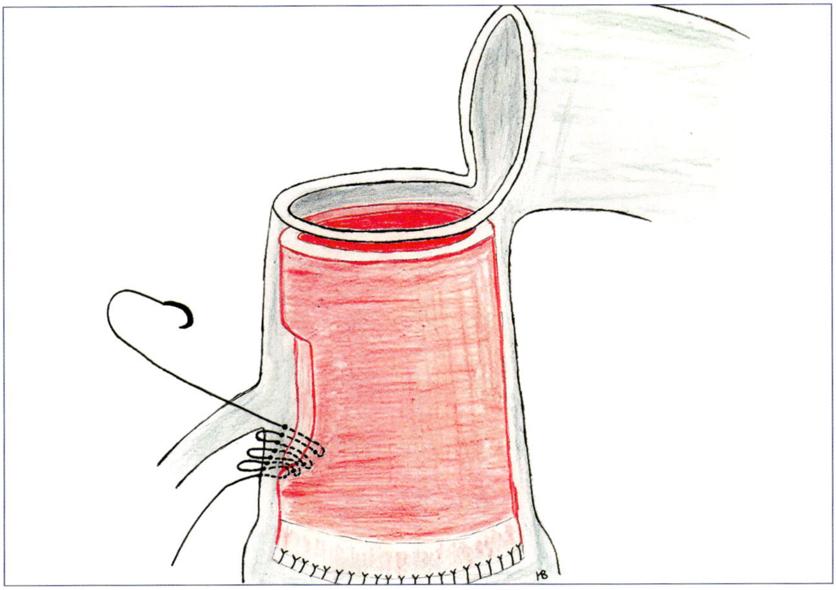

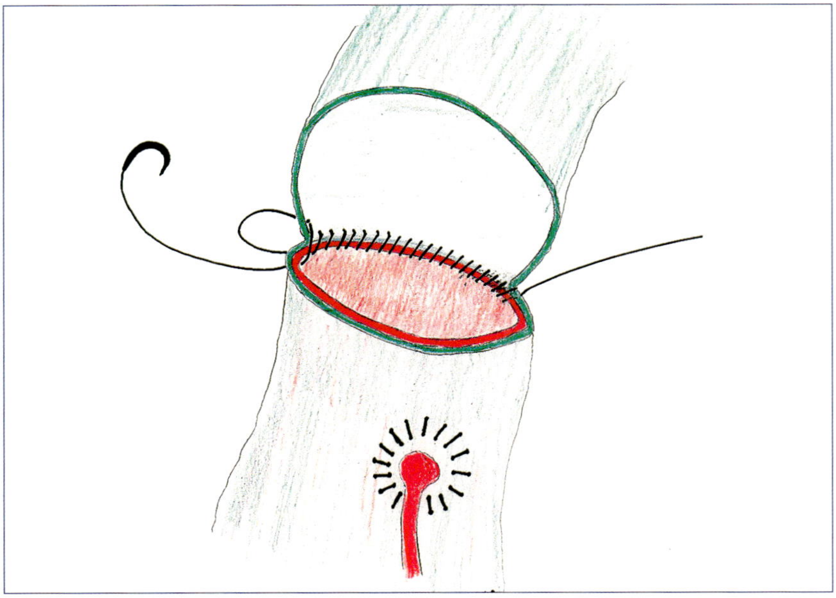

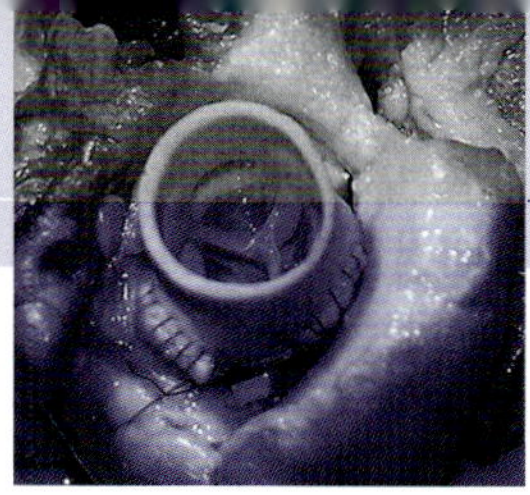

Root inclusion technique:
The basal sutures are done as previously explained and shown. Large holes are then cut into the stentless prosthesis for the coronary arteries. The stentless prosthesis is then fixated around the coronary ostiae by 5-0 prolene sutures, either continously running or singles ones, that take full thickness of the aortic wall and the prosthesis.

Finally, the prosthesis needs to be fixated proximally by an continuous running suture (4-0 or 5-0 prolene).

References

1. Bach DS, Cartier PC, Kon ND, Johnson KG, Deeb GM, Doty DB. for the Freestyle Valve Study Group. Impact of implant technique following freestyle stentless aortic valve replacement. Ann Thorac Surg 2002; 74: 1107–13
2. Binot JP, Carpentier A, Langlois J. Clinical use of heterografts for replacement of the aortic valve. J Thorac Cardiovasc Surg 1968; 55: 23–42
3. Cutrara CA, Goldman BS, Christakis GT. Preferred method for insertion of the Toronto Stentless Porcine Valve. J Card Surg 1998; 13: 408–11
4. David TE, Ivanov J, Eriksson MJ, Bos J, Feindel CM, Rakowski H. Dilation of the sinutubular junction causes aortic insufficiency after aortic valve replacement with the Toronto SPV bioprosthesis. J Thorac Cardiovasc Surg 2001; 122: 929–34
5. Doty DB, Doty JR. Stentless aortic valve replacement: bioprostheses. In: Cardiac Surgery in the Adult. Cohn LH, Edmunds Jr. H. (Hrsg.). 2nd ed. Chapter 35. McGraw-Hill, New York, 2003: 889–898
6. Doty DB, Cafferty A, Kon ND, Huysmans HA, Krause Jr. AH, Westaby S. Medtronic Freestyle aortic root bioprosthesis: Implant techniques. J Card Surg 1998; 13; 369–75
7. Goldman BS, Mallidi H. Update on stentless valves. In: Advanced Therapy in Cardiac Surgery. Franco KL, Verrier. ED (Hrsg.). 2nd ed. Chapter 21. BC Decker, Hamilton. Canada, 2003: 196–206
8. Grunkemeier GL, Li HH, Naftel DC, Starr A, Rahimtoola SH. Long-term performance of heart valve prostheses. Curr Probl Cardiol 2000; 25: 75–154
9. Huysmans HA, David TE, Westaby S (Hrsg.). Stentless bioprostheses. 2nd ed. Isis Medical, Oxford, UK 1999

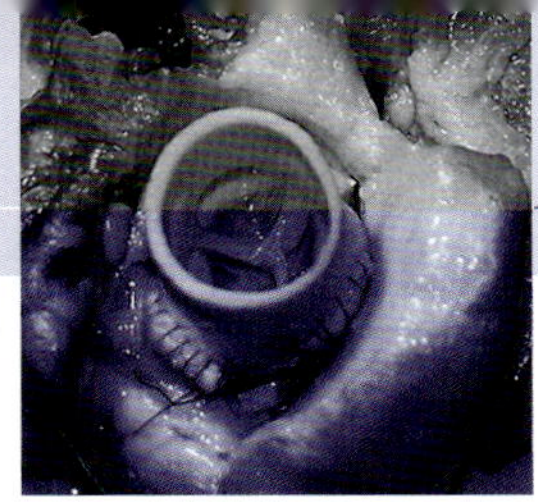

10. Kalangos A, Trigo-Trindade P, Vala D, Panos A, Faidutti B. Aortic valve replacement with the freestyle stentless bioprosthe sis with respect to spacial orientation of the patient coronary ostia. J Thorac Cardiovasc Surg 2000; 119: 1185–93
11. Massetti M, Bruno P, Babatasi G, Le Page O, Neri E, Veron S, Saloux E, Khayat A. Aortic root remodeling with the "cuff" technique for stentless valve implantation. Ann Thorac Surg 2001; 71: 1053–5
12. Nötzold A, Scharfschwerdt M, Thiede L, Huppe M, Sievers HH. In-vitro study on the relationship between progressive sinotubular junction dilatation and aortic regurgitation for several stentless aortic valve substitutes. Eur J Cardiothorac Surg 2005; 27: 90–3
13. O'Brien MF. Implantation technique of the Cryolife-O'Brien stentless xenograft aortic valve. The simple, rapid, and correct way to implant and the errors to avoid. Semin Thorac Cardiovasc Surg 1999; 11 (Suppl. 1): 121–5
14. Quigley RL. The use of a rigid instrument prior to stentles valve implantation facilitates correct alignment of the prosthesis and native aortic valve apparatus. J Heart Valve Dis 2003; 12: 436–8
15. Reardon MJ, Conklin LD, Estrera AL. Technical aspects of implanting the St. Jude Toronto stentless porcine valve. Tex Heart Inst J 1999; 26: 278–82
16. Sievers HH, Lange PE, Bernhard A. Implantation of a xenogeneic stentless aortic bioprosthesis. First experience. Thorac Cardiovasc Surg 1985; 33: 225–6
17. van Nooten G, Ozaki S, Herijgers P, Segers P, Verdonck P, Flameng W. Distortion of the stentless porcine valve induces accelerated leaflet fibrosis and calcification in juvenile sheep. J Heart Valve Dis 1999; 8: 34–41
18. Westaby S, Jin XY, Vaccari G, Katsumata T. The Sorin stentless pericardial valve: implant technique and hemodynamic profile. Sem Thorac Cardiovasc Surg 1999; 11 (Suppl. 1): 62–8

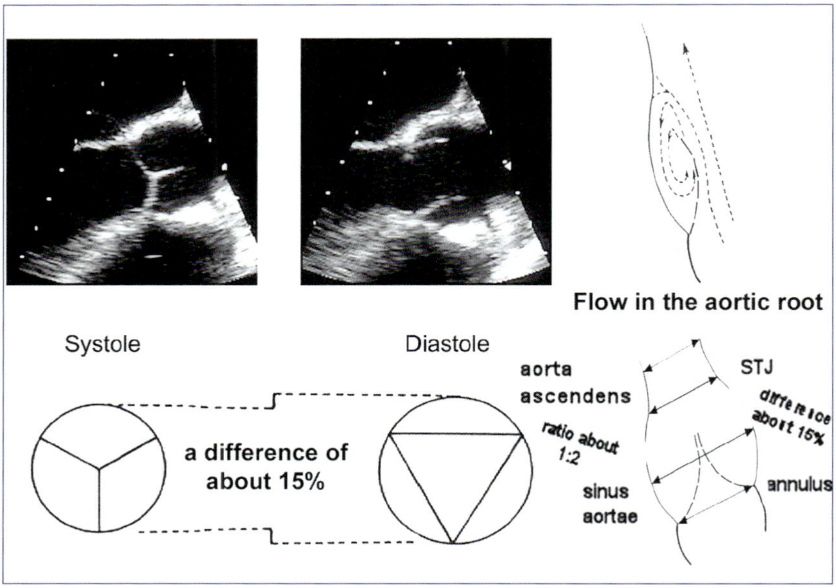
Flow in the aortic root
Systole
Diastole
a difference of
about 15%
aorta
ascendens
STJ
ratio about
1:2
sinus
aortae
annulus

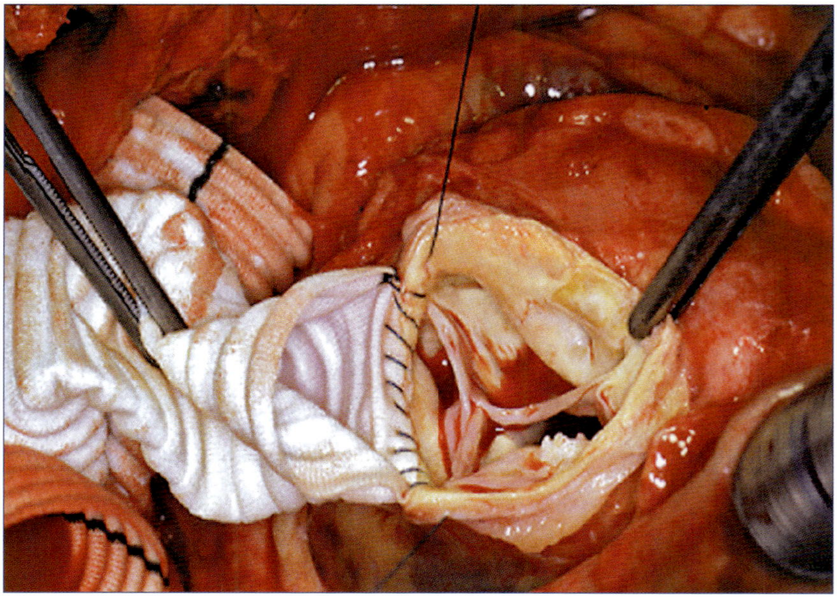

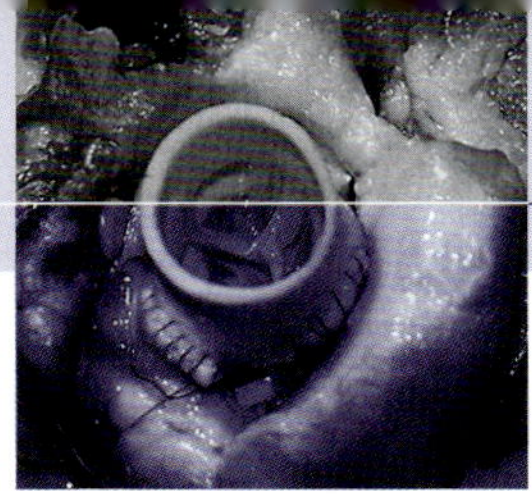

1 2 3 4 5 6 7 8 9 10 11 12 13 14 15

Anatomy of the aortic root:

The aortic root is an extremely sophisticated functional unit, and a harmonic dynamic interaction between its different components (annulus – ventriculo-aortic junction, sinuses of Valsalva, sinotubular junction [STJ] and cusps) is essential for a physiologic performance under varying hemodynamic demands. Definite anatomic relations between these components govern this interaction (1,2).

The principles of all valve-sparing procedures are based upon correction of the STJ alone or in combination with reduction of the annulus, replacement of one or more of the sinuses and/or reconstruction of the leaflets (3).

Supracommissural replacement:

Isolated correction of the sinotubular junction:

In non-ectatic aortic roots with normal annular dimensions dilatation of the STJ results in an outward displacement of the commissures with loss of central cusp coaptation. Hence, adequate cusp coaptation and valve competence can be restored by an isolated correction of the STJ. This is achieved by a supracommissural replacement of the ascending aorta with a prosthesis of 10-15 % smaller diameter than the annulus. The graft is fixed to the STJ with a continuous suture of 3-0 prolene. The diameter of the annulus is determined using Hegar dilators or proper valve sizers (2,4).

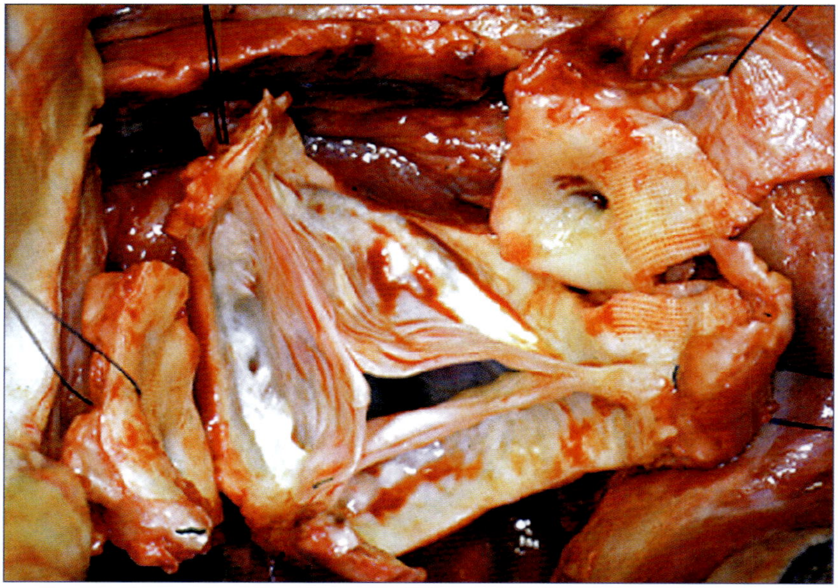

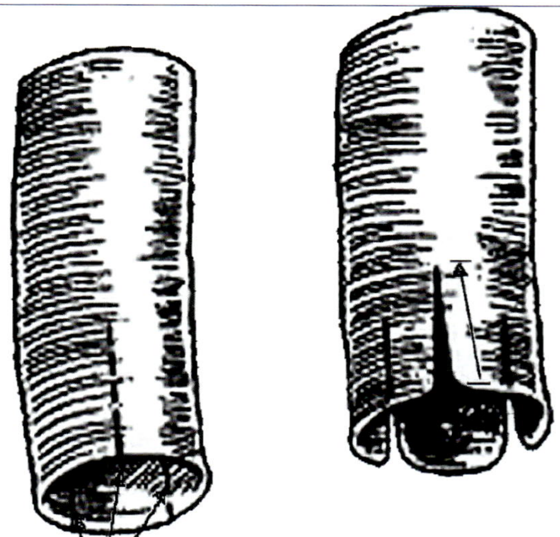
120 ° appart
equalls 1.5 times the
hight of the commissures

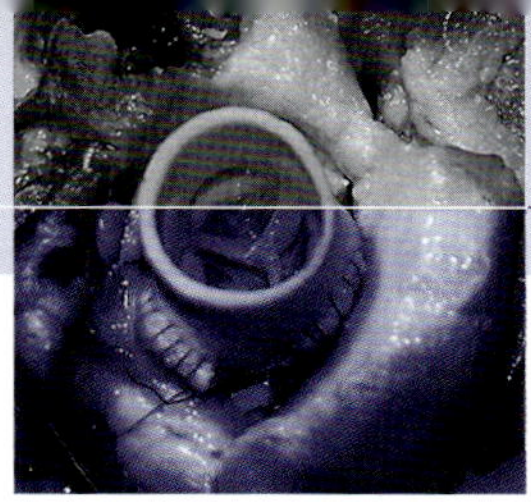

Valve-sparing aortic root replacement:
In presence of an ectatic aortic root valve-preservation mandates a valve-sparing replacement of the aortic root. The ascending aorta is transected about 2 cm above the STJ and the valve inspected to determine whether or not it can be preserved. Thereafter, the sinuses are resected leaving a 2-3 mm rim of the aortic wall adjacent to the fibrous aortic annulus while the coronary ostia are excised as buttons. Thereafter, the commissures and the coronary buttons are suspended by stay sutures. Further action will depend on the type of root replacement chosen. Principally two basic techniques exist, both of which aim at restoration of the STJ with or without routine stabilization of the aortic annulus:

Remodeling technique according to Yacoub (5):
STJ reconstruction with sinus reconstruction:
The average distance between the commissures at which an optimal leaflet coaptation can be achieved is determined. As this represents 1/3 of the circumference at the STJ and as the diameter of a tube approximately equals 1/3 of its circumference, a graft of corresponding diameter is chosen. Three vertical slits 120° apart are cut into one end of the graft thereby producing three tongues designed to replace the sinuses. The width of each tongue thus corresponds to one third of the circumference while the length should initially equal one and a half times the depth of the original sinuses thereby, facilitating the later trimming of the excess Dacron to the remaining rim of the sinuses.

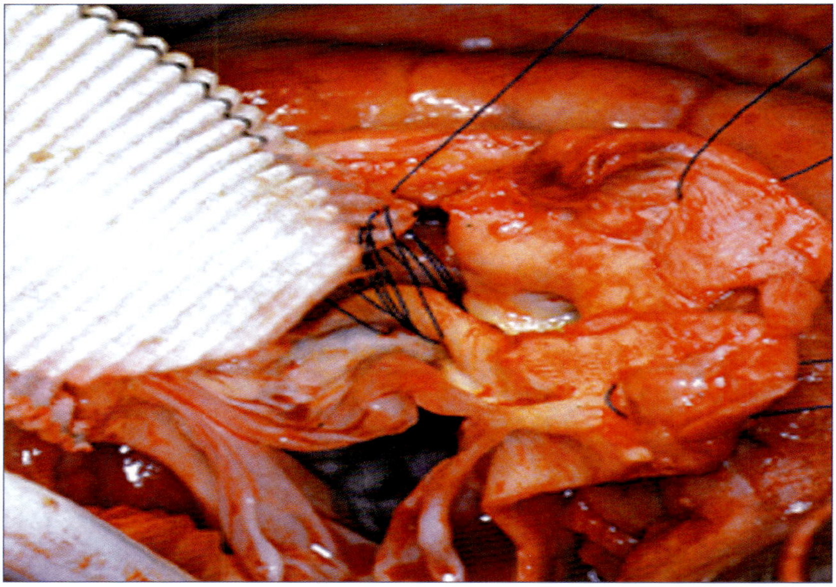

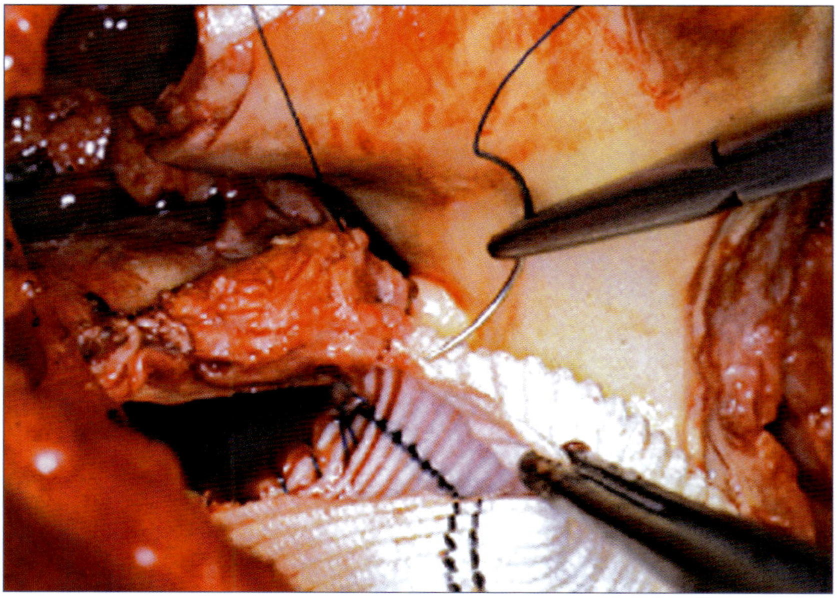

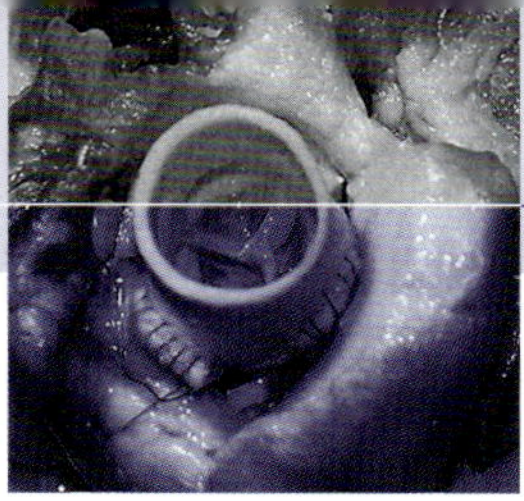

Next the tongues are cut in a configuration that resembles the corresponding sinus curve. The reshaped proximal end of the prosthesis is then fixed to the aortic annulus at the line of attachment of the cusps with continuous 4-0 prolene sutures starting at the centre of the sinuses. Alternatively, the top of the commissures are first sutured to the bottom of the corresponding grooves on the prosthesis followed by trimming and fixation of the tongue-shaped extensions to the corresponding rim of the resected sinuses.

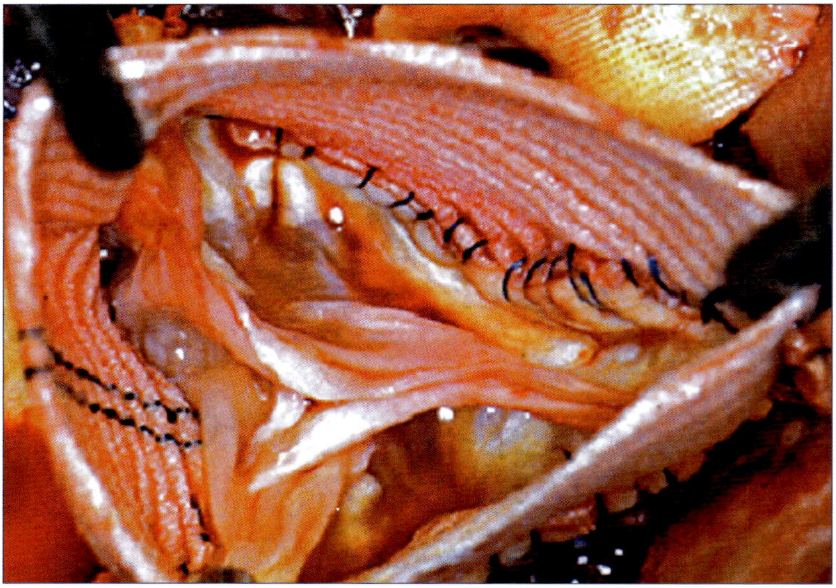

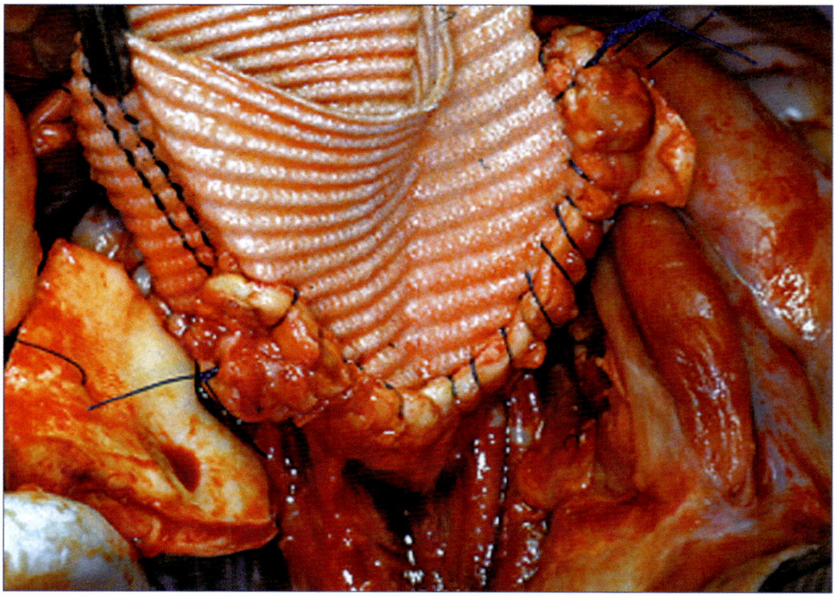

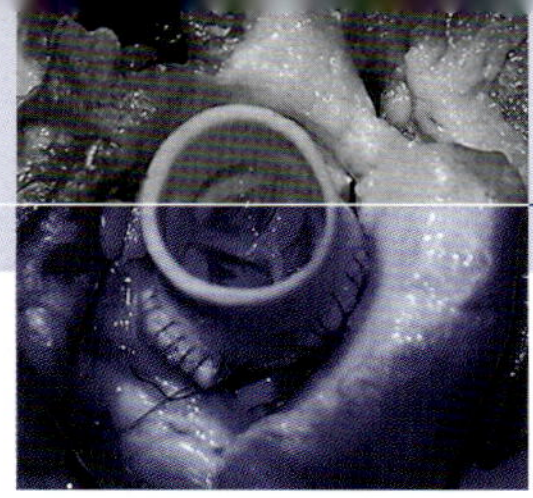

Inspection of the valve as well as testing leaflet coaptation by filling the new aortic root with saline reveals whether further surgical intervention involving the cusps is required.

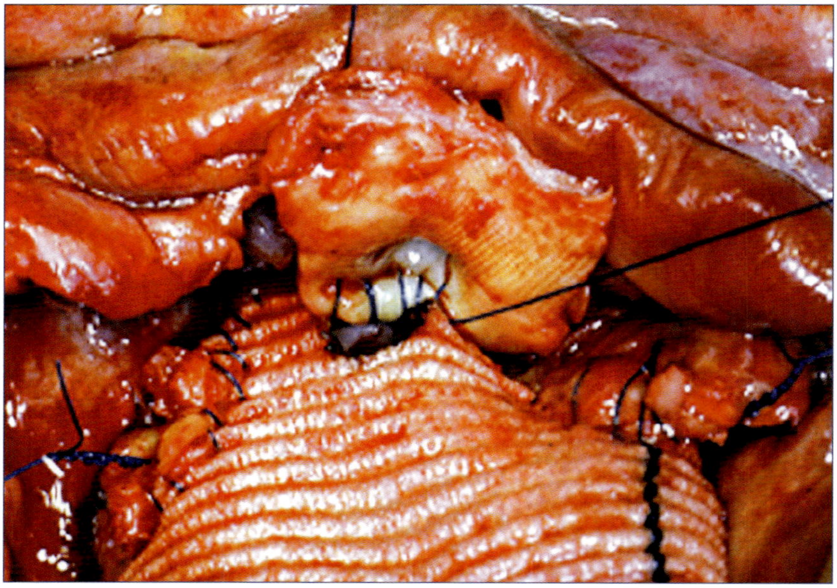

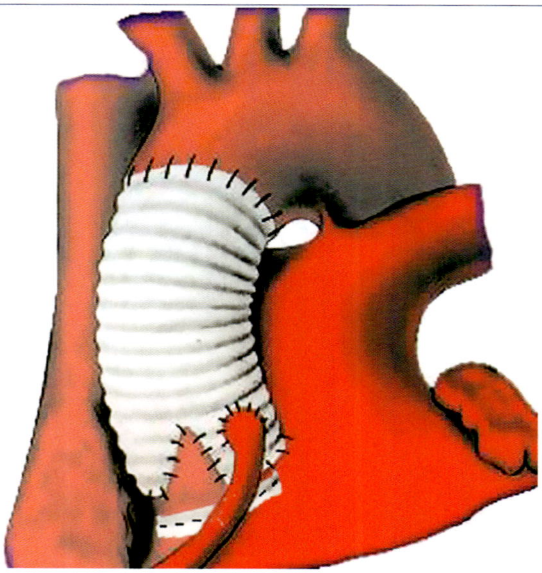

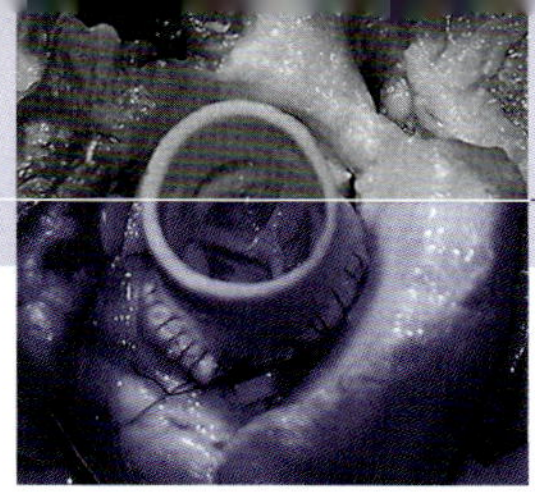

The coronary buttons are then mobilised and reimplanted into the newly fashioned sinuses with continuous 5-0 prolene sutures. Utmost care must be taken to avoid any tension or torsion on reimplantation.

To stabilize the annulus the technique can be modified by attaching a 4–5 mm strip of Dacron to the outside of the left ventricular outflow tract just below the aortic valve. Stitches being placed beginning below the midpoint of the right sinus and progressing counterclockwise to the commissure between the noncoronary and right coronary sinus. This places the stitches on 5/6 of the circumferences, avoiding alteration of the conducting system (6).

When using the remodelling technique in type A aortic dissection it is possible to replace only the dissected sinuses while preserving the intact ones.

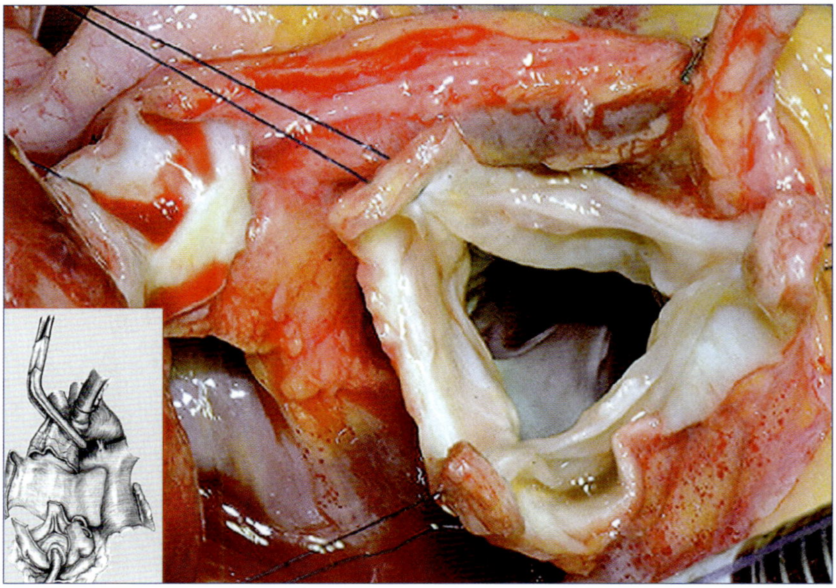

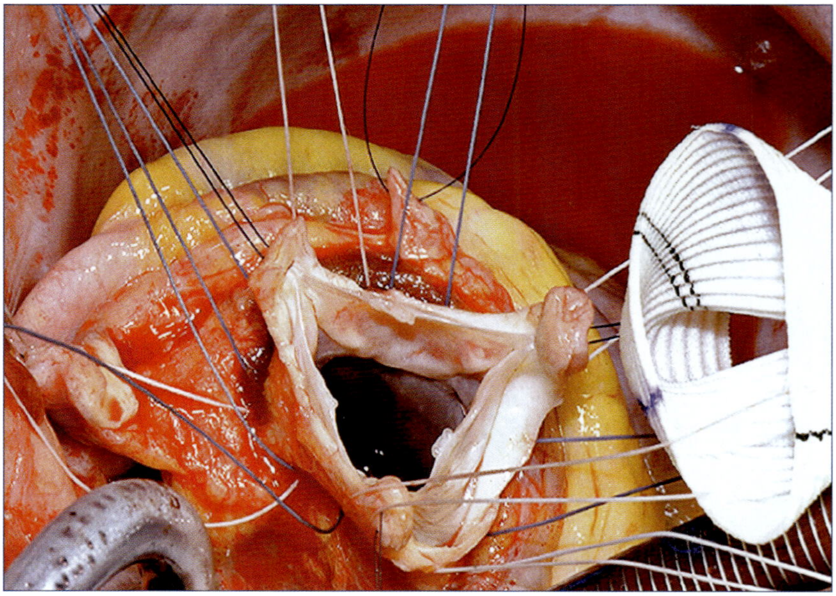

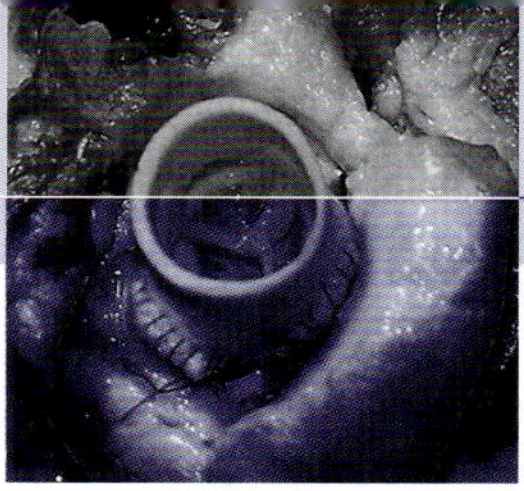

Reimplantation technique according to David (7):

STJ reconstruction with annulus stabilization:

Following excision of the sinuses, the aortic root is extensively mobilized to the level of the ventriculo-aortic junction. The size of the Dacron graft chosen should correspond to that of the ST junction at which an ideal coaptation of the leaflets is achieved. This can be measured using proper valve sizers. According to our experience valve coaptation is ideal when 30 – 40 % of the cusp area is involved. In general a prosthesis of 28 - 32 mm Diameter is used. Three vertical lines 120° apart are drawn onto the proximal end of the graft to mark the approximate position of the commissural suspension.

Next the proximal anastomosis that will anchor the prosthesis to the ventriculo-aortic junction – just below the annulus – is prepared. Therefore 12 transmural horizontal mattress sutures of 3-0 coated polyester are placed circumferentially just beneath the annulus from inside out, following a horizontal plane just below the nadir of the sinuses. One suture corresponding to each commissure and three in-between. These sutures are then passed in a similar fashion through the proximal end of the graft.

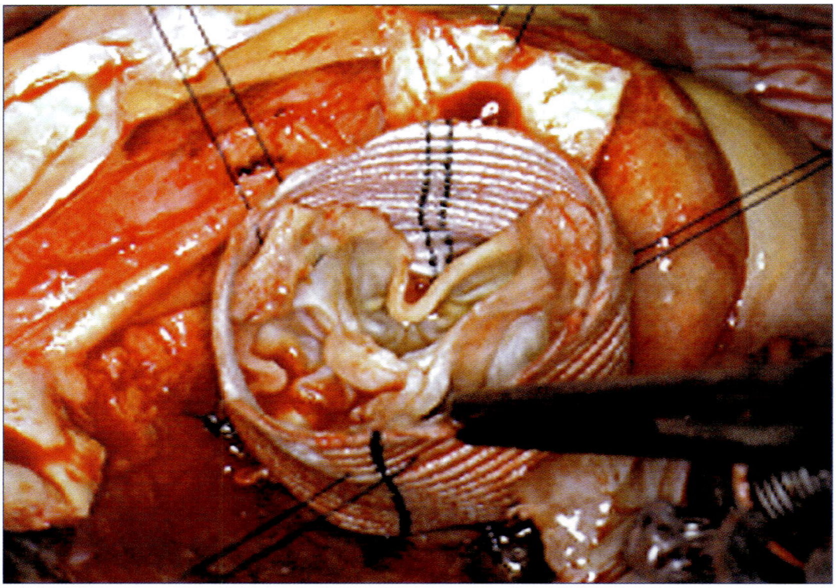

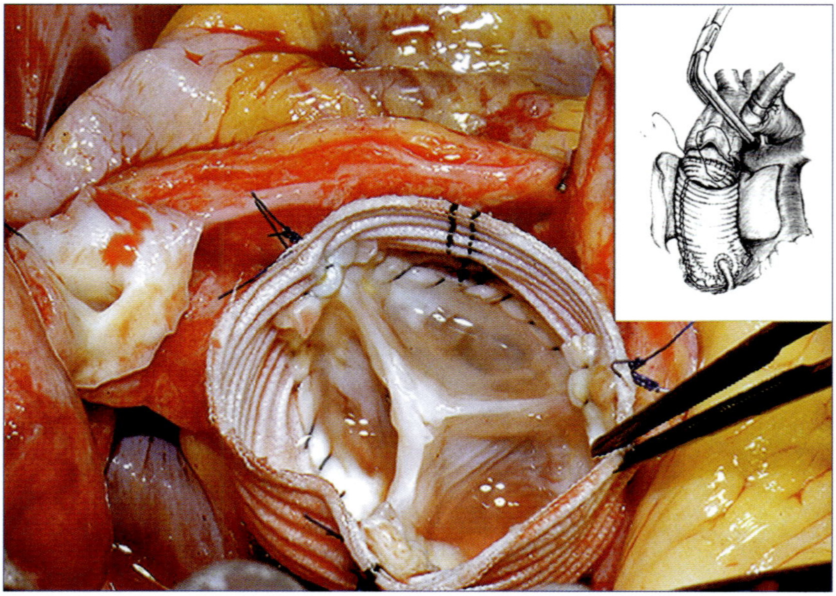

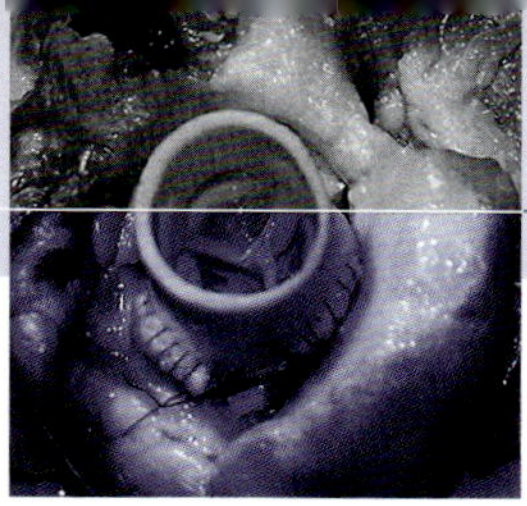

The stay sutures of the commissures are now pulled up through the lumen of the graft and the graft parachuted over the skeletonized aortic root. The sutures are then knotted gently, thereby completing this step of the operation.

The commissures are now resuspended by passing their stay sutures according to their new position through the graft. They are used to hold the commissures in position and are not yet knotted. The valve is then reimplanted into the prosthesis using three continuous horizontal mattress sutures of 4-0 prolene running along the rim of the sinuses. Each beginning as a U stitch at the centre of a sinus and passing to the apices of the neighbouring commissures. After all three sutures are completed they are tightened as are the holding sutures of the commissures. Stretching the prosthesis while reimplanting the valve has to be avoided as it would result in an insufficient height of commissural suspension and subsequently cusp prolapse.

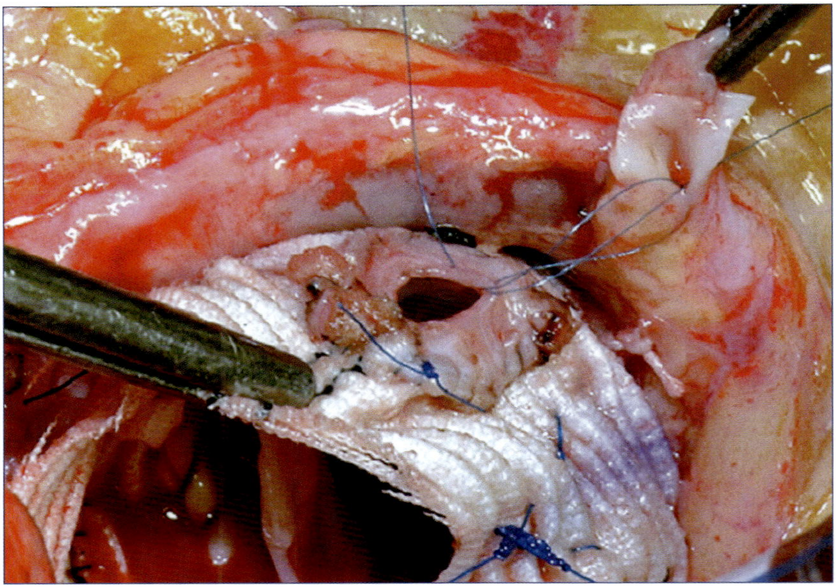

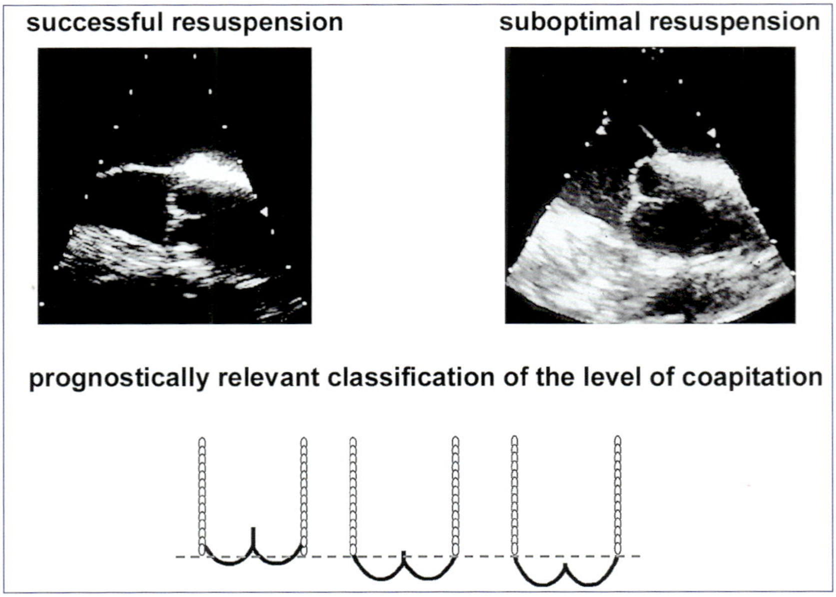
successful resuspension
suboptimal resuspension
prognostically relevant classification of the level of coaptation

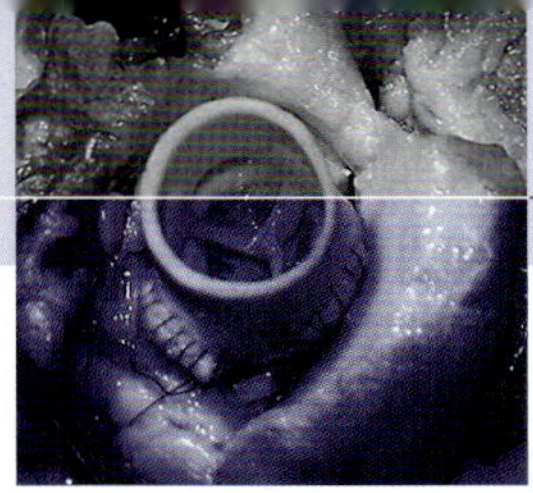

Reimplantation of the coronary buttons completes the procedure. The indirect Reimplantation of an aberrant right coronary artery that originated from the left coronary sinus and passed intramurally between the aorta and the pulmonary artery to the right ventricle is illustrated. A patch of autologous pericardium was first sutured into the targeted position and then the mobilised coronary artery is implanted into the patch.

Utmost care needs to be taken to achieve correct cusp geometry and sufficient height of commissural suspension within the prosthesis, thereby ensuring a proper level of coaptation of the cusps. The level of coaptation should lie above the annulus and hence inside the prosthesis as this has a high prognostic significance for the longevity of the valve repair (8).
Intraoperative echocardiography is therefore an essential instrument of quality control allowing early detection of an insufficient or prognostically unfavourable reconstruction. In our experience any residual insufficiency exceeding a minimal insufficiency is unacceptable and necessitates reevaluation of the reconstruction or even a valve replacement.

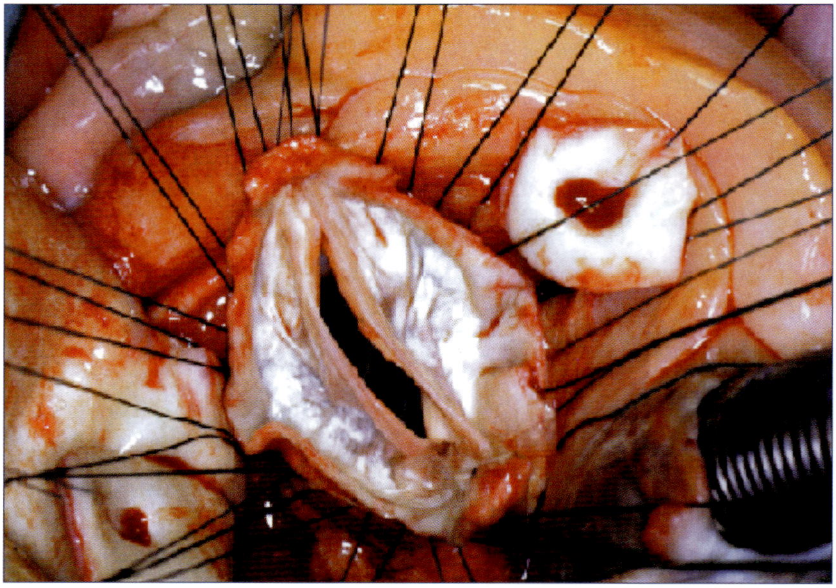

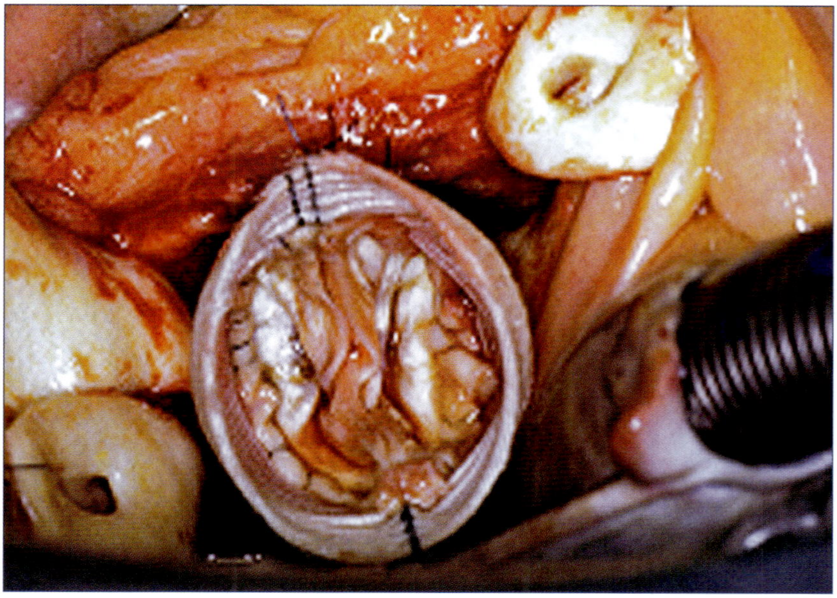

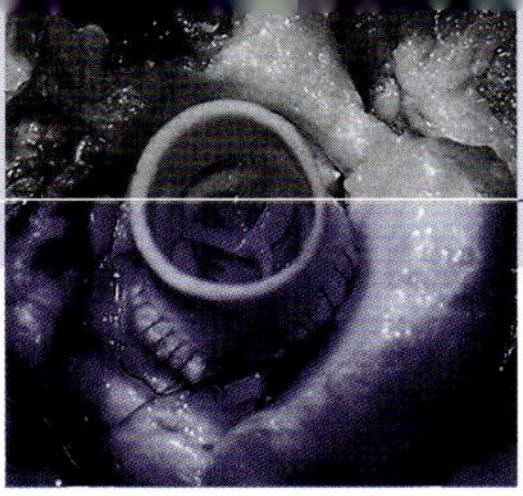

The previously mentioned techniques can also be successfully applied in patients with bicuspid aortic valves showing no or minimal structural changes. However, additional procedures involving the leaflets are frequently needed to ensure a secure and wide coaptation.

Leaflet reconstruction (9–11):

The aim is a correction of leaflet prolapse. Suspending the cusps by a temporary stitch of 6-0 prolene that joins the corpora arantii, a so called Frater stitch (not illustrated) facilitates the assessment of the relative length of the free margins of the leaflets and may give guidance to the type and extent of correction needed. Several techniques addressing cusp prolapse have been described, and the choice of the appropriate one still presents a challenge to surgical judgement:

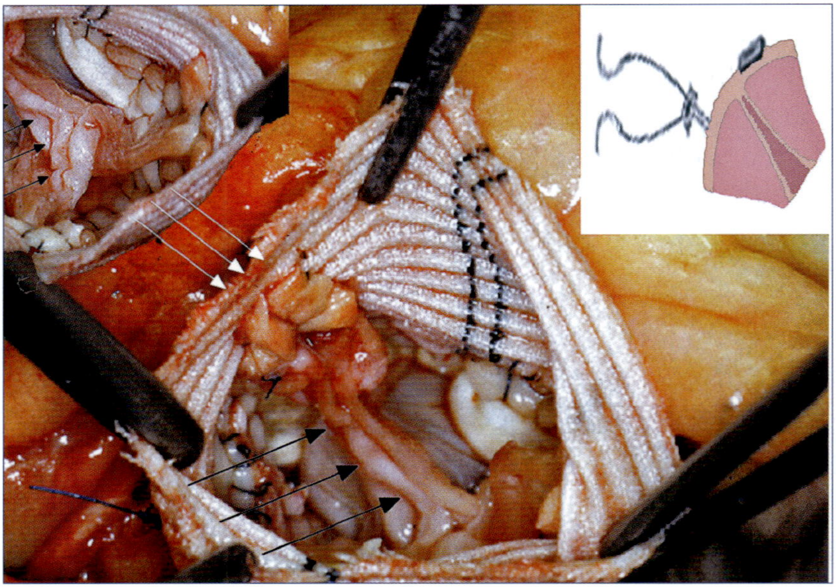

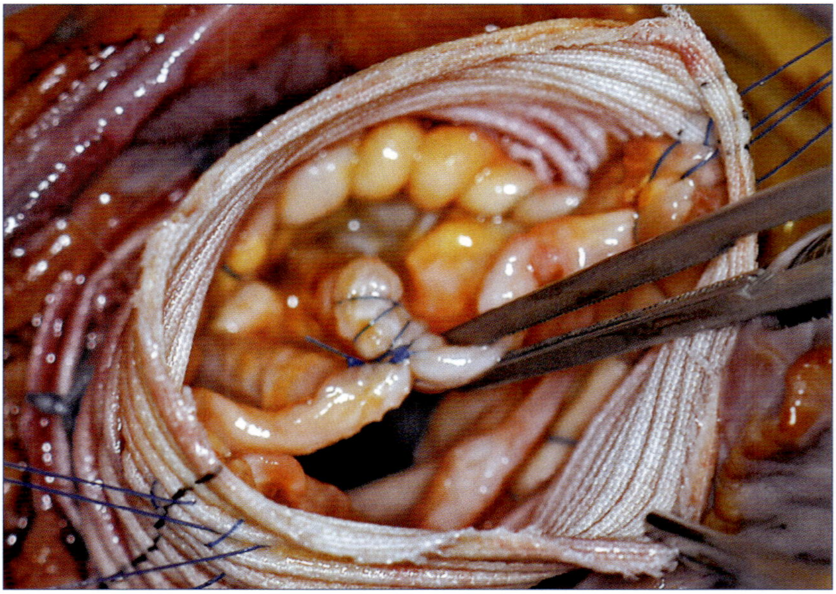

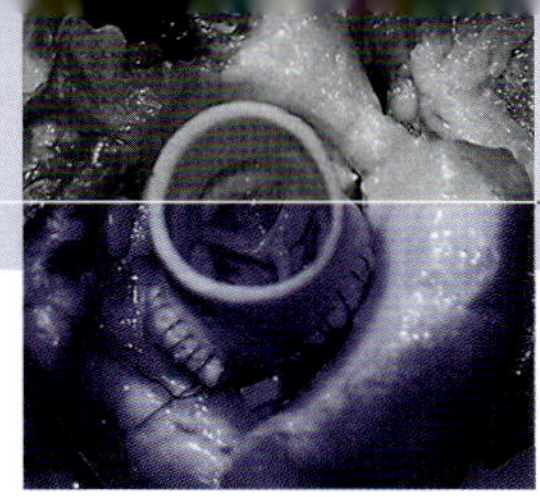

Reduction annuloplasty (small diagram):
Horizontal mattress sutures of 4-0 prolene buttressed with Teflon felt or autologous pericardium are placed through the annulus on each side of the commissure and tied. This reduces the circumference of the annulus and increases leaflet coaptation. The lower the sutures are placed the greater the amount of leaflet coaptation.

Trusler stitch (juxta commissural plication of the free leaflet margin):
The length of the free margin of the prolapsing cusp is adjusted to equal that of the adjacent margins of the normal leaflets. This length is maintained by fixing the appropriate point on the leaflet margin by a stitch to the adjacent leaflet at one or both commissures. The excess tissue is then folded at the commissure and sutured to the aortic wall with 2 or 3 mattress sutures reinforced with Teflon felt.

Triangular plication of the central free leaflet margin:
Here the free margin is plicated in its middle portion with interrupted sutures of 5-0 or 6-0 prolene. Thereby shortening the redundant leaflet margin to desired length and elevating it to coapt with the non prolapsing cusps.
Strengthening the free leaflet margin: (not illustrated)
When the free margin is thinned and overstretched, it can be reinforced and shortened with a single or double continuous horizontal suture of 6-0 Gore-Tex running parallel to the free leaflet margin and anchoring it to the commissures. Alternatively the suture can be woven along the free edge of the cusp.

Aortic Valve Repair

A. El-Essawi • W. Harringer

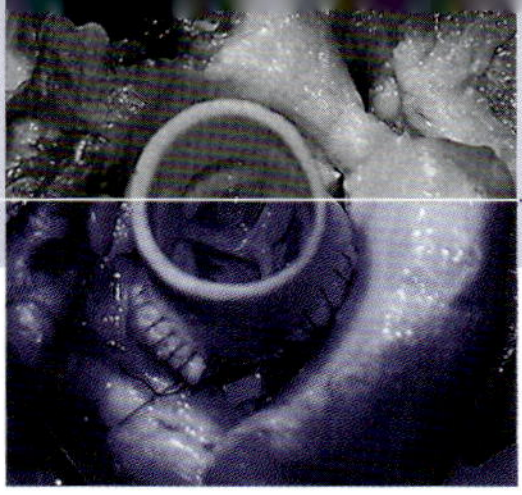

Reduction annuloplasty (small diagram):
Horizontal mattress sutures of 4-0 prolene buttressed with Teflon felt or autologous pericardium are placed through the annulus on each side of the commissure and tied. This reduces the circumference of the annulus and increases leaflet coaptation. The lower the sutures are placed the greater the amount of leaflet coaptation.

Trusler stitch (juxta commissural plication of the free leaflet margin):
The length of the free margin of the prolapsing cusp is adjusted to equal that of the adjacent margins of the normal leaflets. This length is maintained by fixing the appropriate point on the leaflet margin by a stitch to the adjacent leaflet at one or both commissures. The excess tissue is then folded at the commissure and sutured to the aortic wall with 2 or 3 mattress sutures reinforced with Teflon felt.

Triangular plication of the central free leaflet margin:
Here the free margin is plicated in its middle portion with interrupted sutures of 5-0 or 6-0 prolene. Thereby shortening the redundant leaflet margin to desired length and elevating it to coapt with the non prolapsing cusps.
Strengthening the free leaflet margin: (not illustrated)
When the free margin is thinned and overstretched, it can be reinforced and shortened with a single or double continuous horizontal suture of 6-0 Gore-Tex running parallel to the free leaflet margin and anchoring it to the commissures. Alternatively the suture can be woven along the free edge of the cusp.

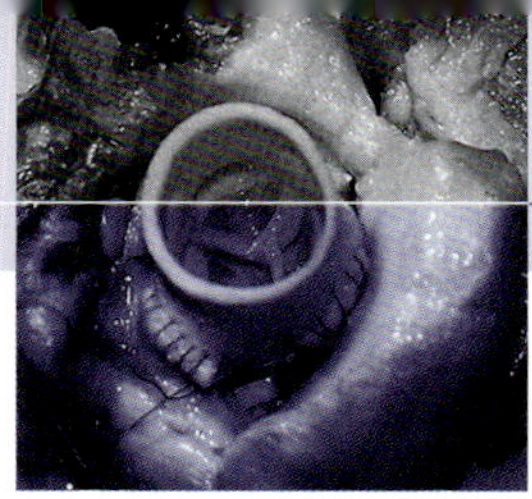

1 2 3 4 5 6 7 8 9 10 11 12 13 14 15

References

1. Angiology In: Williams PL, Warwick R, Dyson M, Bannister LH. (editors). Gray´s Anatomy. 37th ed. Chirchill Livingstone; Edin burgh London Melbourne and New York, 1989: 711–712.
2. Kunzelmann KS, Grade KJ, David TE, Cochran RP, Verier ED. Aortic root and valve relationschip: impact on surgical repair. J Thorac Cardiovasc Surg 1994; 107: 162–170.
3. Harringer W, Kallenbach K, Haverich A. Aortenklappenrekonstruktion mit Aorta-ascendens-Ersatz: Indikation, Technik, und Ergebnisse. Z Kardiol 2001; 90(Suppl 6): VI/85–VI/91.
4. Frater BW. Aortic valve insufficiency due to aortic dilatation: corrected by sinus rim adjustment. Circulation 1986; 74(Suppl I): 136–142.
5. Sarsam MA, Jacoub M. Remodeling of the aortic valve annulus. J Thorac Cardiovasc Surg 1993; 105: 435–438.
6. David TE, Feindel CM. An aortic valve-sparing operation for patients with aortic incompetence and aneurysm of the ascending aorta. J Thorac Cardiovasc Surg 1992; 103: 617–621.
7. David TE. Aortic valve-sparing operations in pateients with ascending aortic aneurysm. Curr Opinion in Cardiology 1997; 12: 391–395.
8. Yacoub MH, Gehle P, Chandrasekaran V, Birks EJ, Child A, Radley-Smith R. Late results of a valve-preserving operation in patients with aneurysms of the ascending Aorta and Root. J Thorac Cardiovasc Surg 1998; 115: 1080–1090.
9. Doty DB, Arcadi JM. Methods for graft size selection in Aortic valve sparing operations. Ann Thorac Surg 2000; 69: 648–650.
10. Pethig K, Milz A, Hagel C, Harringer W, Haverich A. Aortic valve re-implantation in ascending aortic aneurysm: risk factors for early failure. Ann Thorac Surg 2002; 73: 29–33.
11. Cosgrove DM, Rosenkranz ER, Hendren WG, Bartlett JC, Stewart WJ. Valvuloplasty for aortic insufficiency. J Thorac Cardiovasc Surg 1991; 102: 571–577.
12. David TE, Armstrong S, Ivanov J, Webb G. Aortic valve sparing operations: An update. Ann Thorac Surg 1999; 67: 1840–1842.
13. David TE. Aortic valve repair and aortic valve- sparing opera tions. In Cohn LH, Edmunds LH Jr (editors). Cardiac Surgery in the Adult. Mc Graw-Hill, New York, 2003: 811–824.

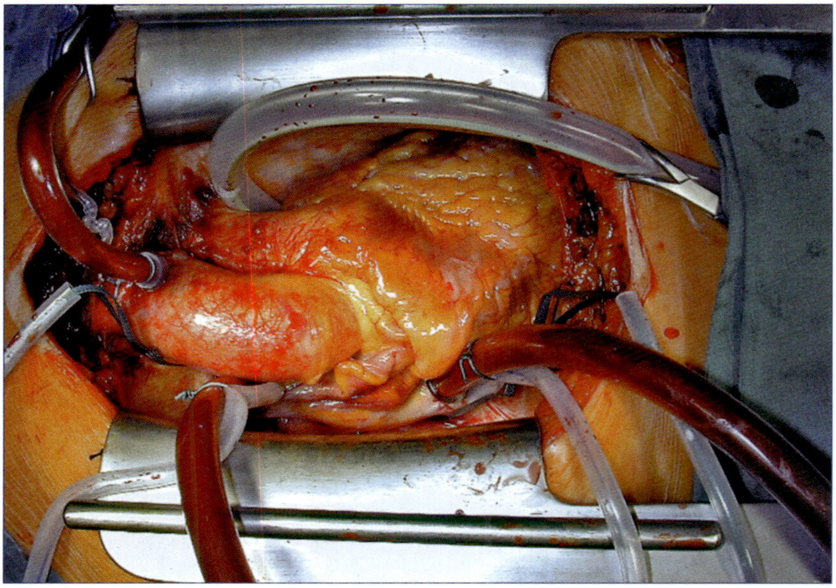

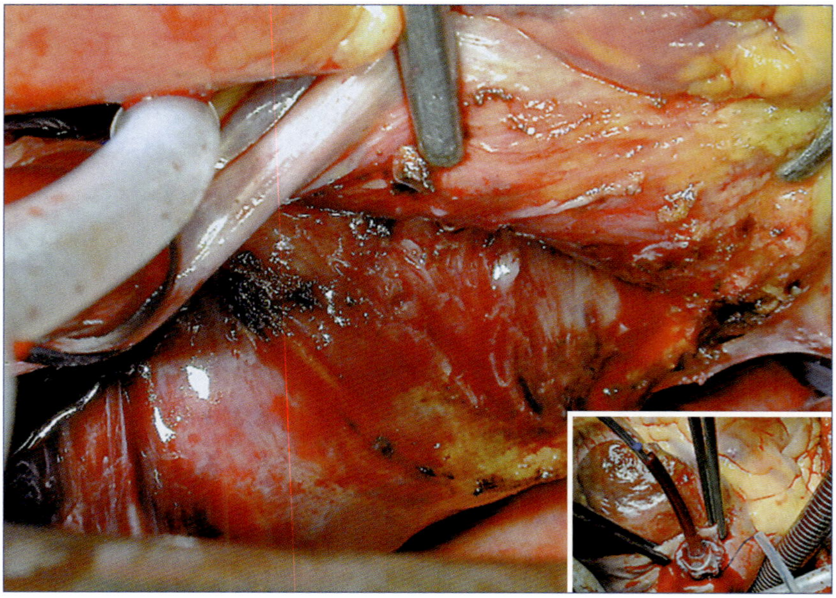

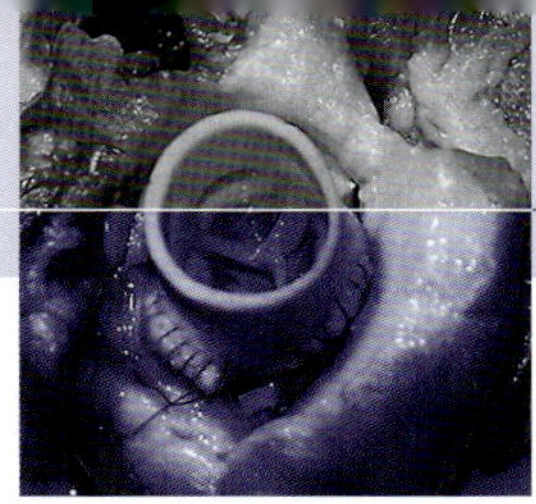

Mitral Valve Replacement: Implantation of a Mechanical Prosthesis

Operative situation after sternotomy. Establishment of cardiopulmonary bypass. Cooling to 32 °C. Application of antegrade or retrograde cardioplegia. Double cannulation of the heart by securing both caval veins. If necessary, the superior vena cava (SVC) is mobilized 2 cm cranially for improved exposition. Alternatively, mitral replacement is performed by application of a single venous cannulation of the right atrium. However, this technique is not recommended as it might be difficult to dissect the interatrial groove appropriately. Furthermore, in case of accidental opening of the right atrium an "air-block" of the extracorporeal circulation might result in poor venous drainage. For general protection of air emboli, CO2 insufflation into the pericardium is highly recommended due to the fact that CO2 is easily reabsorbed into the blood as compared to room air. A specific mitral valve retractor application (i.e. Cosgrove, as displayed) is beneficial and provides stable and durable exposition of the mitral valve.

Standard Access to the Mitral Valve

Dissection of the interatrial groove, while the first assistant pulls the right atrium ventrally. Starting at the upper right pulmonary vein, the interatrial groove is dissected in caudal direction. The more the interatrial groove can be exposed towards the first assistant, the more the later exposure of the mitral valve will be enhanced. Thereafter, a retrograde cardioplegic catheter is inserted through the free wall of the right atrium (small image). It is advantageous to perform this cannulation relatively close to the upper right margin of the right atrial apendage as this offers an improved insertion angel into the coronary sinus. A major benefit of retrograde cardioplegia administration is that it allows for repetitive dosages of cardioplegia without need for release of the mitral retractor who otherwise alters the geometry of the aortic root with a resulting aortic insufficiency and improper application of antegrade cardioplegia.

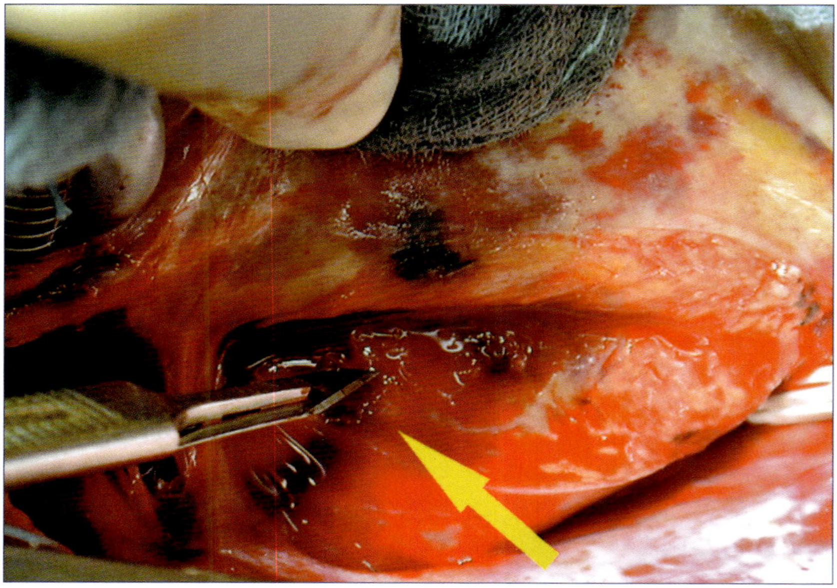

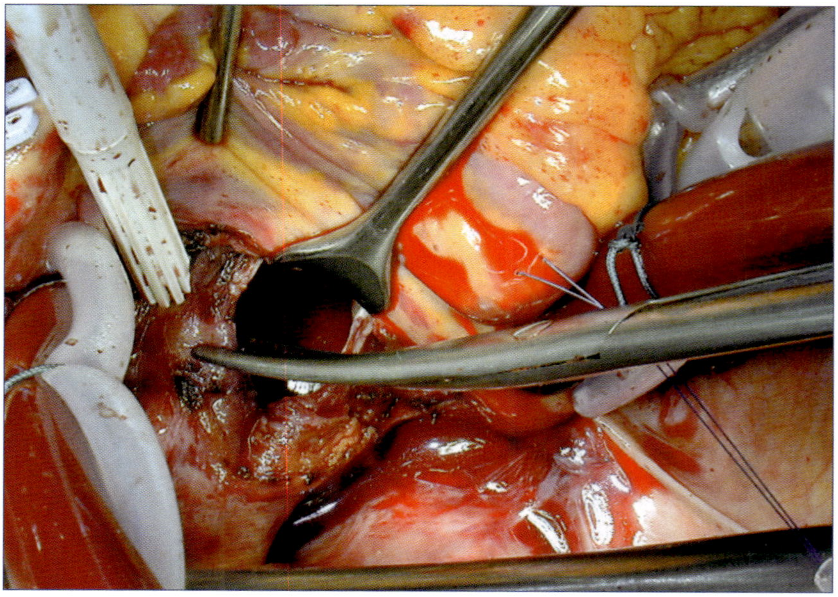

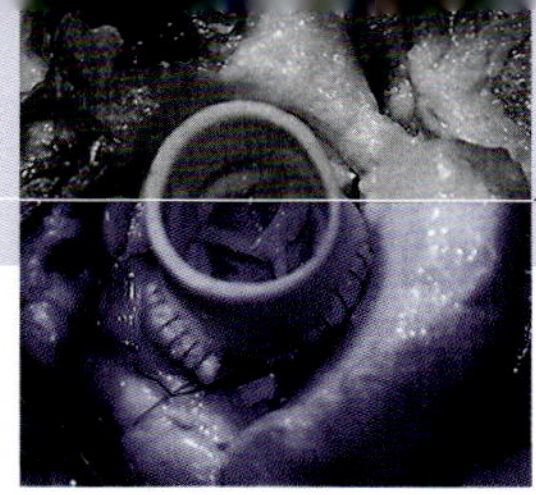

Incision of the Left Atrium

During the antegrade or retrograde cardioplegia administration, a small incision of the left atrium is performed. Approximately 5 mm should be left as a free margin towards the first assistant.

Left Atrial Incision I

Enlargement of the primary stitch incision leftwards, towards and below the superior caval vein.

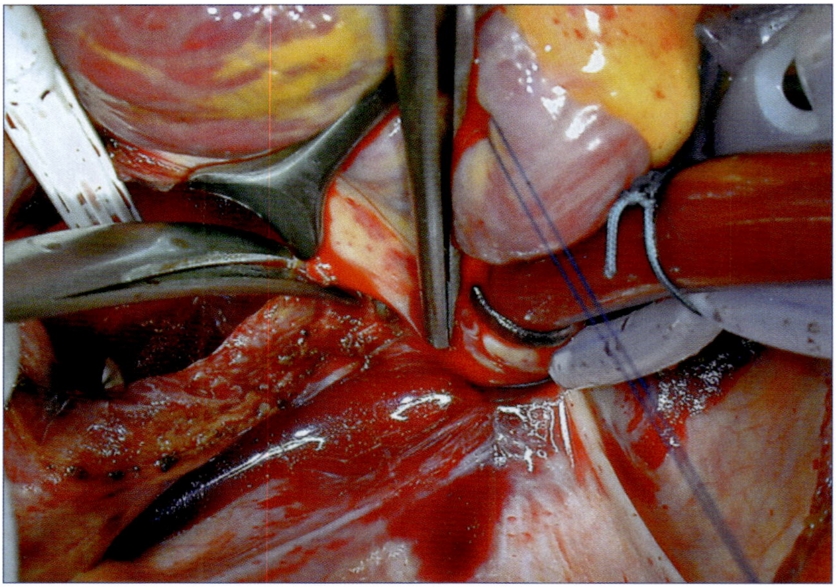

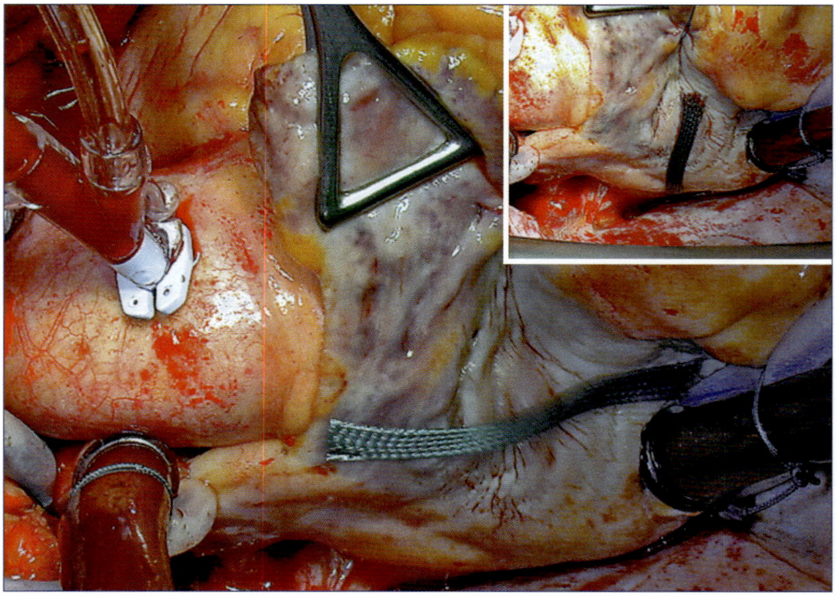

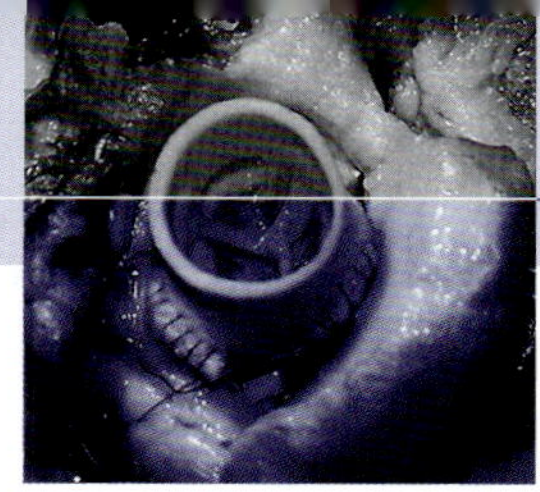

Left Atrial Incision II

Enlargement of the incision towards the right is performed with special attention to the inferior caval vein and is then extended towards the mitral valve

Alternative Access Approaches

Alternatively, an access through the right atrium can be performed. The incision line is shown in this figure. Following the right atrial incision, a stitch incision opens the foramen ovale. Thereafter, this stitch incision is extended by 3-5 cm and a retractor is inserted. The Dubost access offers a different approach, which describes a combination of the interatrial groove access and an access through a perpendicular incision of the right atrial wall at the septum. Additional access approaches, which should be reserved to the experienced surgeon, are through the atrial roof including a transection of the SVC or the aorta, if necessary.

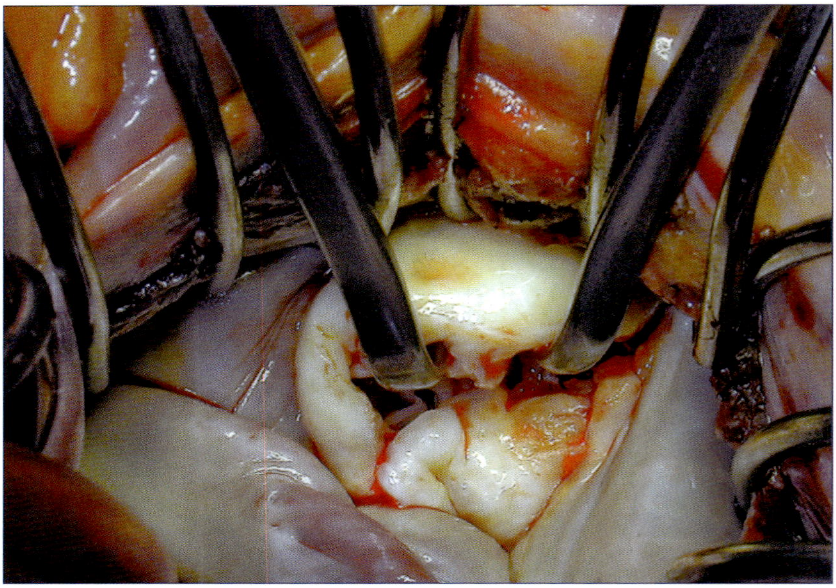

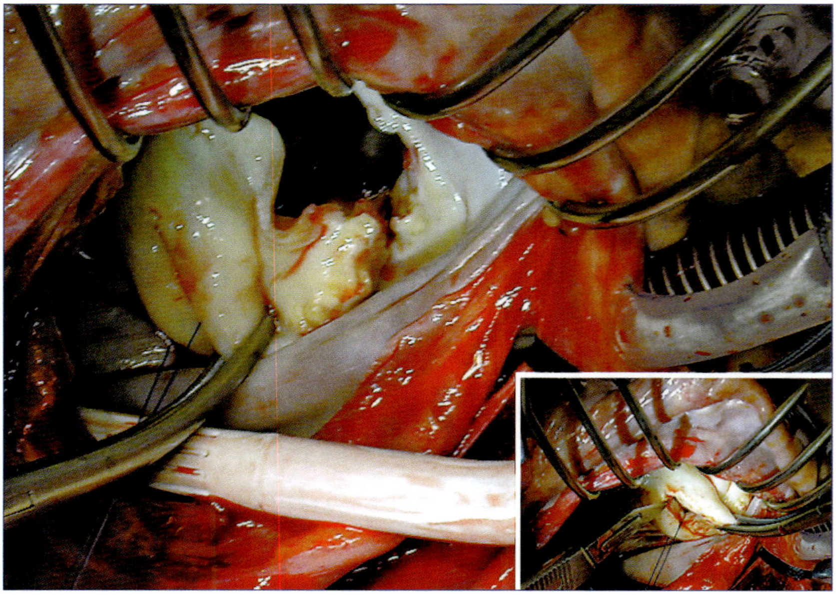

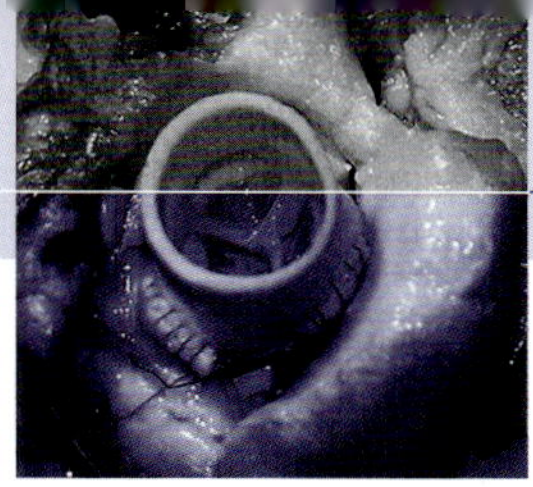

Inspection of the Mitral Valve

First, up to three retractors are inserted into the left atrium in order to facilitate optimal exposure of the mitral valve. The valve itself is examined using special hooks. The figure displays a case of mitral stenosis with retracted and thickened leaflets and a restrictive subvalvular apparatus.

Excision of the Valve Leaflets

Initially, a 3-0 auxiliary suture was placed into the anterior leaflet in order to displace it towards the surgeon. Severe calcifications were present; hence, a complete resection of the leaflet was performed to enable a prosthesis implantation.

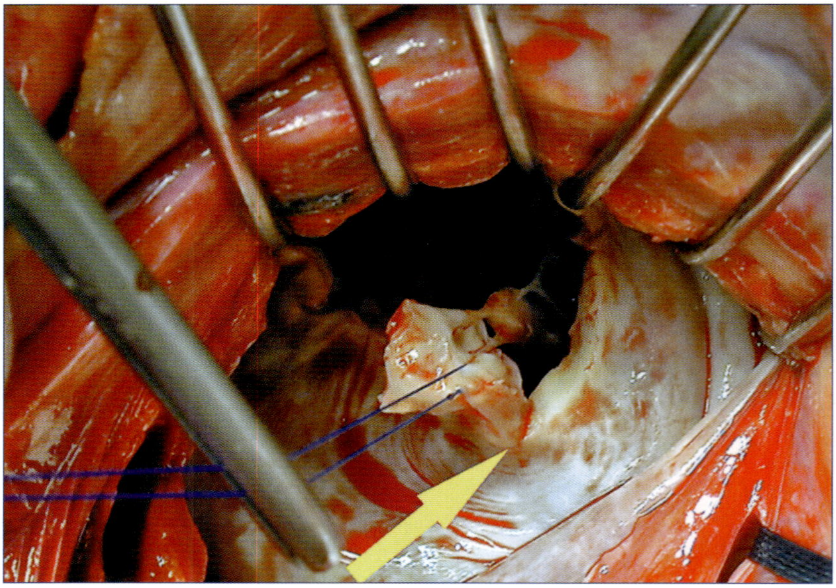

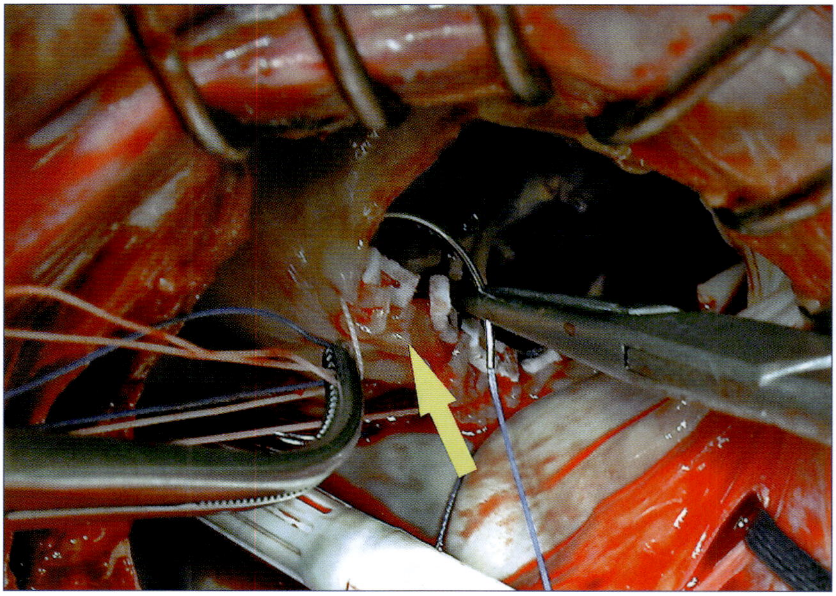

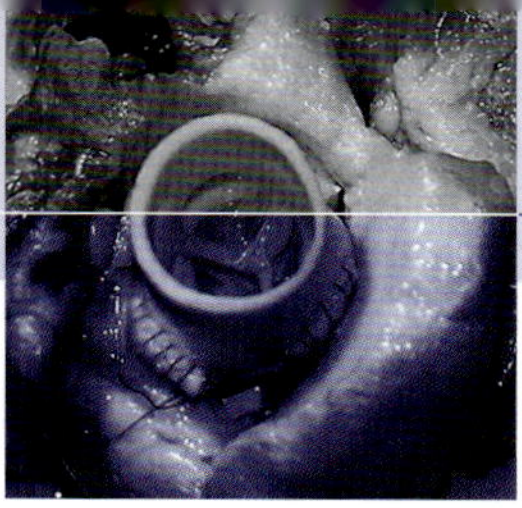

1 2 3 4 5 6 7 8 9 10 11 12 13 14 15

Resection of the Posterior Leaflet

Extensive mitral valve stenosis may require resection of both leaflets, including the subvalvular apparatus. However, a functional impairment of the left ventricle may result as a long term effect. Consequently, complete resection should be preferably avoided. In the presented case, the leaflet thickening is effectively visible.

Valve Sutures I

Valve sutures can be placed both from the ventricle (epi-annular) or from the atrium (intra-annular). The epiannular technique allows the attachment of the preserved subvalvular apparatus to the base of the prosthesis which, by preservation of the ventriculo-annular continuity, results in improved long term results.

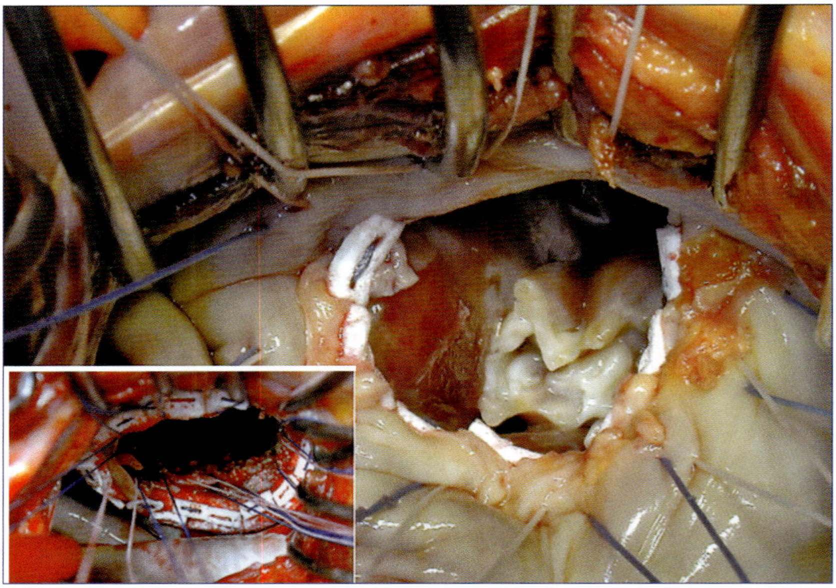

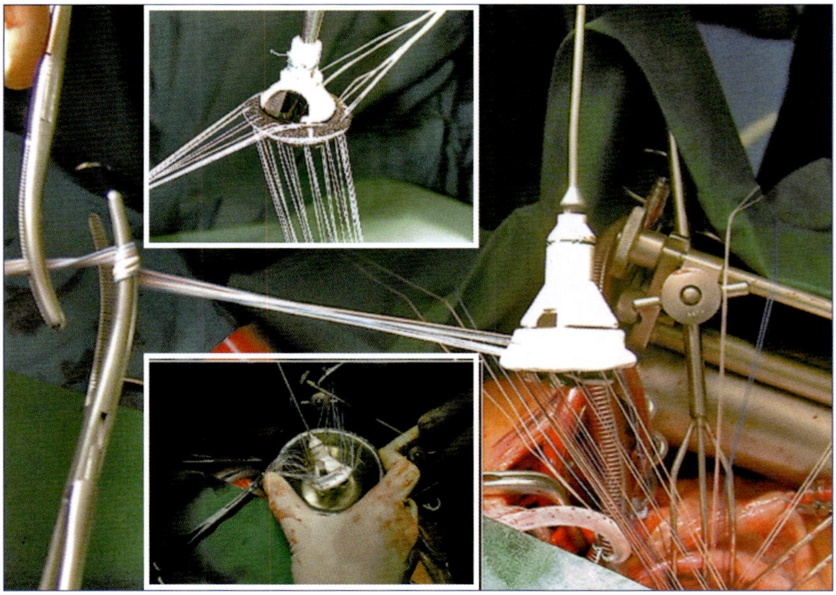

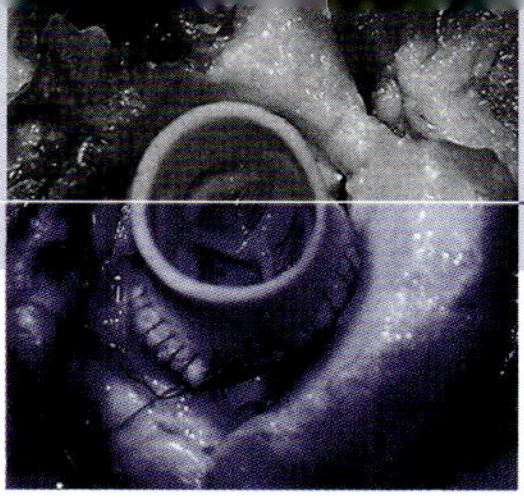

Valve Sutures II

Completion of the epiannular valve sutures. Typically, 2-0 Teflon reinforced sutures are applied. The small image illustrates the intraannular stitch technique. Frequently, a somewhat more extended atrium eversion results as compared to epiannular techniques, which can be especially problematic in patients with severe calcifications of the annulus.

Preparation of the Valve Prosthesis for Implantation

Depending on the chosen prosthesis type, approximately 10–15 stitch pairs are threaded through the prosthesis ring. By varying the placement of the sutures, a variable width under the prosthesis ring can be achieved and may gain special importance regarding the anchoring of the subvalvular apparatus. Additionally, in order to avoid endocarditis, the valve may be immersed in an antibiotic solution, which also facilitates the insertion of the prosthesis, if the sutures are wet.

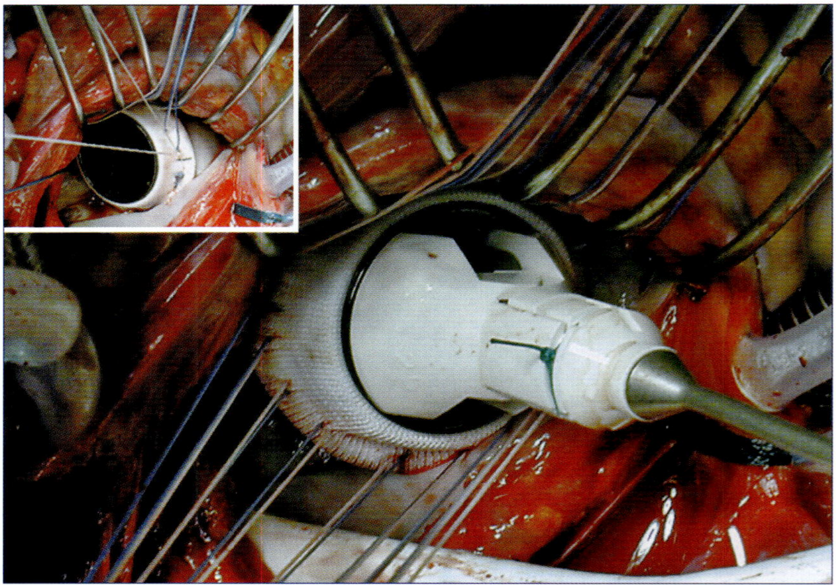

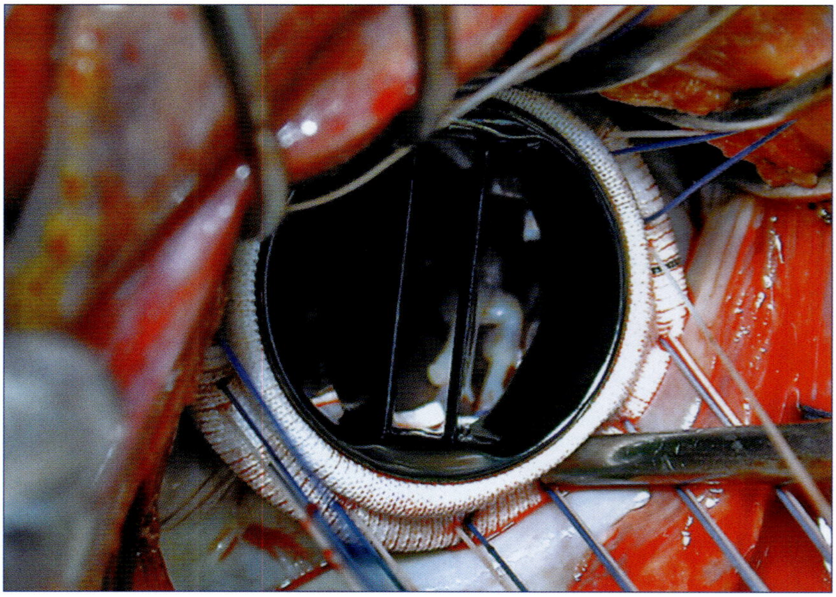

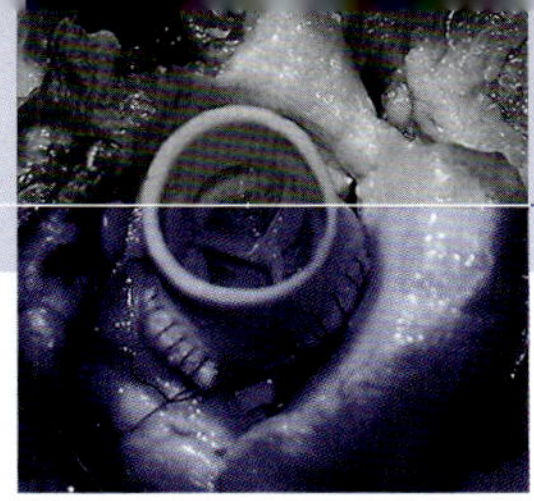

Insertion of the Valve Prosthesis

The prosthesis is introduced using its corresponding holder. When implanting a biological prosthesis, occasionally, it is recommended not to remove the valve holder until the first three sutures at the commissures are tied, because the struts may get trapped in the ventricle wall or the subvalvular apparatus. Implantation starts in the most accessible region. If necessary, the already tied sutures can be used to displace the prosthesis for exposure of those sutures which are not easily visible to the surgeon (small Figure).

Fixation of the Valve

In the figure displayed, the mechanical valve prosthesis is anti-anatomically rotated first. One must confirm secure attachment of the suture ring to the atrial tissue.

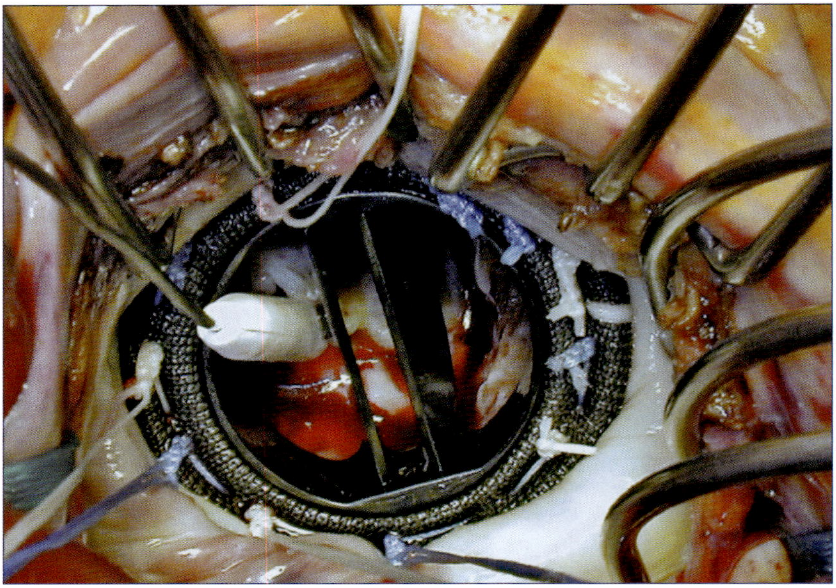

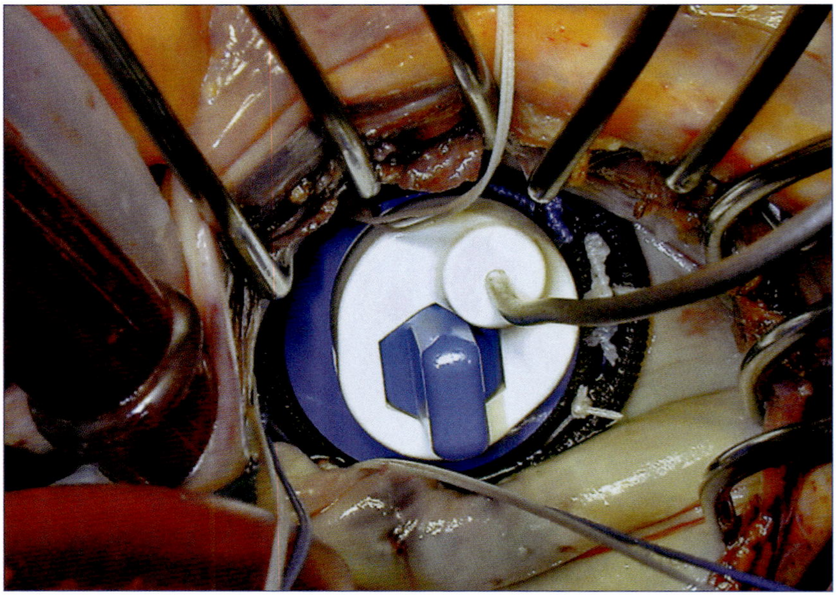

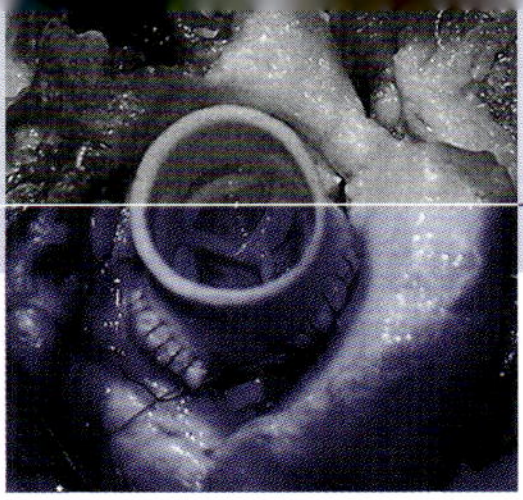

Inspection of the Valve Prosthesis
After complete implantation, the prosthesis is inspected by means of a soft tip to confirm free and unobstructed leaflet motion. In this open leaflet position, the subvalvular area can be inspected with superb visual quality.

Rotating of the Prosthesis
Periodically, valve prosthesis rotation is essential to achieve unhindered motion of the leaflets. Consequently, the valve prosthesis is directed anatomically (i.e., transverse) or anti-anatomically. Both adjustments are viable. Animal experiments have demonstrated marginal advantages of the anti-anatomical position for bi-leaflet prostheses.

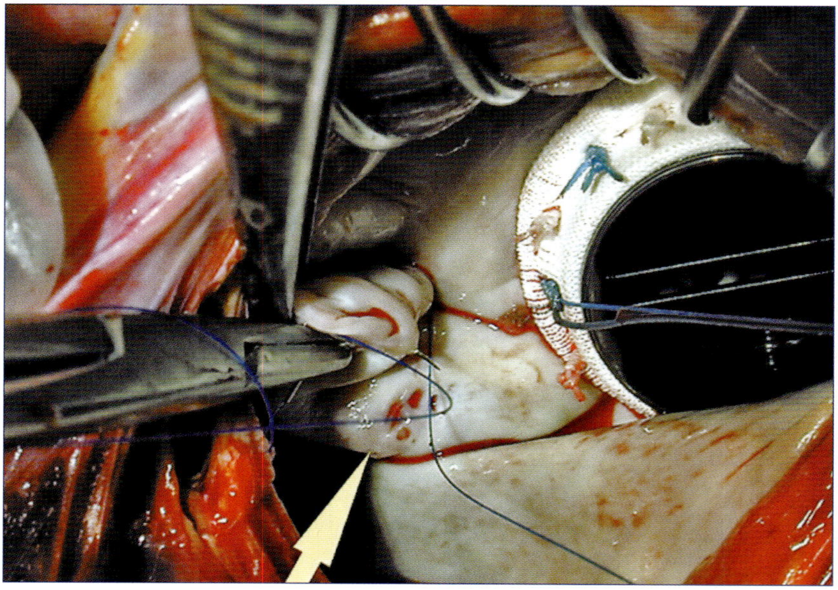

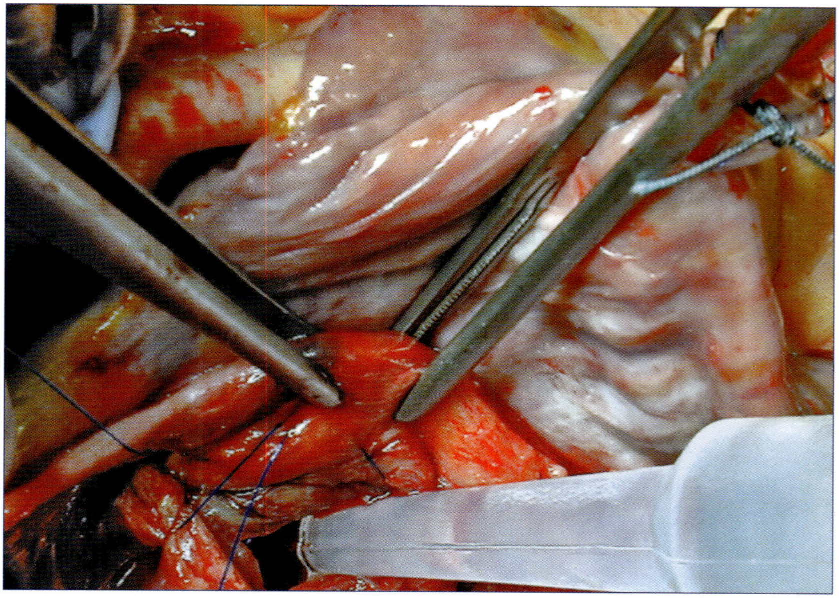

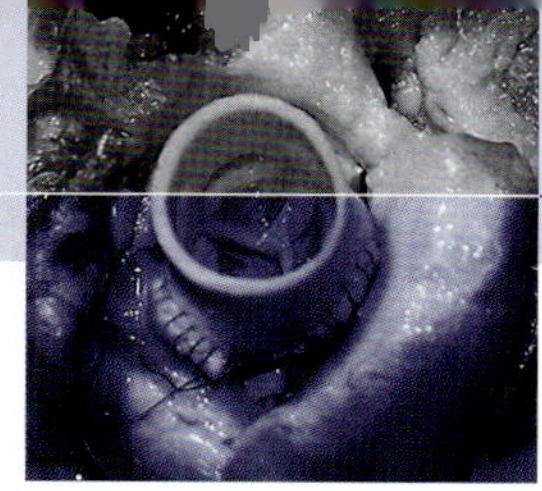

Occlusion of the Left Atrial Appendage

The left atrial appendage (LAA) occlusion is performed using 3-0 prolene suture with an SH needle. Occluding the LAA reduces embolic events significantly in spite of sinus rhythm. It is helpful to use the valve sutures to achieve better exposure by pulling in a helpful dirction.

Closure of the Atriotomy

For atriotomy closure, 3-0 prolene sutures are applied starting at the left and right corner, respectively, towards the middle. It is imperative to include the entire atrial wall into this suture. The left atrium and the pulmonary veins are de-aired using saline with the lungs inflated prior to completion of the suture.

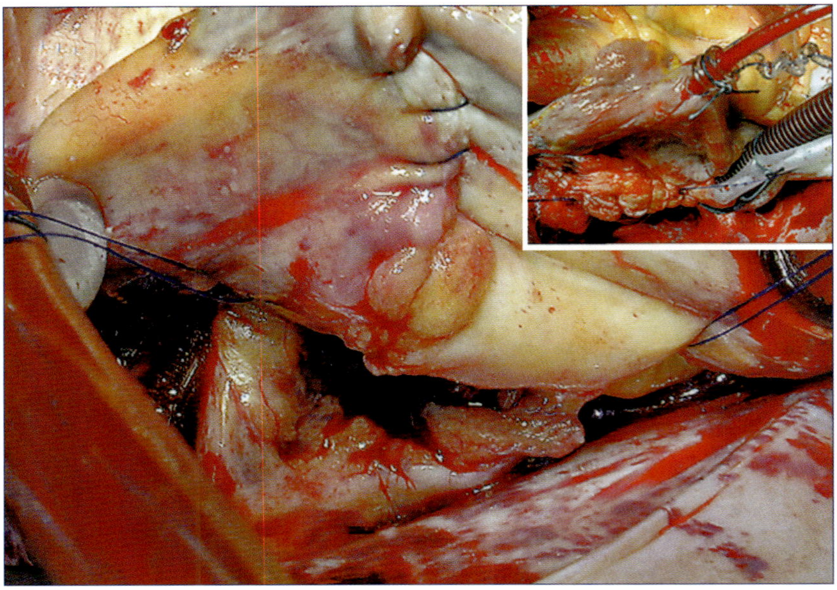

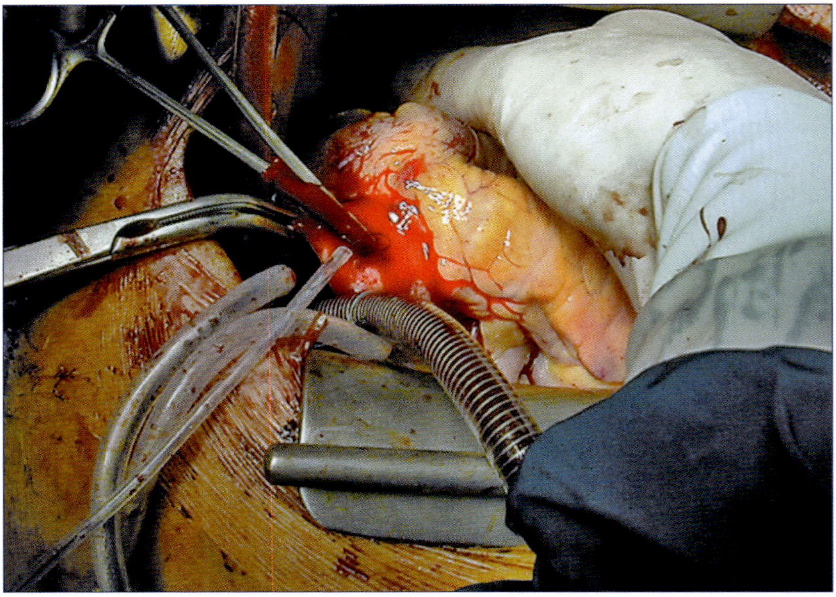

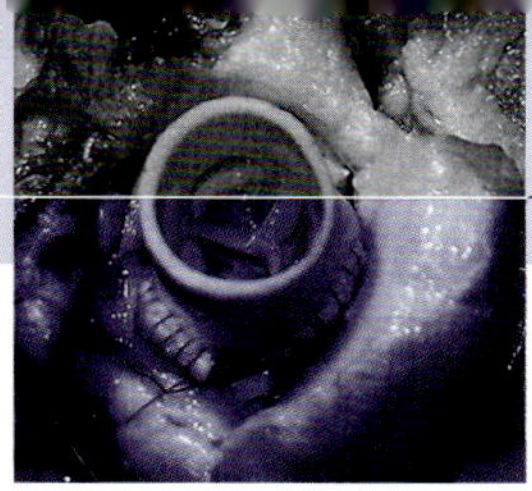

Atrial Closure after the Dubost Approach

If access to the left atrium is initially supplemented by a perpendicular, transseptal approach (according to Dubost), an adequate re-approximation starting with the perpendicular incision is essential. The small figure illustrates the removal of the retroplegia catheter and the transition to partial cardiopulmonary bypass by loosening the tourniquets around both caval veins.

De-airing of the Heart

The heart is de-aired antegradely by reducing venous drainage while repetitive lung ventilation with full tidal volume is performed by the anesthesiologist. Hereby, the heart is compressed manually. The heart must not be displaced too much, since the valve prosthesis may act as a hypomochlion and can increase rupture risk of the ventricular site. The aortic cross clamp is released in Trendelenburg position and patient reperfusion occurs after defibrillation.

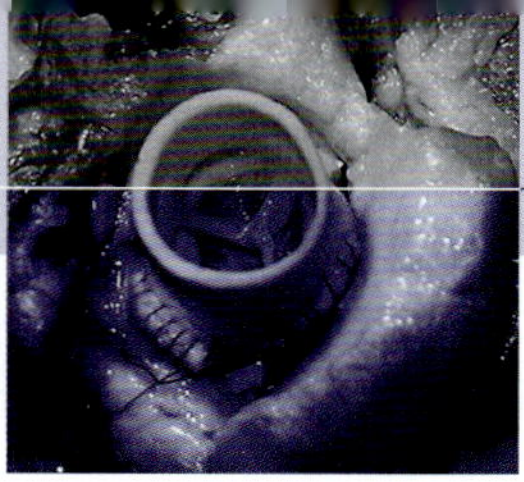

References

1. Carabello BA. Indications for mitral valve surgery. Journal of Cardiovascular Surgery 2004; 45(5): 407–18.
2. Chen SX, Xi EP, Zhang WX. Preservation of the entire mitral subvalvular apparatus during mitral valve replacement in patients with mitral stenosis. Hunan Yi Ke Da Xue Xue Bao 2003; 28(6): 615–8.
3. Iida H, Mochizuki Y, Matsushita Y, Mori H, Yamada Y, Miyoshi S. A valve replacement technique for heavily calcified mitral valve and annulus. J Heart Valve Dis 2005; 14(2): 209–11.
4. Kayacioglu I, Ates M, Sensoz Y, Gorgulu S, Idiz M, Kanca A. Comparative assessment of chordal preservation versus chordal resection in mitral valve replacement for mitral stenosis (long-term follow-up: 8 years). Tohoku Journal of Experimental Medicine 2003; 200(3): 119–28.
5. Raman J, Shah P, Seevanayagam S, Cheung J, Buxton B. Mitral regurgitation: comparison between edge-to-edge repair and valve replacement. Asian Cardiovascular & Thoracic Annals 2003; 11(2): 131–4.
6. Sasaki H, Ihashi K. Chordal-sparing mitral valve replacement: pitfalls and techniques to prevent complications. European Journal of Cardio-Thoracic Surgery 2003; 24(4): 650–2.
7. Thompson MJ, Behranwala A, Campanella C, Walker WS, Cameron EW. Immediate and long-term results of mitral prosthetic replacement using a right thoracotomy beating heart technique. European Journal of Cardio-Thoracic Surgery 2003; 24(1): 47–51; discussion 51.
8. Walkes JC, Reardon MJ. Status of mitral valve surgery. Current Opinion in Cardiology 2004; 19(2):117–22.
9. Yilmaz AT, Oz BS, Kucukaslan N, Gunay C, Yilmaz M. Preservation of anterior leaflet chordae with modified miki technique: how to do it. Card Surgery 2005; 20(1): 70–2.
10. Yoshikai M, Ito T, Murayama J, Kamohara K. Mitral annular reconstruction. Asian Cardiovascular & Thoracic Annals 2002; 10(4):344–5.

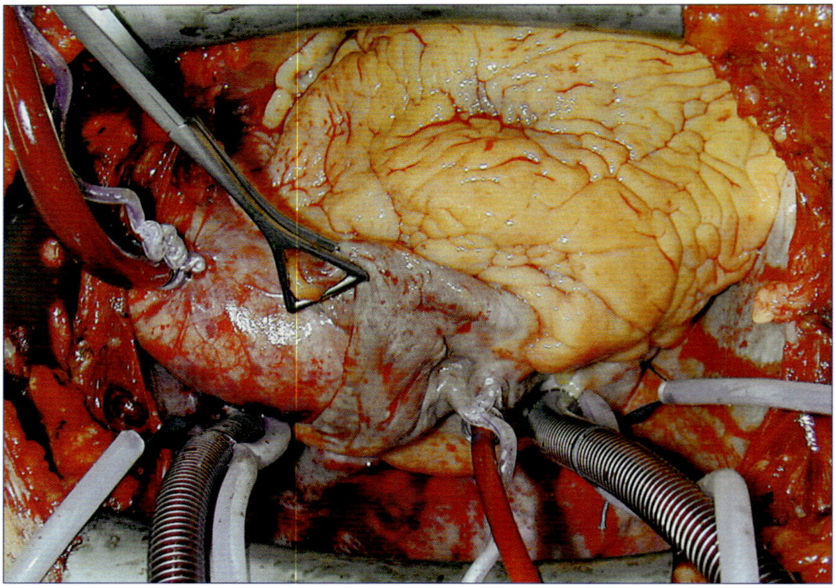

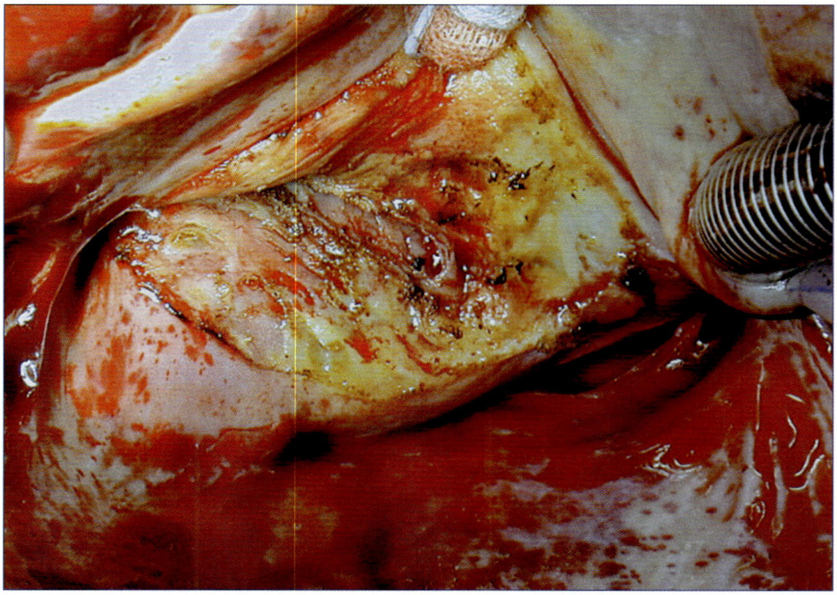

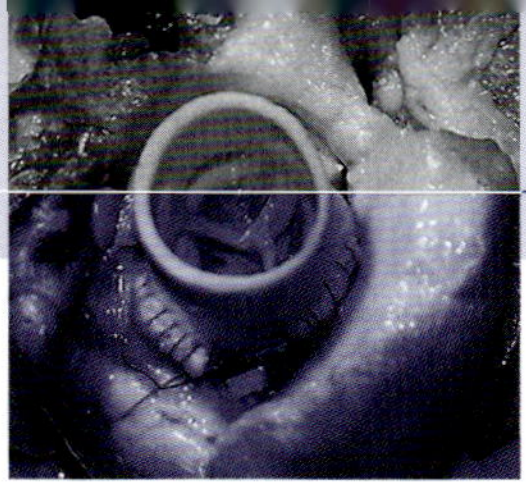

Cannulation

The most suitable approach for mitral valve repair is accomplished by the establishment of total cardiopulmonary bypass with selective cannulation of both caval veins. In difficult anatomical situations, this approach allows extension of the atrial incision in any direction. By applying tension to the inferior caval vein tourniquet, additional optimisation of exposure can be achieved. Placement of a transatrial catheter into the coronary sinus (coronary sinus catheter) allows for repetitive administration of cardioplegia at any time. When applying cardioplegia via the aortic route, in general, the entire exposure of the left atrium must be released, since the retractor often causes aortic valve incompetence. After establishment of extracorporeal circulation, all tubing lines are brought to the patient's left side.

Access

Usually, access to the mitral valve is easily achieved through the inter-atrial groove (Watson's groove) ventrally to the right pulmonary veins. After incision of the epicardium, the right and left atrium can be separated using scissors or a HF coagulator over a distance of 3–6 cm. This preparation provides a significantly improved view as well as sufficient options for further dissection maneuvers. Any injury to the right atrium should be avoided and immediately repaired as continuous bleeding alters the following mitral valve repair. Alternative access using the transatrial approach through the interatrial septum as well as the approach via the left atrial roof after dissection of the superior caval vein should be reserved for patients with very small atria.

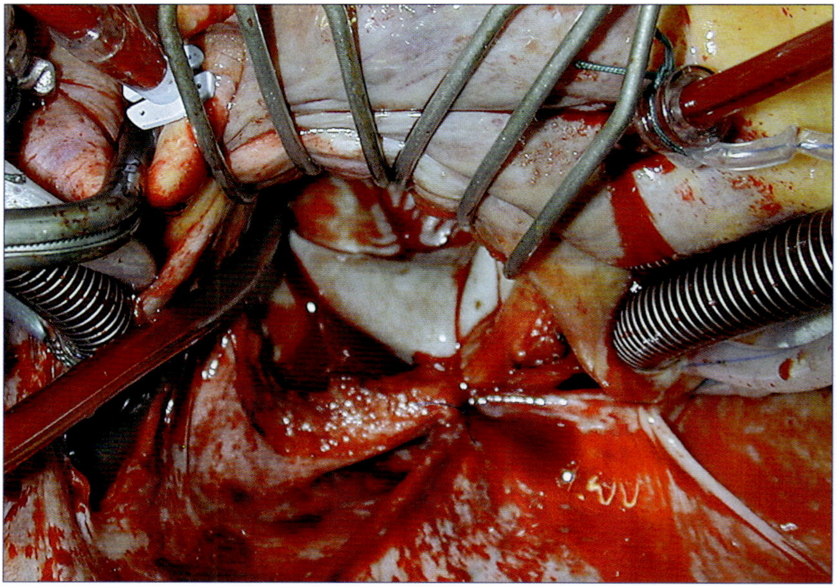

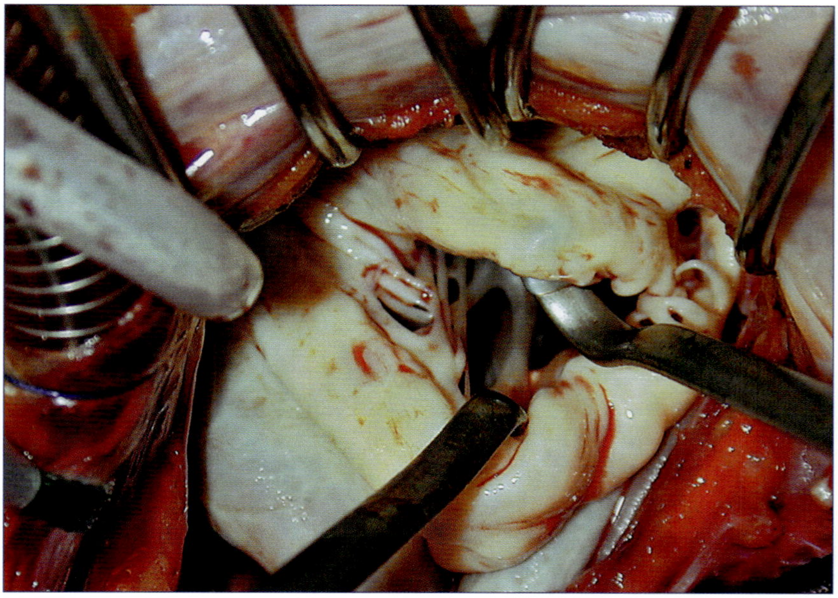

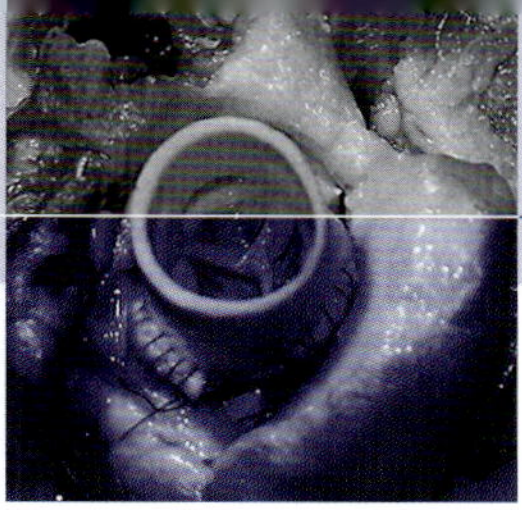

Atrial retraction

Left atrial incision should be long enough to avoid uncontrolled rupture at the edges after positioning of the retraction hooks. If the access to the mitral valve is complicated the incision can be extended cranially into the roof of the left atrium and inferiorly into the myocardium caudally of the right inferior pulmonary vein. The time required for the optimal visualization of the mitral valve is a good investment. A gauze placed adjacent the left atrial appendage behind the left ventricle displaces the mitral valve towards the surgeon and can improve exposure significantly. A stay suture from the free edge of the left atrium to the pericardium might further stabilize the view.

Exploration of the mitral valve

The first step in mitral valve repair is the determination of valve pathology, i.e. the mechanism which causes valve insufficiency. In this function test, the left ventricle is filled with Ringer's solution applicated using a large syringe, and backflow through the mitral valve indicates the location of the valve defect. Subsequently, each part of the valve should be examined separately using fine mitral hooks. According to Carpentier's classification of the mitral valve the hight of the coaptation line of complementary segments of both anterior and posterior leaflet should be defined (A1–P1, A2–P2, A3–P3).

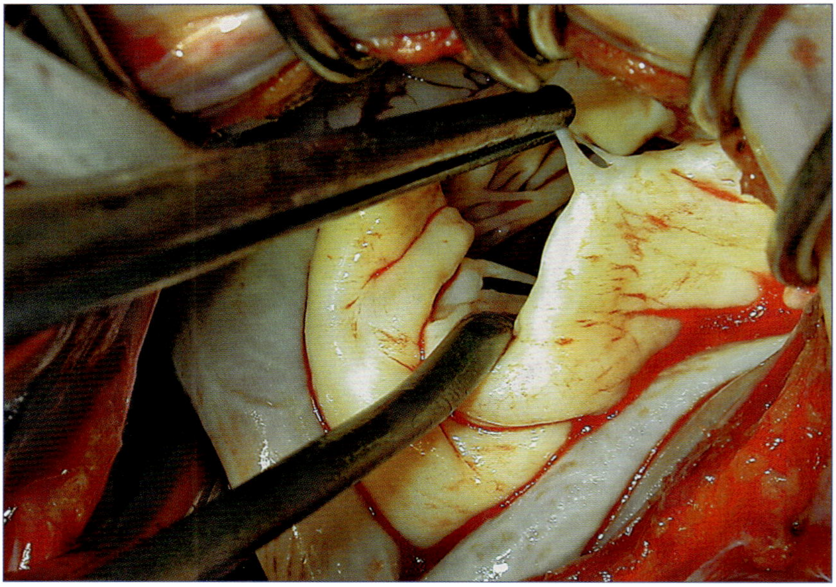

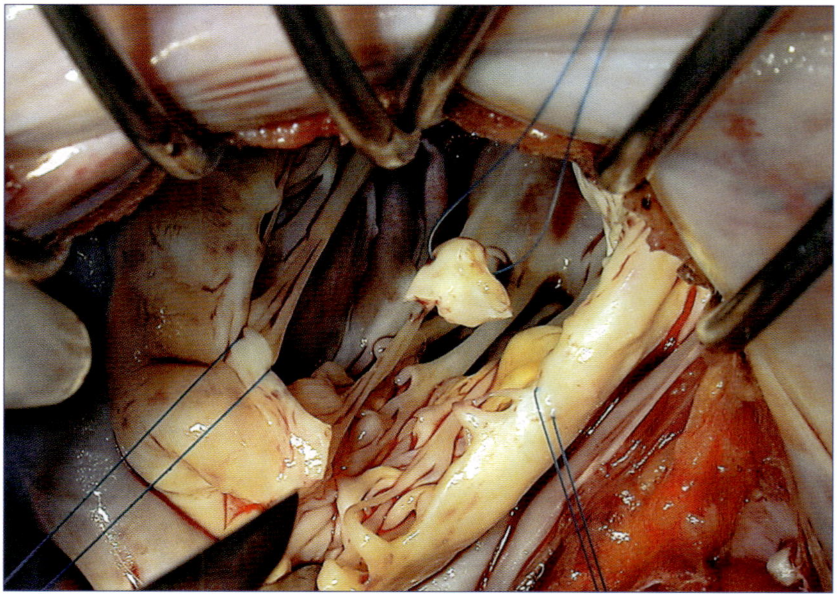

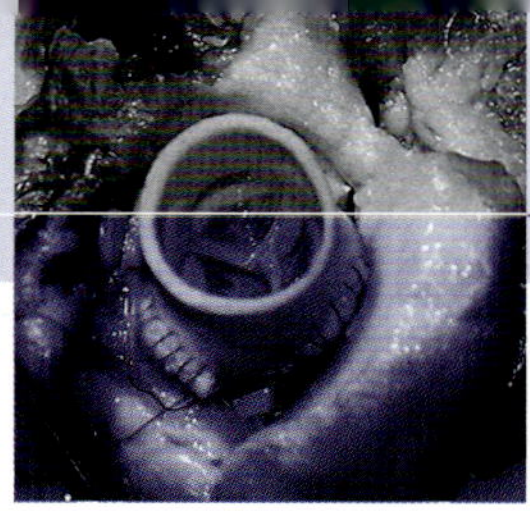

Determination of the mitral valve pathology

After valve exploration, the underlying pathology which results in mitral incompetence must have been clearly determined. The most common defect which results in isolated valve incompetence is the mitral valve prolaps. Due to the increasing tension at the free edge, chordal rupture may occur preferentially at the P2 segment of the posterior leaflet. Although an elongation typically affects both valve leaflets, the defect can be corrected by an isolated repair of the posterior leaflet in most cases. The figure shows chordal rupture at the junction between the P2- and the P3-segment which is best visualised by the above mentioned function test.

Determination of the extent of tissue resection

Once a quadrangular resection is chosen, the resection dimensions and margins must be defined. Commonly the whole P2 segment can be removed. In cases of very small or affected P1- and/or P3-segments the described technique has to be modified. The two closest and most robust first order chords (which is attached to the free margin of the valve) next to the P2-segment are marked by a fine suture (e.g. Prolene® 5/0, Ethicon). In case of anterior leaflet prolaps it is advantageous to prepare and secure one bundle of chordae from the free edge of the P2 segment with an additional suture for later chordal transposition. The length of the annular basis of the resected P2 segment might be up to 5 cm.

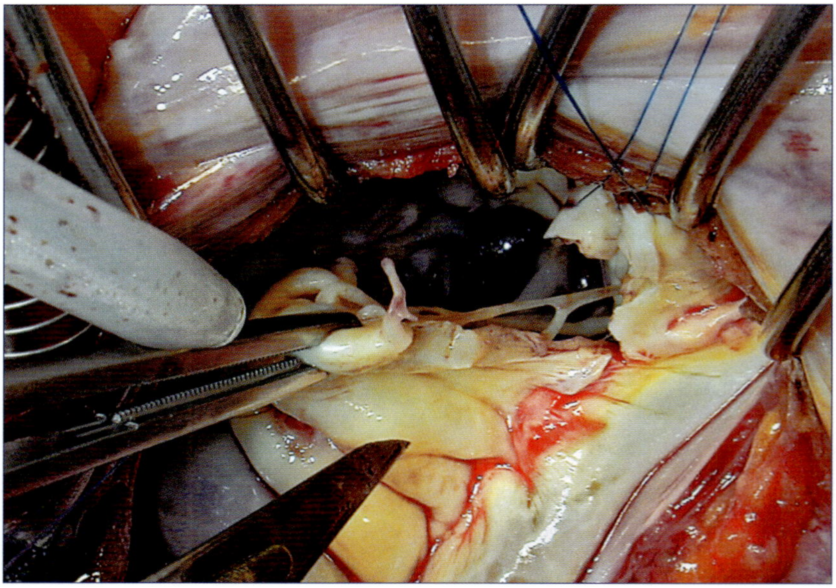

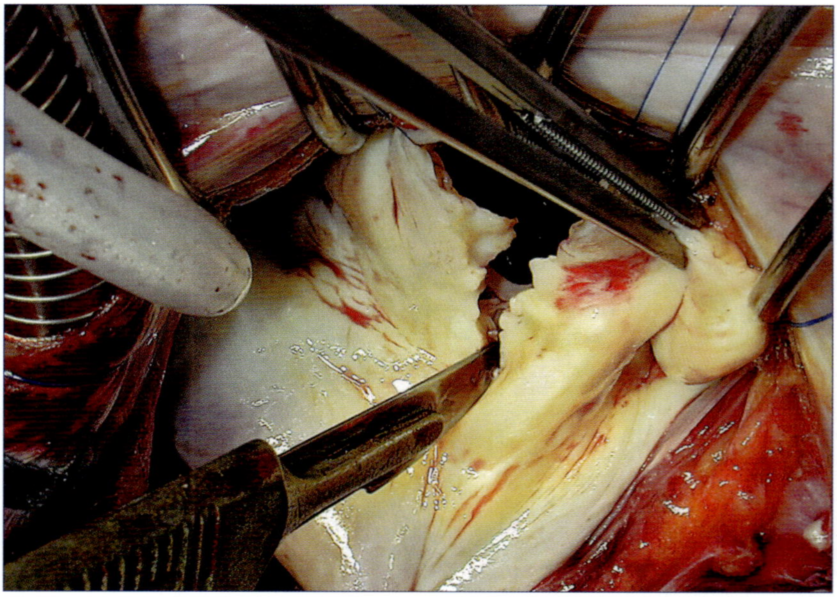

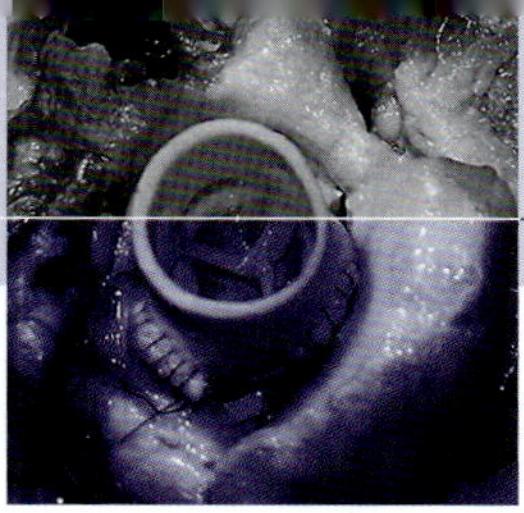

Quadrangular resection I

Using a scalpel the posterior leaflet is incised at the free edge medially from the marking suture at the P3 segment towards the mitral valve annulus. Chordae of the remaining valve segments have to be saved carefully.

Quadrangular resection II

In analogy, the segments P1 and P2 are separated from each other. The base of the P2 segment will also be transsected from the mitral annulus with the explicit understanding that the annulus itself must not be incised too deeply and, in addition, the left ventricular posterior wall must not be injured. The accompanying chordae of P2 are easy to identify and to resect close to the head of the papillary muscle.

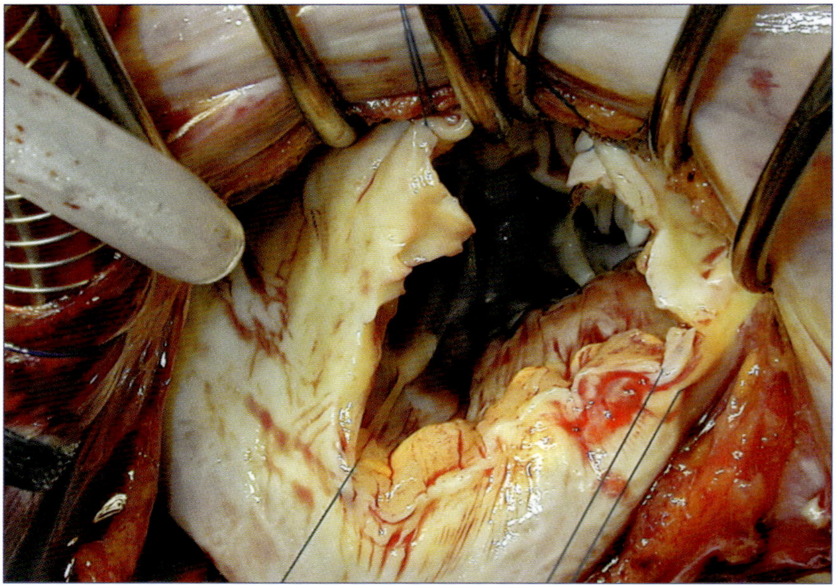

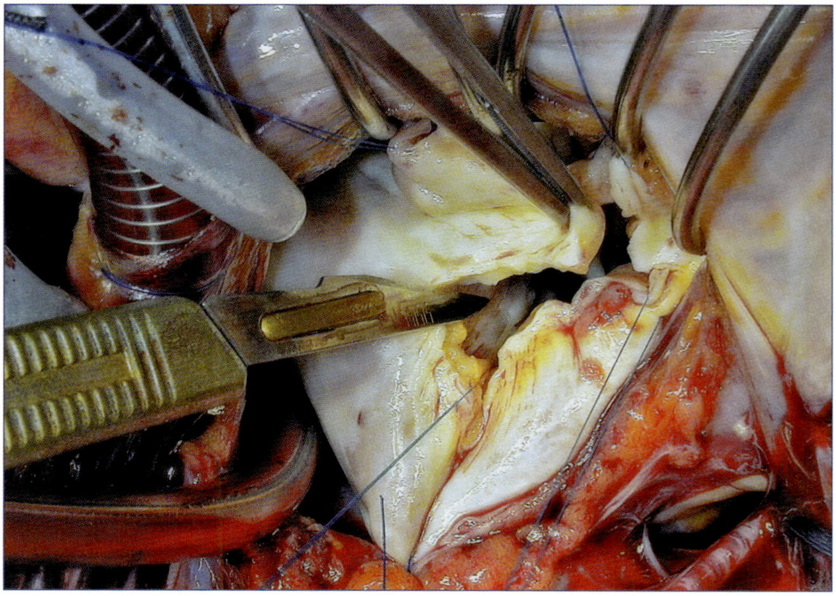

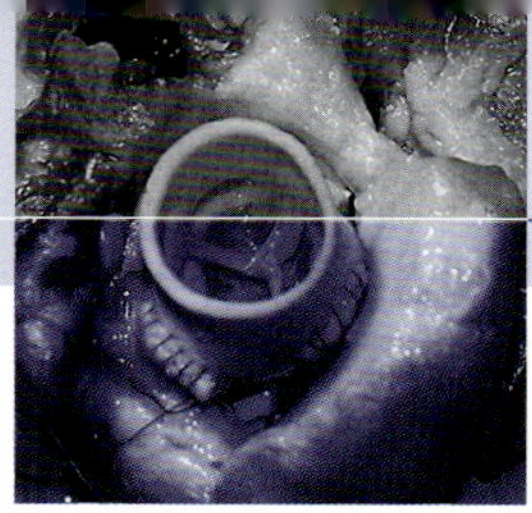

Quadrangular resection III

After quadrangular resection the posterior mitral leaflet appears as shown in the figure. For better illustration of the next repair steps, the positions where the free margins of the residual P1 and P3 segments are anchored at the posterior annulus are marked with additional prolene sutures.

Sliding plasty – P1 incision

The next two steps are performed only when a sliding plasty is necessary. The P1 segment is detached from the base of the posterior annulus. However, this incision which starts at the resection margin of the P2 segment is not completely extended up to the anterior commissure but should ideally measure one third of the length of the resected P2 basis in order to result in a harmonic sliding plasty.

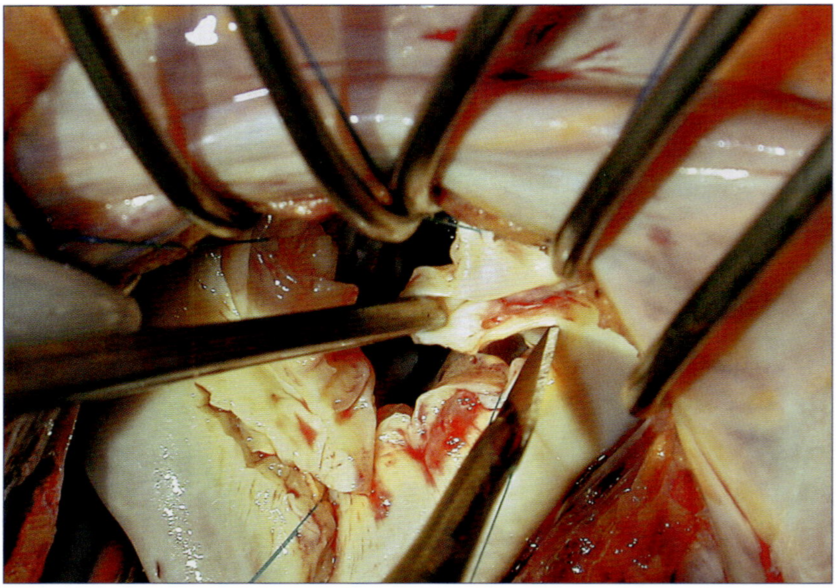

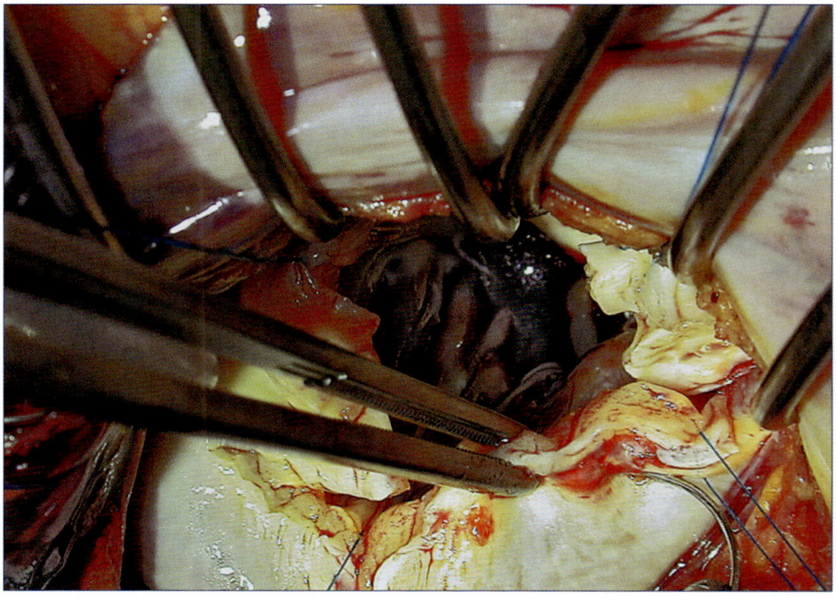

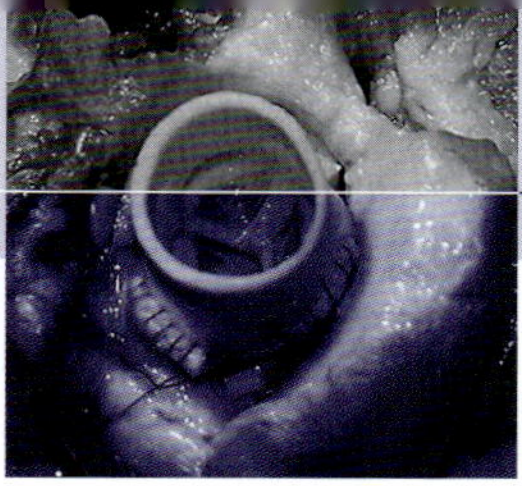

1 2 3 4 5 6 7 8 9 10 11 12 13 14 15

Sliding plasty – P3 incision
The detachment of the P3 segment is performed correspondingly. As a result, a major part of the posterior annulus is freed from the associated leaflet.

Reduction of the length of the posterior annulus (annuloraphy)
The goal of the next maneuver is to shorten the posterior mitral valve annulus as much as possible. Hence, a non-reabsorbable valve suture with Teflon felts is placed tangentially through the mitral annulus. For better orientation this suture should be placed exactly in the middle. Alternatively, the suture can be placed from the cavum of the left ventricle through the posterior annulus. By leaving the ends of this suture temporarily, a better visualization and easier manipulation of the valve might result.

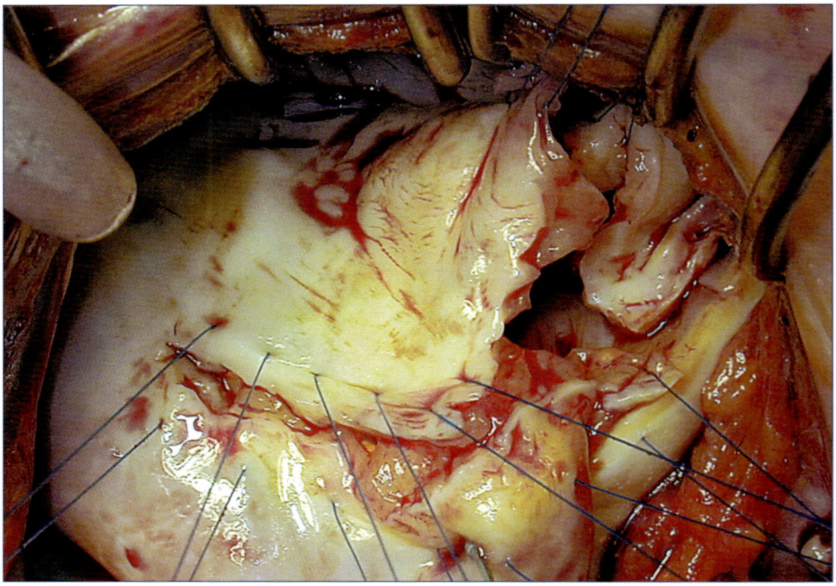

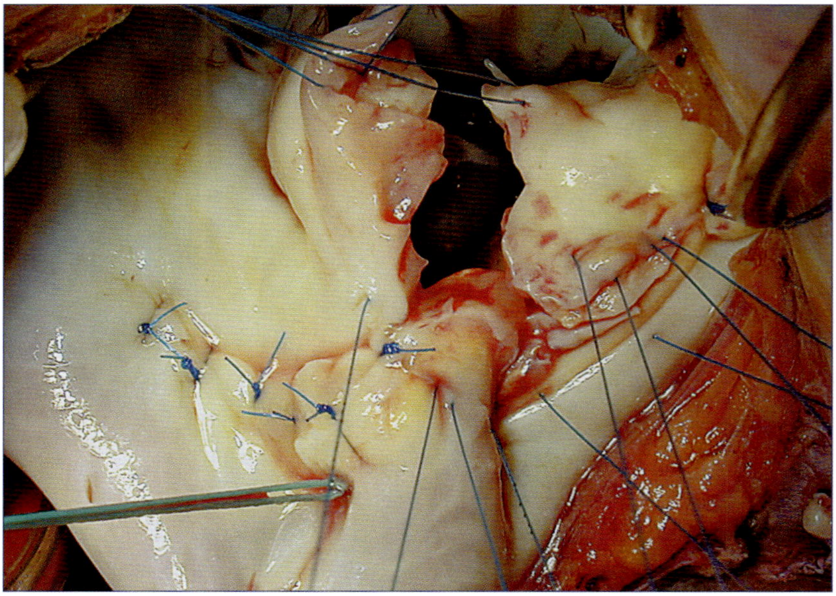

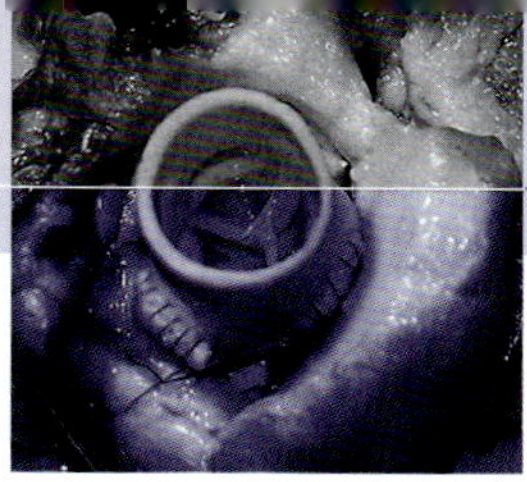

Re-fixation of the P1 segment

For re-fixation of the remaining posterior leaflet a distance between the stitches of approximately 1–2 mm is optimal at the margin of the leaflet. The stitch distance at the annulus, however, might be as large as 5–10 mm depending on the size of the defect which has to be repaired. Using this technique the P1 segment is translocated into the P2 defect. The suture of the medial annuloraphy now serves as a good orientation and illustrates how far the P1 segment has to be translocated. It is crucial that enough leaflet tissue is included into the stitch row.

Re-fixation of the P3 segment

The re-fixation of the P3 segment is performed correspondingly Occasionally, the valve tissue is very fragile. As a consequence, sutures can tear though the tissue with a resulting acute mitral incompetence. For these patients, a technique of interrupted single sutures should be preferred which also allows for the correction of some suboptimal stitches in order to achieve an optimal result. Using the technique of running suture, a significant reduction of ischemia time may result. For the re-adaptation of the posterior leaflet, a non-reabsorbable suture should be used (e.g. Prolene® 5/0, Ethicon).

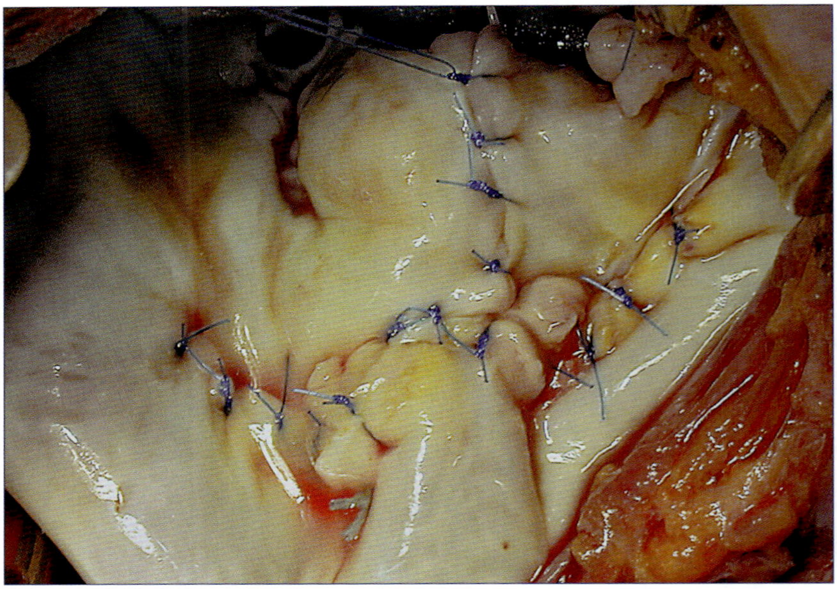

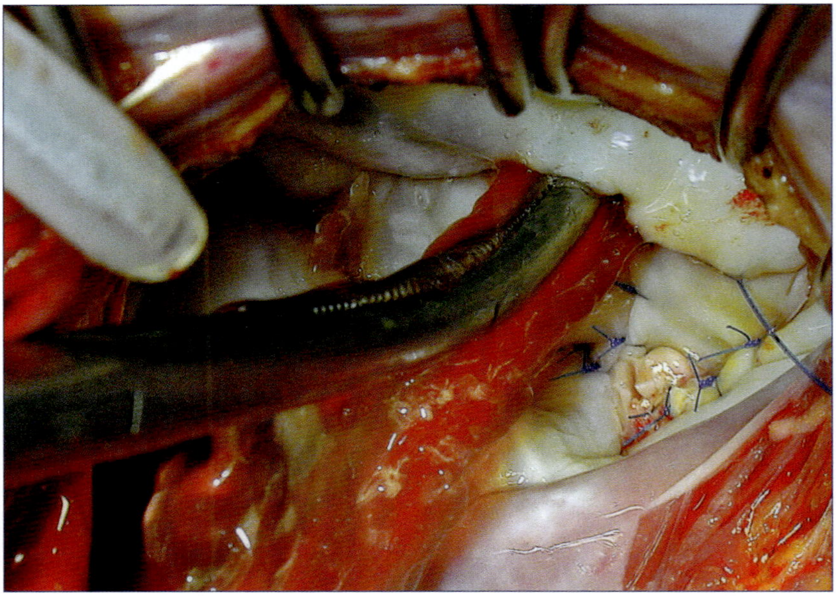

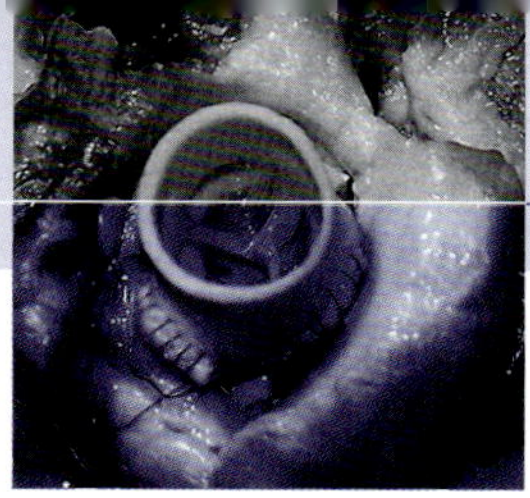

Closure of the cleft

After reconstruction of the posterior annulus the remaining cleft between P1 and P3 has to be closed using interrupted single sutures. A continuous running suture would shorten the height of the posterior leaflet. The first stitch has to connect both edges at the free margin resulting in a harmonic posterior "neo-leaflet". The remaining stitches towards the annulus might correct minimal differences of the height of P1 and P3, respectively. Significant differences between P1 and P3 have to be corrected during the preceeding re-fixation procedure by adjusting the stitch depth into the leaflet.

Testing of the Repair Result

A successful reconstruction must show a satisfactory result prior to annuloplasty. The left ventricle is filled with Ringer´s solution as described above. In case of persisting regurgitation, the underlying reason must be determined and fixed by additional repair maneuvers. The annuloplasty does not improve a poor repair; it only secures the repair result.

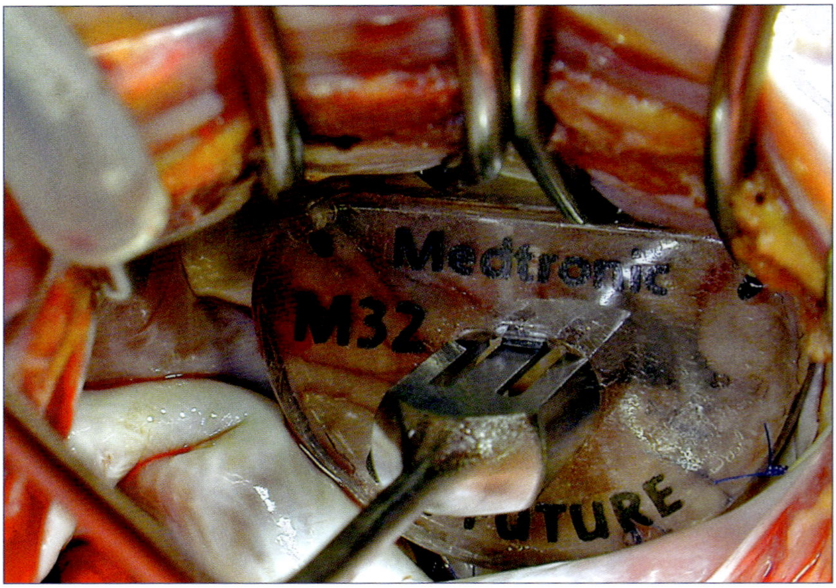
Medtronic
M32
FUTURE

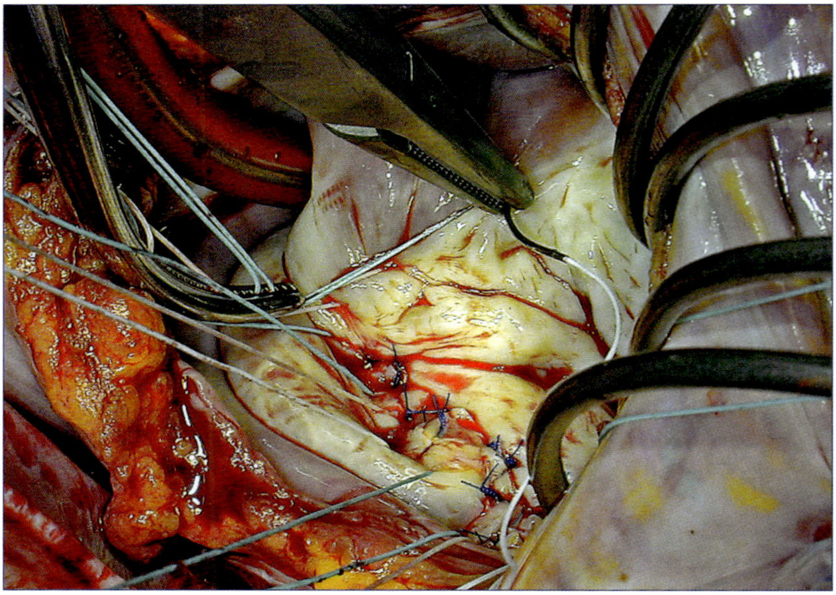

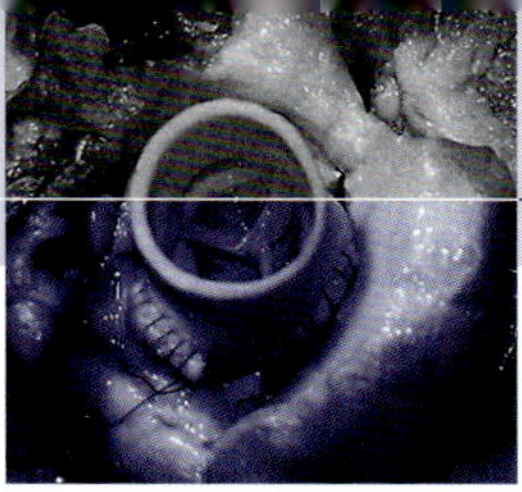

Annuloplasty – Sizing of the ring device

In the own practice an annuloplasty device is used in all patients after mitral valve repair. However, the exact type and/or manufacturer of the annuloplasty device should be chosen according to the experiences and preferences by the specific center.

The first step of annuloplasty is to determine the adequate size of the annuloplasty ring. Downsizing after quadrangular resection makes no sense and endangers the result. However, in case of isolated mitral valve annuloplasty for type I mitral valve incompetence (according to Carpentier), down-sizing is necessary. The measurement of the distance between the two commissures (caused by the insertion of the anterior leaflet at the left ventricular septum) is best suitable for the definition of the correct ring size. These commissures correlate with the markers at the ring sizer.

Annuloplasty – Placement of the sutures

Valve sutures without teflon felts are placed longitudinally through the mitral annulus. It is of significance that the sutures are placed outside (towards the atrium) of the leaflets and the repair region. In the region of P2 and P3, the course of the circumflex artery should be considered to prevent injury to that coronary artery. The difficult stitches in the area of both commissures might be facilitated by pulling down previously placed stitches using an overhold clamp in order to improve the exposure.

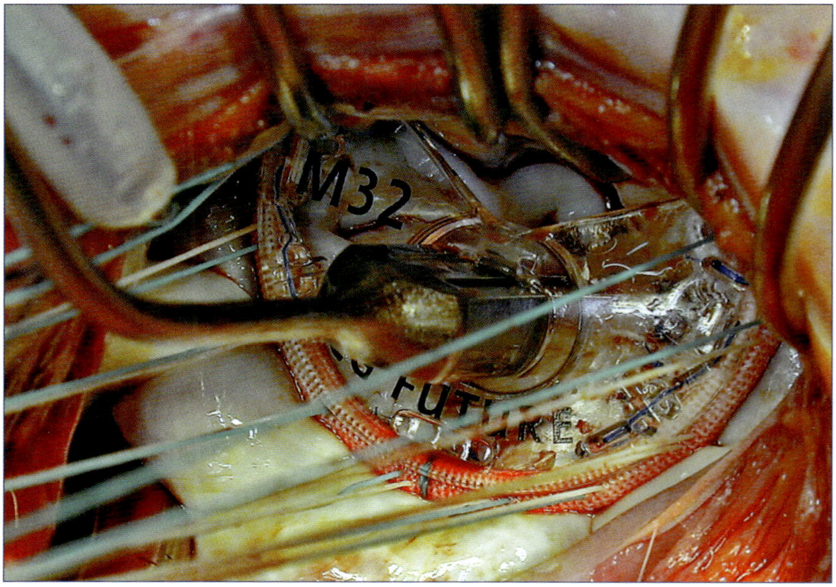
M32

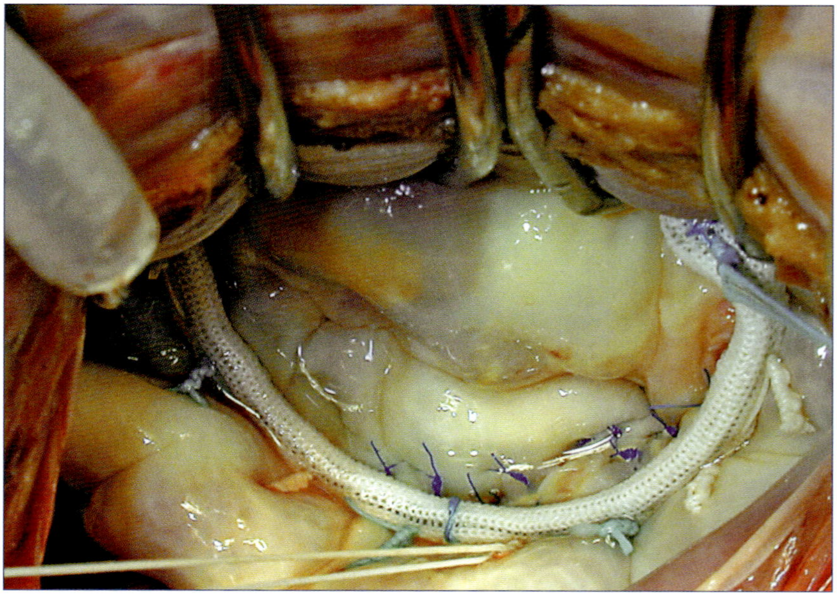

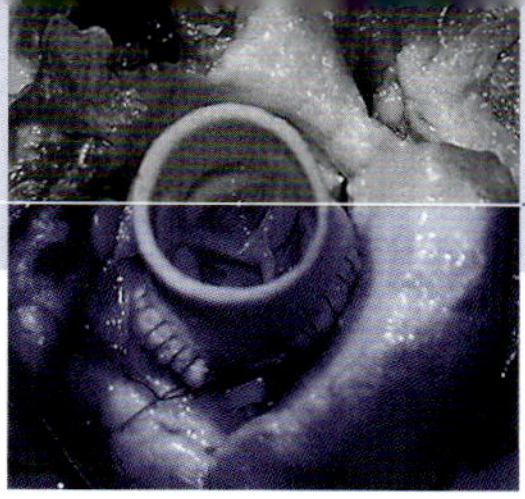

Annuloplasty – Ring implantation

After the sutures are placed through the annuloplasty ring, the ring might be impregnated with an antibiotic prophylactically and is then approximated. Thereafter, the sutures are knotted.

Final testing

The final function test must prove the absolute competence of the repaired mitral valve. The atriotomy is closed using a running suture. After weaning the patient from cardiopulmonary bypass, a structured transesophageal echocardiography control (TEE) is mandatory.
A minimal central mitral regurgitation confined to early systole is tolerable. In addition to the confirmation of valve competence, the transvalvular gradient for exclusion of a functional stenosis should also be determined.

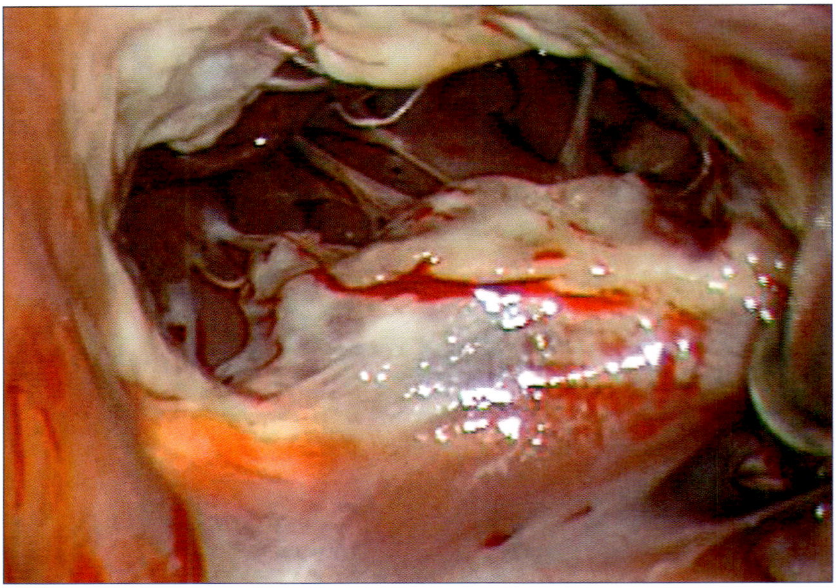

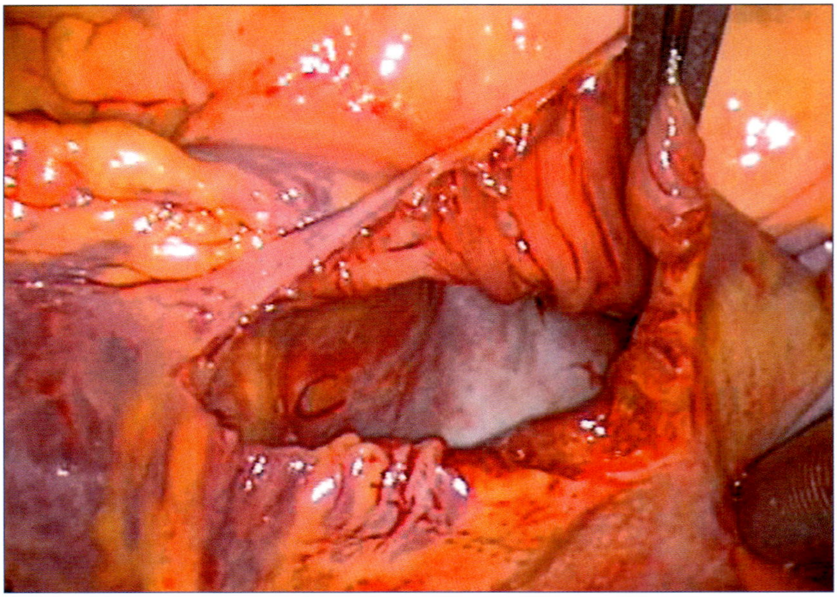

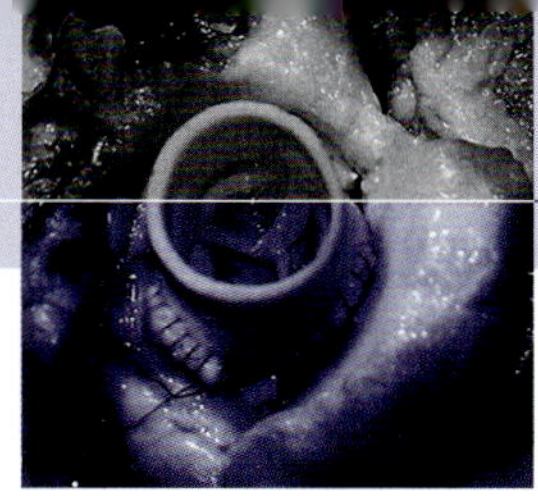

Principles of Tricuspid Valve Repair

P. B. Rahmanian • D. H. Adams

Introduction:

Isolated diseases of the tricuspid valve are rare. Tricuspid valve regurgitation (TR) is usually secondary to left sided valvular heart disease which causes pulmonary hypertension, right ventricular dilatation, and subsequently tricuspid annular dilatation. Leaflet tethering may also occur in the setting of severe right ventricular dilatation. The ACC/AHA 2006 guidelines for the treatment of valvular heart disease list tricuspid valve (TV) repair for severe TR in patients undergoing mitral valve surgery as a class I indication (moderate TR with pulmonary hypertension or tricuspid annular dilatation is a class IIb indication) (1). Many authors, however, now advocate more aggressive application of tricuspid repair techniques in patients with significant tricuspid annular dilatation even if associated with only mild TR at the time of mitral valve surgery (2). Numerous types of tricuspid repair have been described in the literature including suture annuloplasty (DeVega) and prosthetic annuloplasty using various flexible bands and remodeling rings (3-5). Several clinical series suggest the superiority of prosthetic remodeling annuloplasty over other surgical techniques (6).

Approach:

Bi-caval venous cannulation is performed using tourniquets to isolate the right atrium from the venous circulation. The right atrium is assessed through a right atriotomy parallel or at 60 degree angle to the atrioventricular groove.

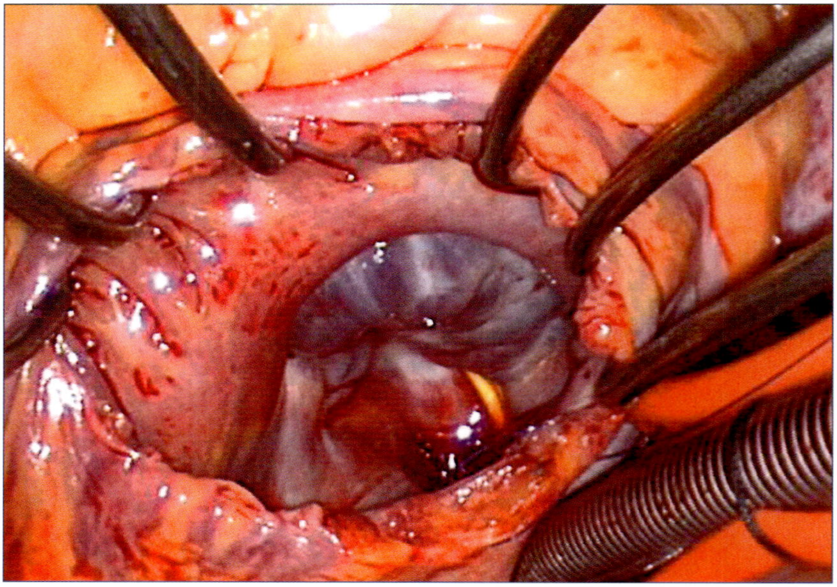

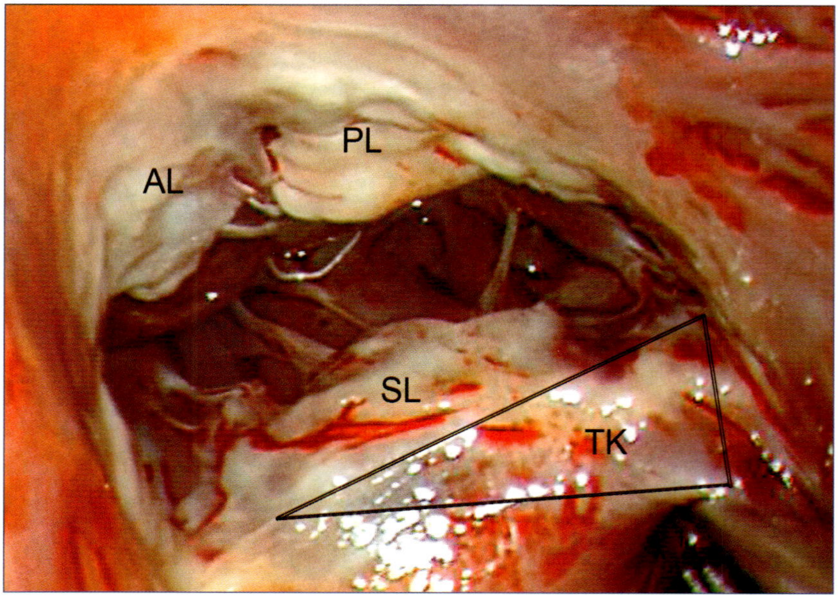
PL
AL
SL
TK

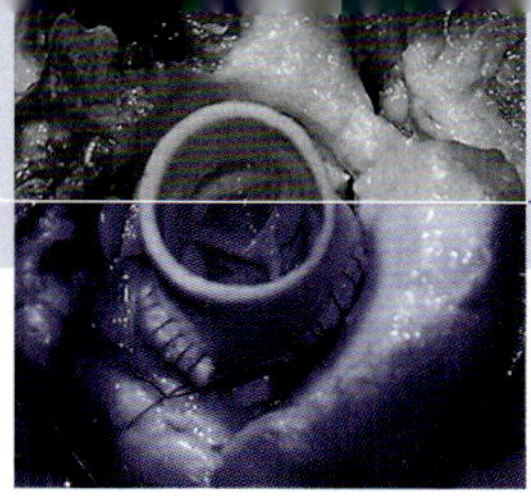

Optimal exposure can be achieved using a self-retaining mitral valve retractor placing 1 blade superior and 1 blade lateral to the tricuspid valve. Alternatively stay-sutures can be placed in the right atrial wall to optimize exposure.

Surgical anatomy/ valve analysis

This is the case of a patient with degenerative mitral regurgitation (Barlow's disease) and secondary TR due to severe annular dilatation. AL: anterior leaflet, PL: posterior leaflet, SL: septal leaflet. The dilatation predominantly involves the annulus around the base of the posterior leaflet, with the septal leaflet portion of the annulus relatively spared (7). The triangle of Koch (TK) is an important anatomical landmark visualized by imaginary lines between the coronary sinus, and the septal commissures. It is important because the AV nodal bundle is located near its apex in the region of the membranous septum, and thus suture placement in this area is to be avoided.

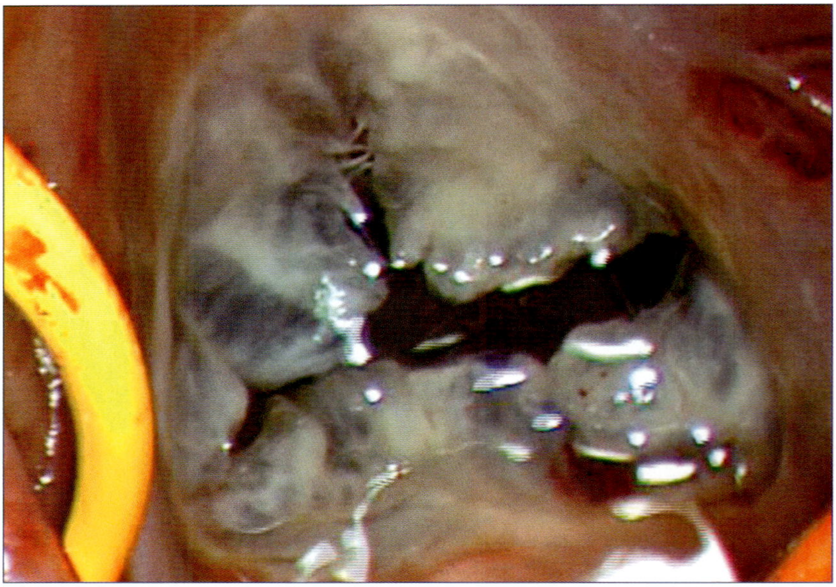

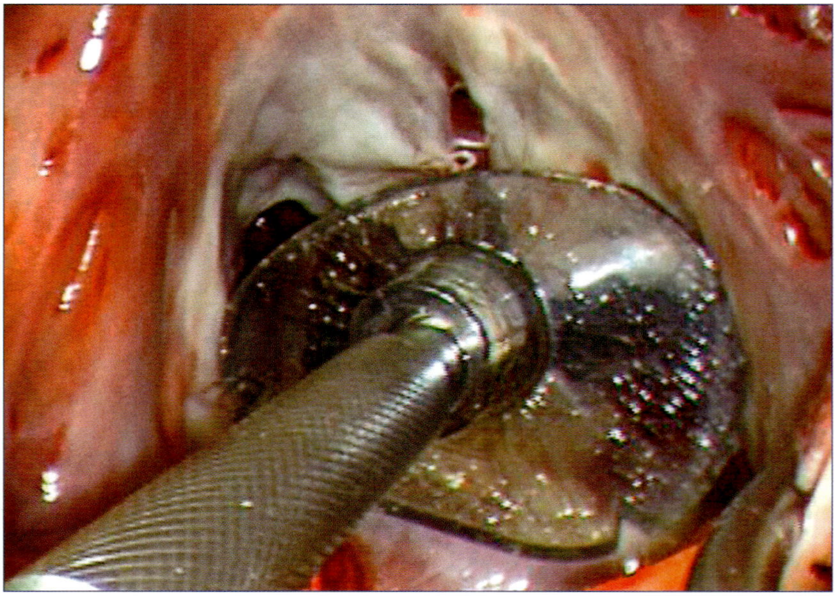

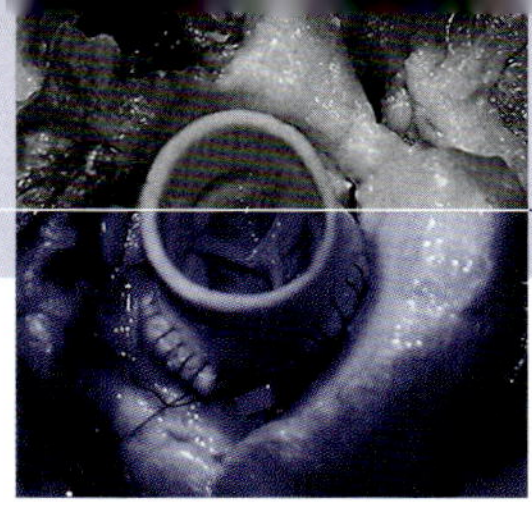

A saline test reveals the loss of coaptation between all three leaflets due to annular dilatation, particularly between the posterior and the septal leaflets. Note the swan ganz catheter has been removed from the RV outflow tract and will be repositioned at the completion of the repair.

Sizing:

Sizing of the tricuspid valve is based on two measurements:

1. The inter-comissural distance of the septal leaflet
2. The surface area of the anterior and posterior leaflets.

First the inter-commissural (inter-trigonal) distance of the septal leaflet is measured.

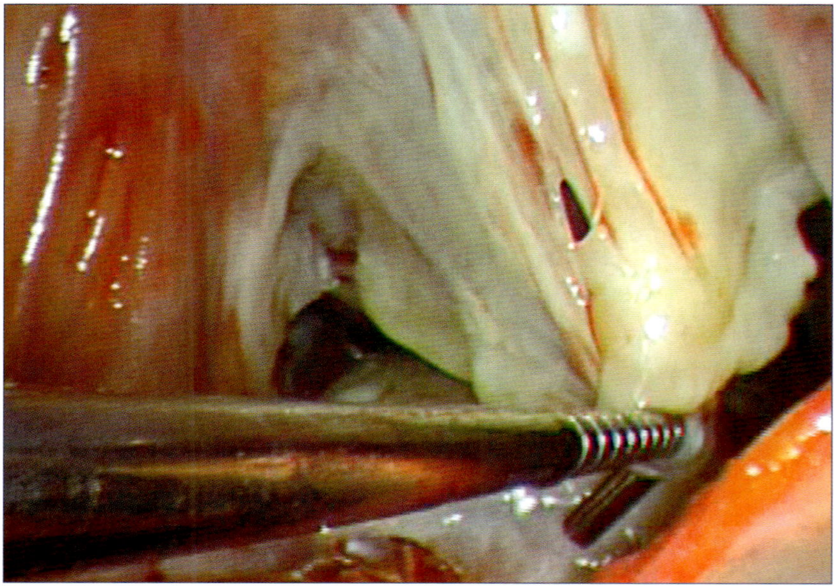

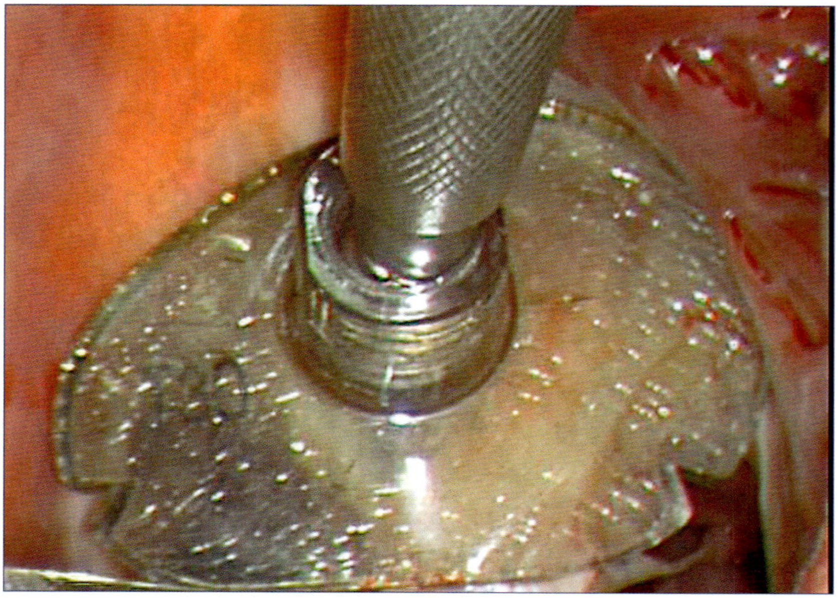

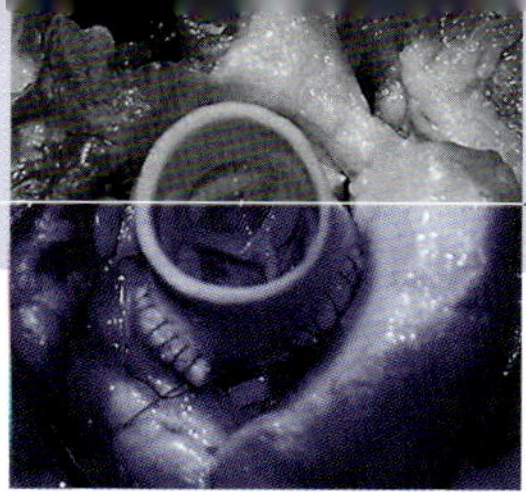

1 2 3 4 5 6 7 8 9 10 **11** 12 13 14 15

Using a valve hook, primary chordae of the anterior and posterior leaflets arising from the anterior papillary muscle are secured at the margin of the leaflets and pulled down to expose the surface area of these two leaflets.

The surface area of the anterior and posterior leaflet is measured using the plane of the sizer. If the inter-commissural distance and surface area measurement result in different sizes, the ring size is chosen in favor of the surface area of the leaflets. In general, we also tend to pick a smaller ring if between sizes.

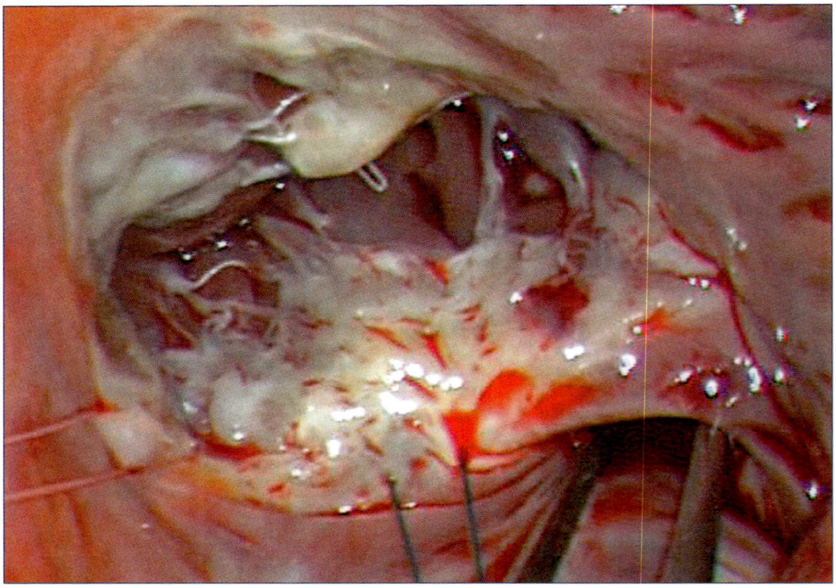

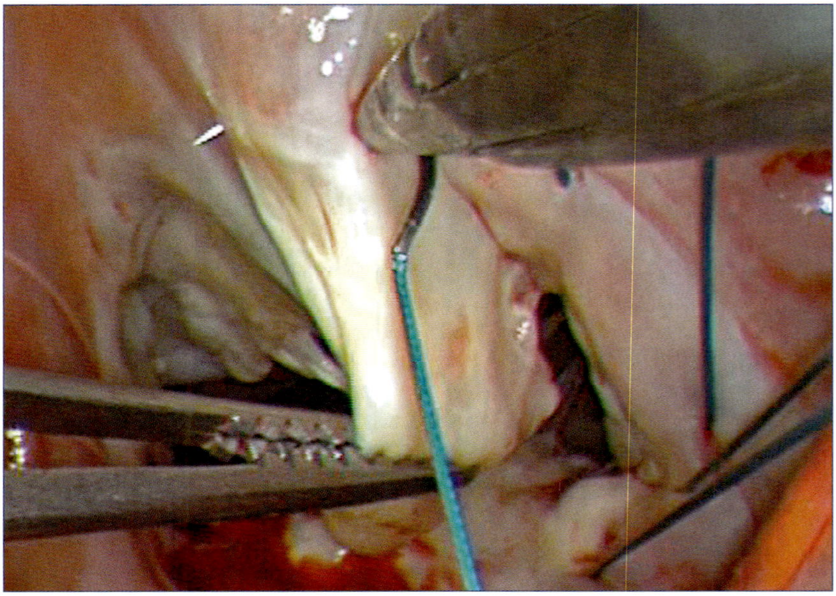

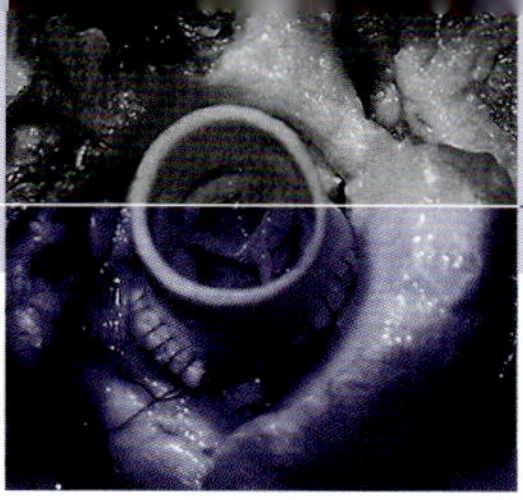

Ring implantation

Ring implantation is performed by placing a series of 8 to 10 simple 2-0 Vicryl mattress sutures through the tricuspid annulus around the orifice. As previously mentioned, particular attention needs to be directed to avoid injury of the intracardiac conduction system. The atrioventricular node is located in the area of the membranous septum. This area is marked by placing the first two sutures on either side of this area.

The remaining sutures are then placed circumferentially around the annulus. The atrio-annular junction is identified by pulling down the anterior and posterior leaflets respectively. The stitches are placed with wide bites in a 1 mm distance from this atrio-annular junction and directed towards the ventricle.

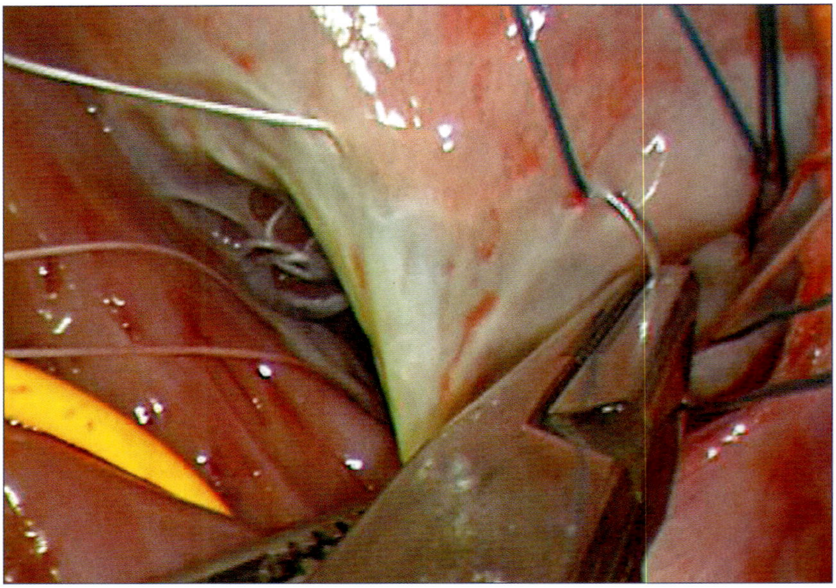

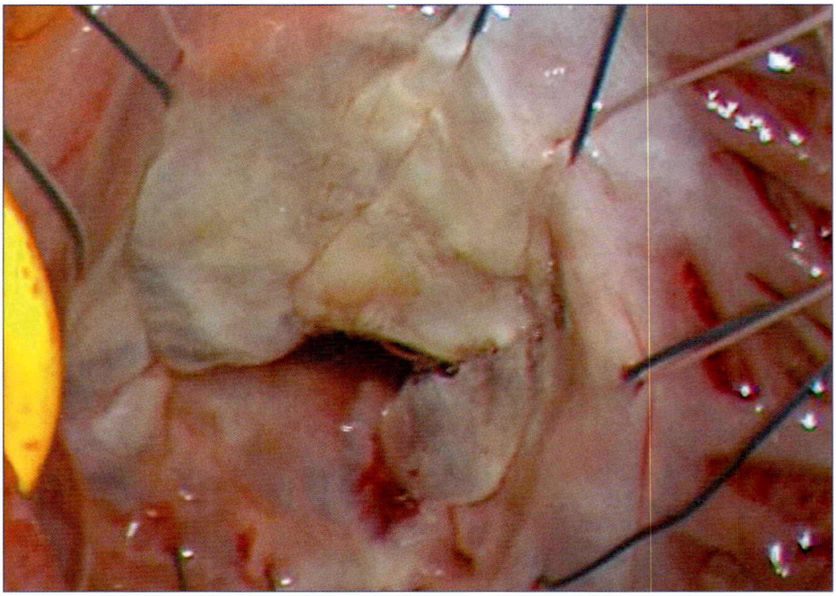

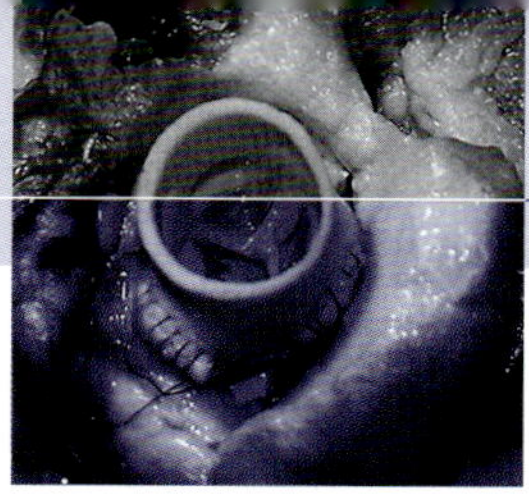

Overlapping of the sutures and smaller corresponding bites through the ring particularly at the posterior leaflet produces a measured annular plication in this region of maximal dilatation.

All of the ring sutures are now in place.

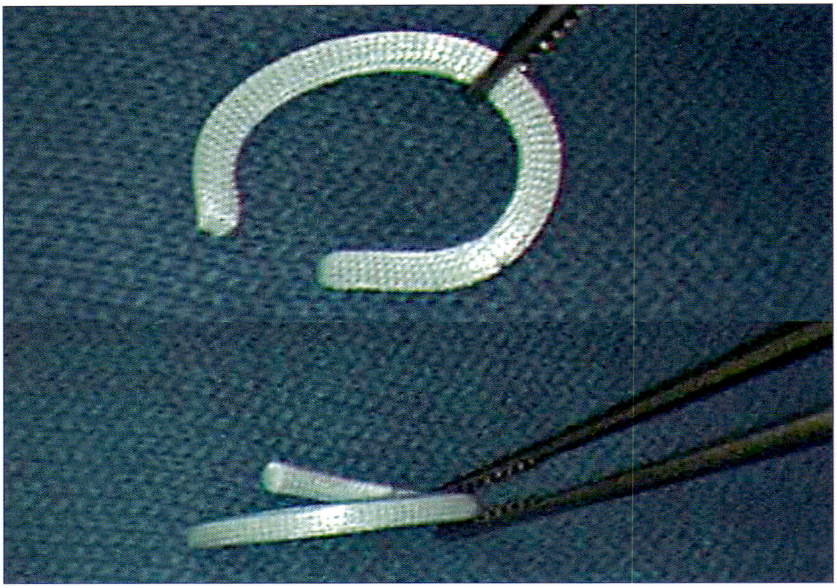

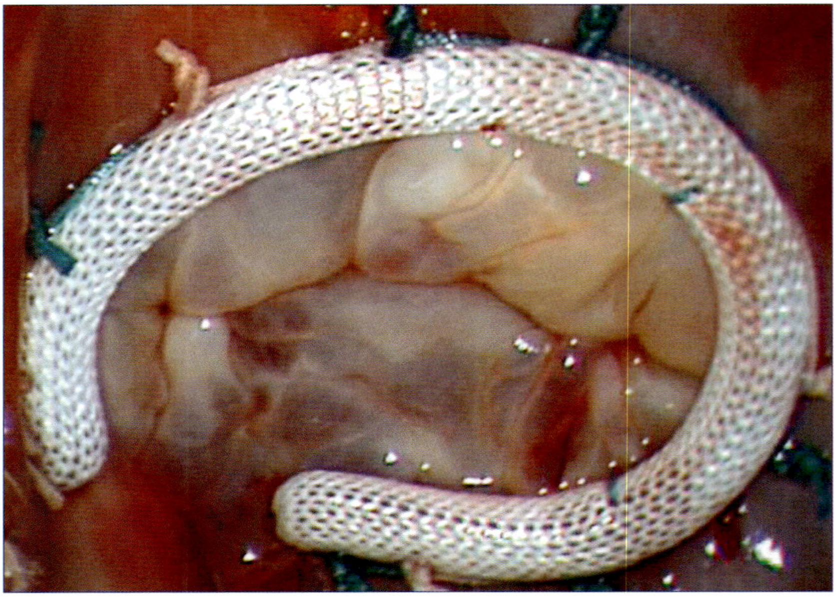

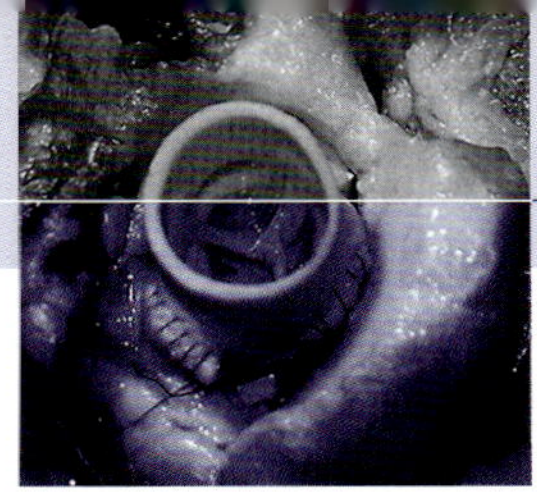

Remodeling annuloplasty ring:

In this case we selected a Carpentier Edwards "Classic" tricuspid semi-rigid ring. Prior to implantation we bent the septal portion slightly inward to create a three dimensional shape which mimics the annular direction along the membranous septum. Newer three dimensional rings are also available now that mimic the shape of the tricuspid annulus (5).

Each arm of the sutures is then passed through the sewing ring of the prosthesis. Next, the ring is lowered into position and tied securely to the annulus. The final saline test shows a competent valve with a good amount of coaptation between all three leaflets.

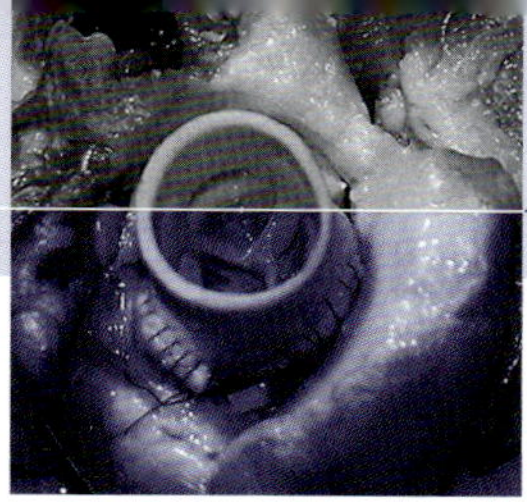

References

1. Bonow RO, Carabello BA, Chatterjee K, de Leon AC, Jr., Faxon DP, Freed MD, et al. ACC/AHA 2006 guidelines for the management of patients with valvular heart disease: a report of the American College of Cardiology/American Heart Association Task Force on Practice Guidelines (writing Committee to Revise the 1998 guidelines for the management of patients with valvular heart disease) developed in collaboration with the Society of Cardiovascular Anesthesiologists endorsed by the Society for Cardiovascular Angiography and Interventions and the Society of Thoracic Surgeons. Journal of the American College of Cardiology. 2006 Aug 1;48(3): e1-148.
2. Dreyfus GD, Corbi PJ, Chan KM, Bahrami T. Secondary tricuspid regurgitation or dilatation: which should be the criteria for surgical repair? The Annals of thoracic surgery. 2005 Jan;79(1):127-32.
3. Matsuyama K, Matsumoto M, Sugita T, Nishizawa J, Tokuda Y, Matsuo T, et al. De Vega annuloplasty and Carpentier-Edwards ring annuloplasty for secondary tricuspid regurgitation. The Journal of heart valve disease. 2001 Jul;10(4):520-4.
4. Carpentier A, Deloche A, Hanania G, Forman J, Sellier P, Piwnica A, et al. Surgical management of acquired tricuspid valve disease. The Journal of thoracic and cardiovascular surgery. 1974 Jan;67(1):53-65.
5. Filsoufi F, Salzberg SP, Coutu M, Adams DH. A three-dimensional ring annuloplasty for the treatment of tricuspid regurgitation. The Annals of thoracic surgery. 2006 Jun;81(6):2273-7.
6. McCarthy PM, Bhudia SK, Rajeswaran J, Hoercher KJ, Lytle BW, Cosgrove DM, et al. Tricuspid valve repair: durability and risk factors for failure. The Journal of thoracic and cardiovascular surgery. 2004 Mar;127(3):674-85.
7. Ton-Nu TT, Levine RA, Handschumacher MD, Dorer DJ, Yosefy C, Fan D, et al. Geometric determinants of functional tricuspid regurgitation: insights from 3-dimensional echocardiography. Circulation. 2006 Jul 11;114(2):143-9.

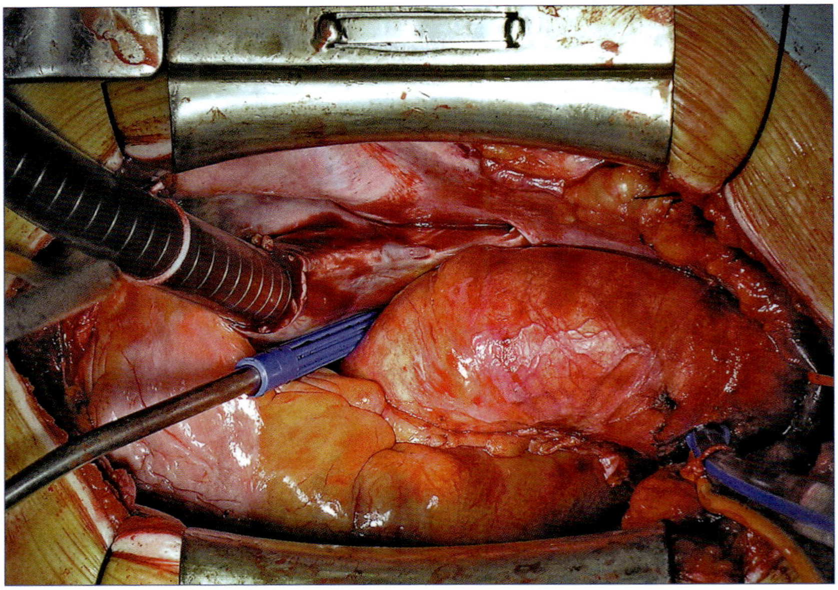

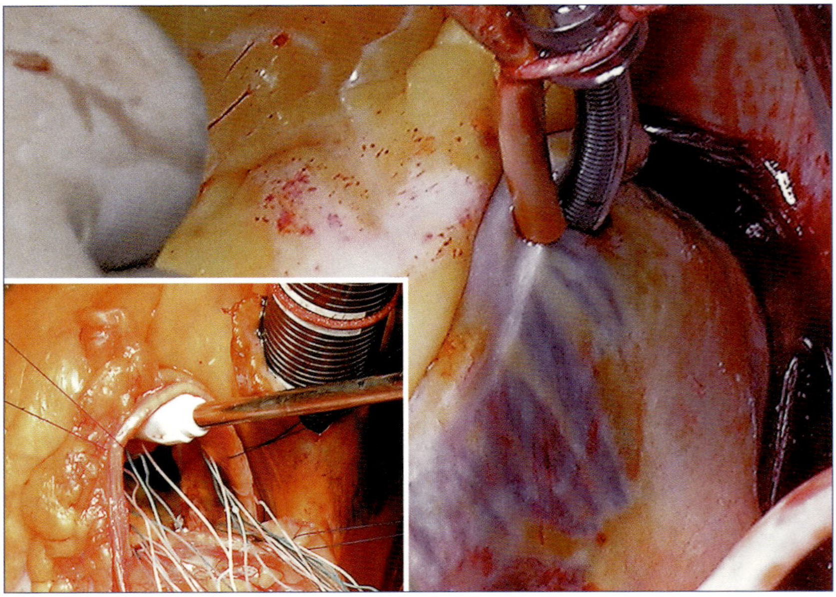

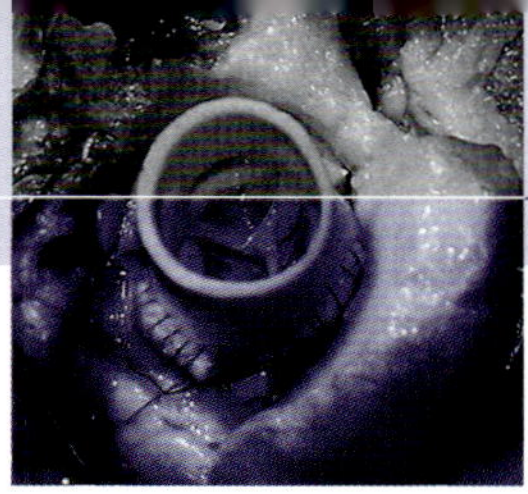

Aortic Valve Replacement and CABG

The combined aortic valve replacement and CABG procedure starts like an isolated CABG with harvesting of the grafts for bypass. When choosing the graft materials one should focus attention to the fact if there is enough space on the ascending aorta for proximal anastomosis. The bypass graft can be placed through the transverse sinus. After valve replacement there is a risk of air embolism into the grafts which causes circulatory depression and rhythm disorder. By choosing a lateral location of the proximal anastomosis this risk can be decreased.
The cannulation of the aorta should be performed more in the proximal arch to keep enough space for the proximal anastomosis and the aortotomy. Different to isolated procedures we choose slightly lower temperatures (28°–30° C) on extracorporal bypass using an LV vent through the right superior pulmonary vein.

In comparison with isolated procedures, in combined ones the single steps must be compatible and an extensive cardioprotective management is potentially needed as these procedures generally take longer cross-clamp times.
With regard to the generally hyperthrophied myocardium associated with aortic valve stenosis combined procedures with longer aortic clamp times need an optimal myocardial protection which can be achieved by using ante- and retrograde blood cardioplegia.

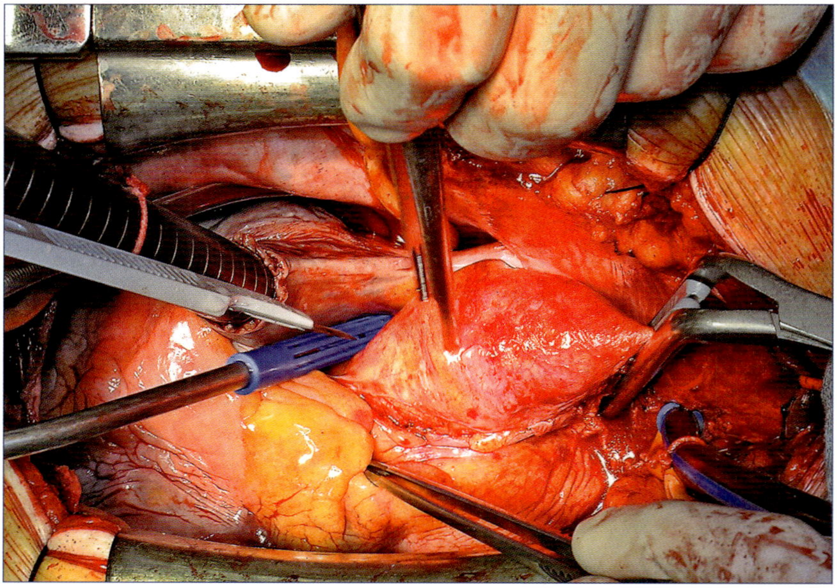

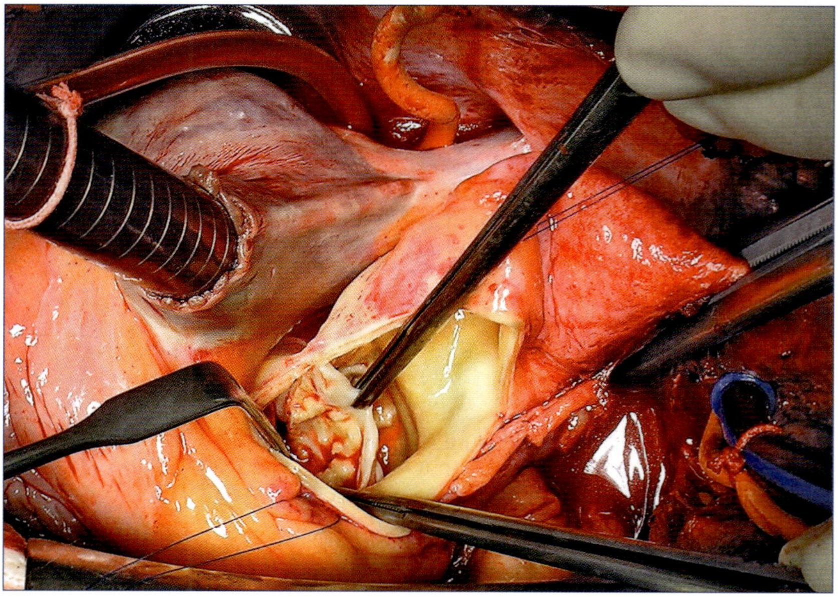

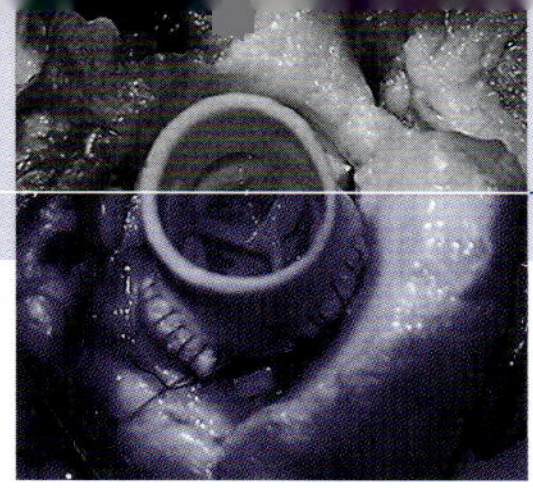

In comparison to isolated aortic valve replacement the incision of the aorta should be done more proximal and towards the pulmonary artery. Mostly, this allows for a secure partial clamping of the aorta at the time of proximal anastomosis of vein grafts without touching the suture line of the aortotomy.

After excision of the valve the aortic annulus has to be carefully decalcified followed by sizing and choosing of the valve prosthesis. While retrograde perfusion of the coronary arteries is carried on, the left ventricle is flushed with saline solution to remove debris .

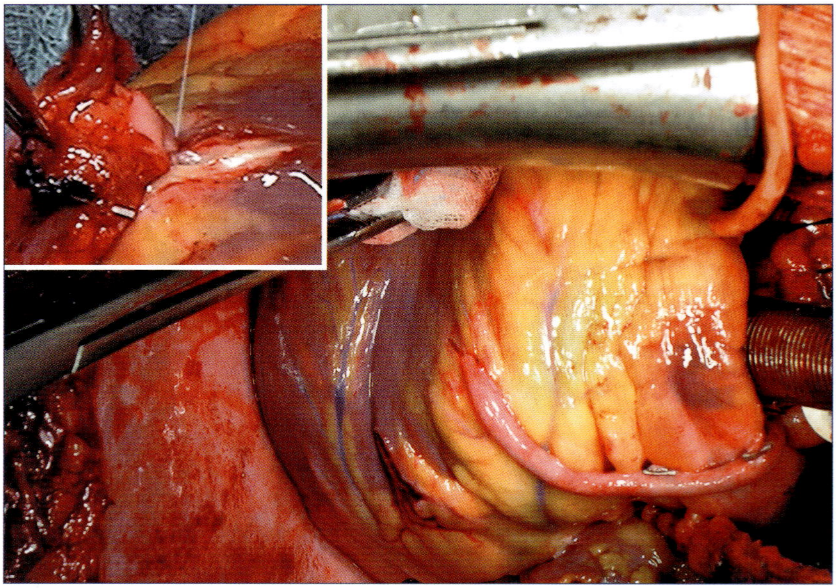

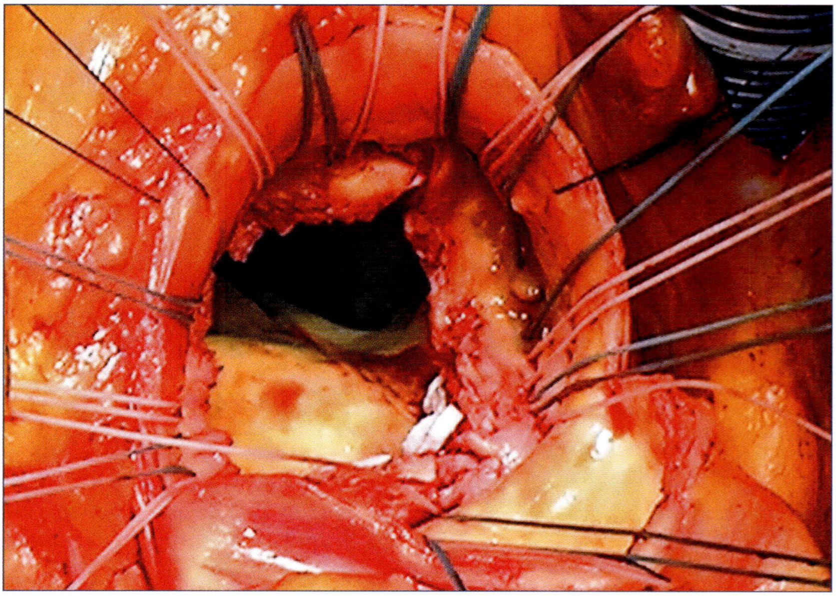

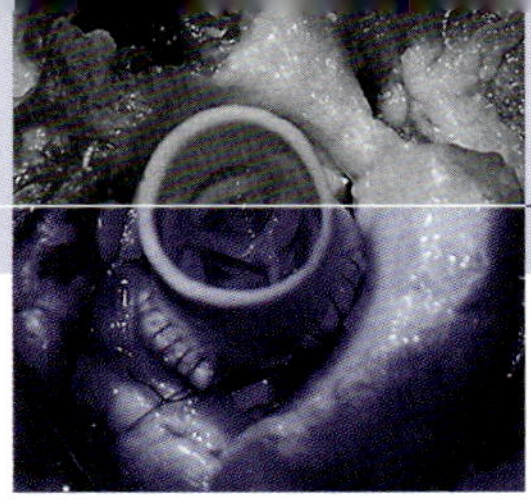

Before implantation of the valve prosthesis the distal anastomosis should be performed in a standard order (posterior wall, lateral wall, anterior wall). The exposition of the lateral and posterior wall is often difficult due to the left ventricular hypertrophy especially in severe aortic stenosis. Opening the right pleura in general helps to expose the obtuse marginal branches in severely hypertrophied left ventricle. In consideration of a higher incidence of re-do surgeries after combined procedures, venous bypasses should be passed around the left ventricle, preventing a location on the right atrium.

The implantation of the valve is performed in a common fashion using U-sutures with pledgets.

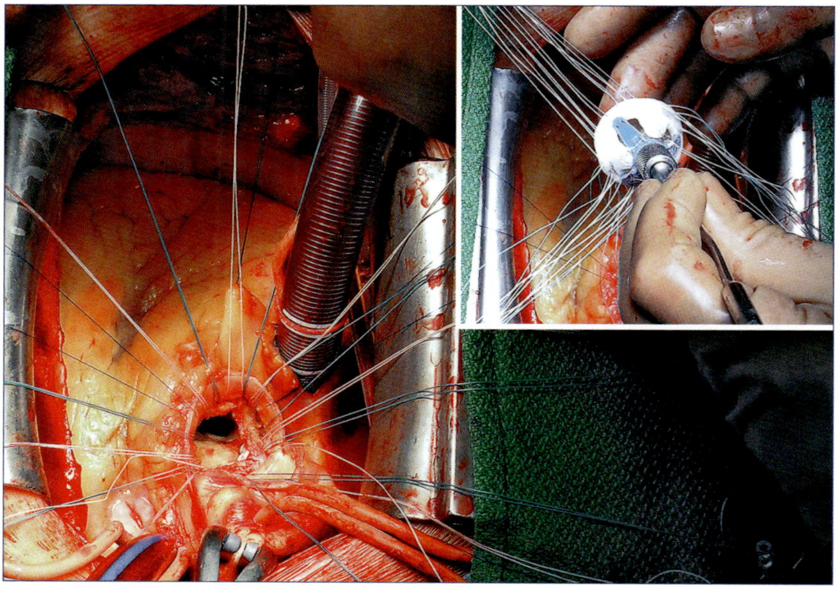

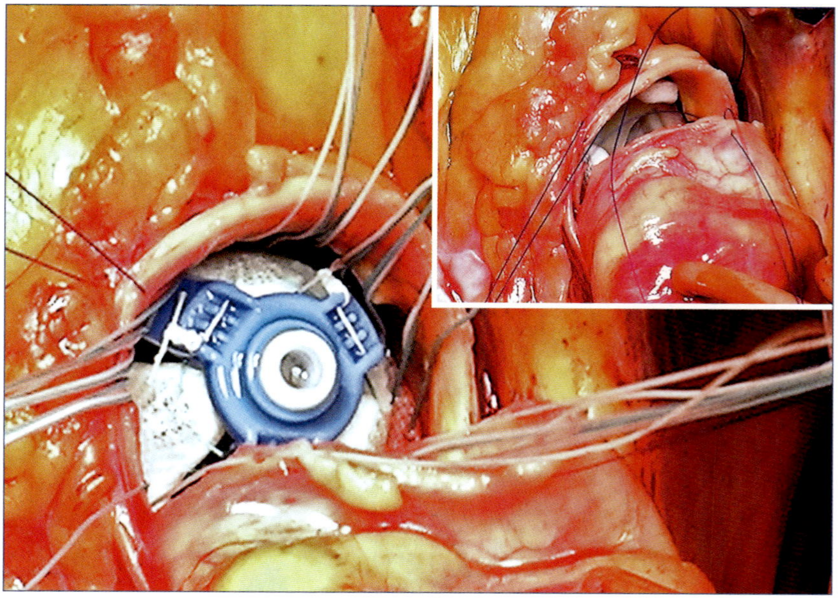

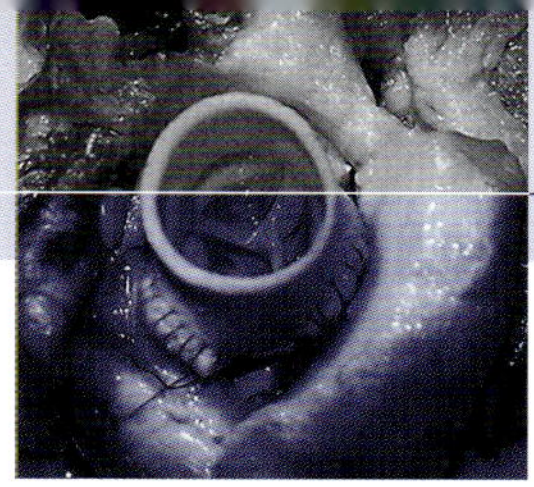

After the implantation of the prosthesis is completed, paravalvular leakage should be ruled out carefully.

The closure of the aortotomy can be done with a combination of an initial "mattress" suture followed by a running suture. Both suture lines should be completed during cross clamp time with most possible exposure of the aortic wall. Generally pledgets are not used, but for suture reinforcement, pericardium or part of the saphenous vein are used as pledgets in alternative.
De-airing is done through an incision on the distal part of the aorta ascendens optionally with combined venting of the left ventricular apex. A control of complete de-airing can be done by echocardiography.

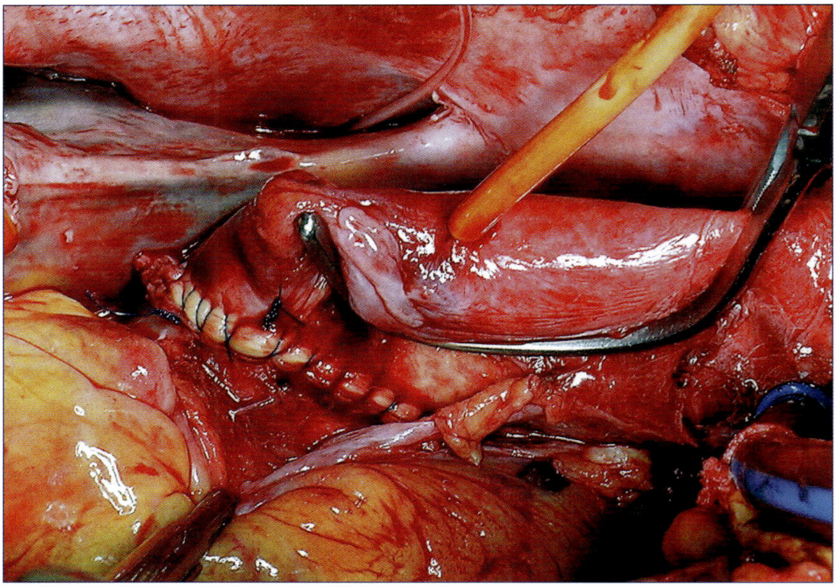

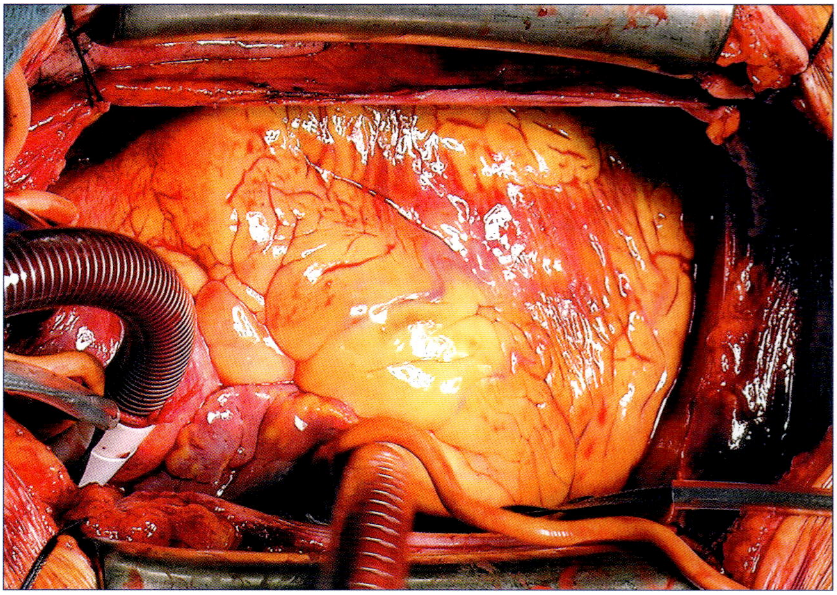

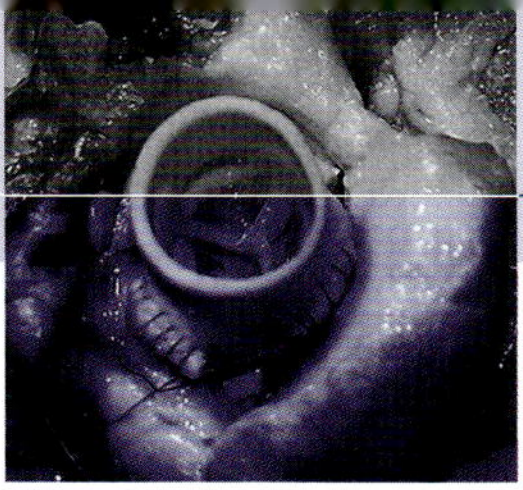

If the aorta is short, one can proceed with proximal anastomosis during single cross clamp time to avoid sheer stress on the aortotomy. In case of side clamping for proximal anastomosis, the Satinski or Cooley-clamp should not be placed on the aortotomy. A lateral positioning of proximal anastomoses is beneficial in order to prevent air embolism into the bypass grafts. During reperfusion the distal anastomoses and the aortotomy can be controlled and if necessary be corrected on pump. Lifting the heart after extracorporeal circulation should be avoided, as the implanted valve prosthesis can work as a lever to the aortic base which in extreme cases can lead to aorto-ventricular dehiscence.

Mitral Valve Repair and CABG

First steps are similar to the combined aortic valve replacement. For extracorporeal circulation bicaval cannulation is carried out using snears around the cannulas.

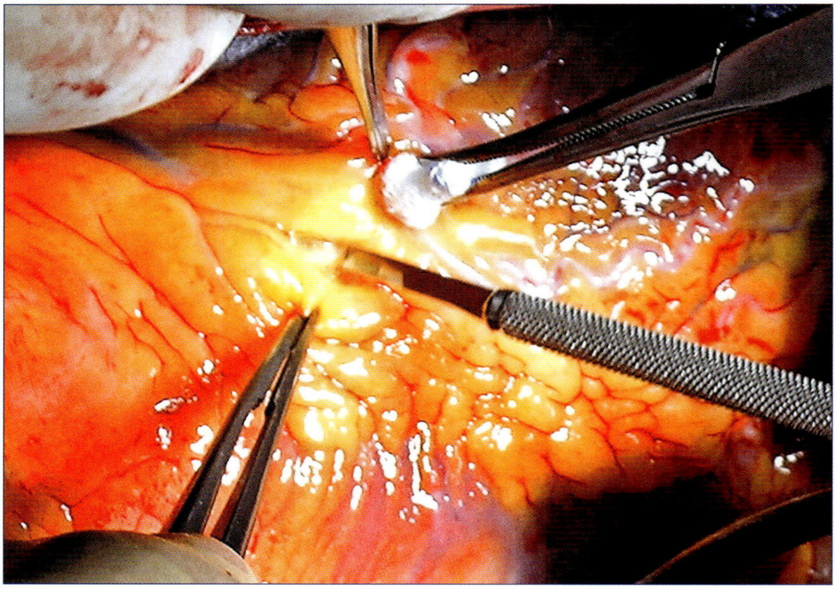

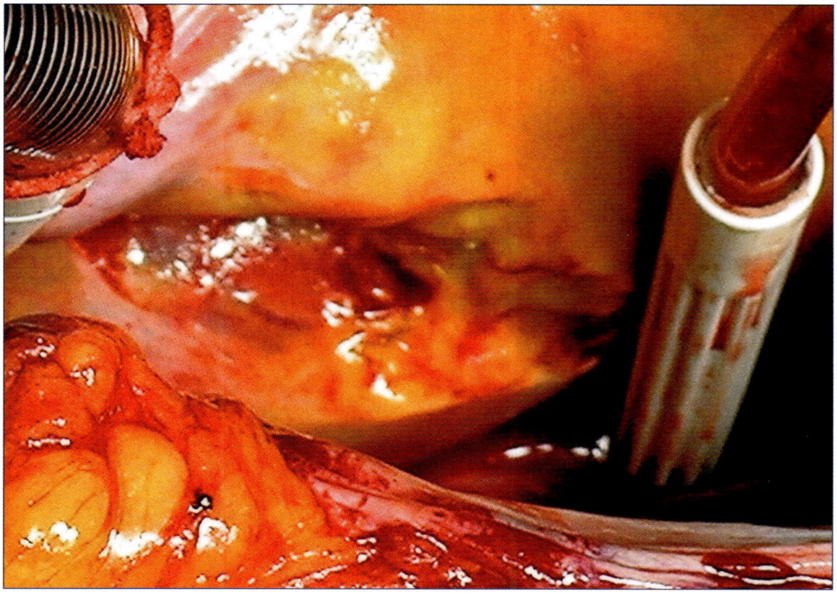

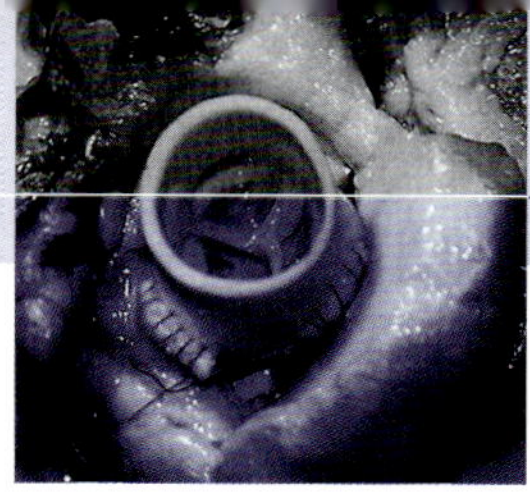

Generally the coronary arteries are prepared on partial bypass. In case of heavily calcified mitral annulus it is helpful to open the right pleural space to simplify the exposure of the lateral wall.
Also the combined procedure with mitral valve surgery needs extensive myocardial protection.

For the combined procedure the preferred approach at our institution is through Sonnegerd Grove (sulcus interatrialis) into the left atrium.

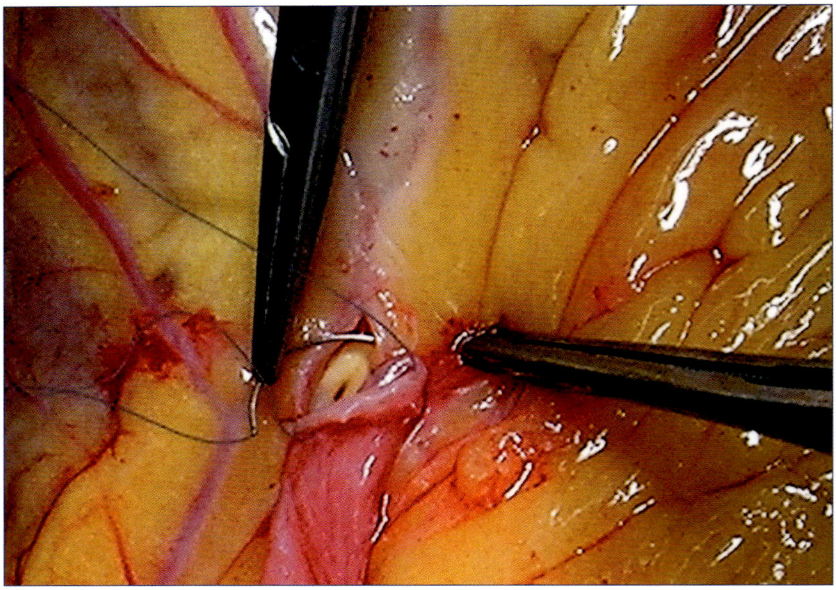

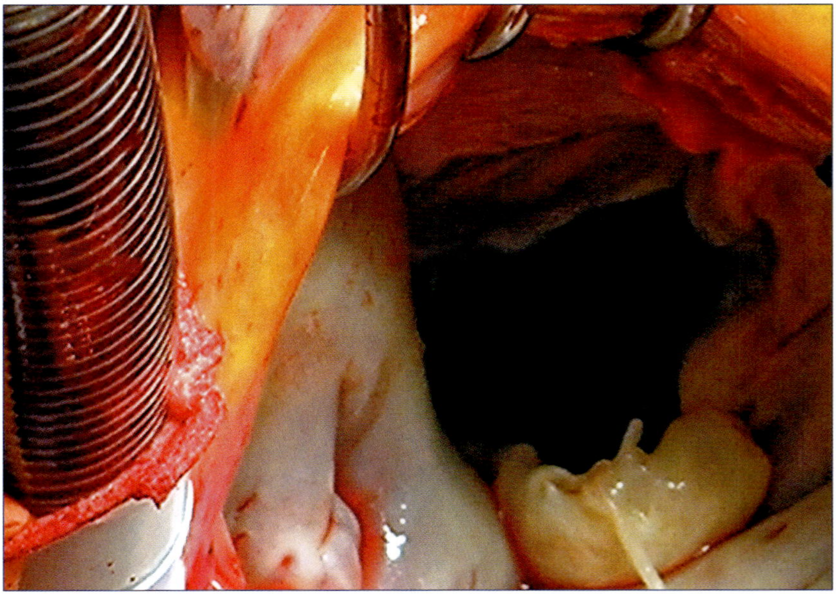

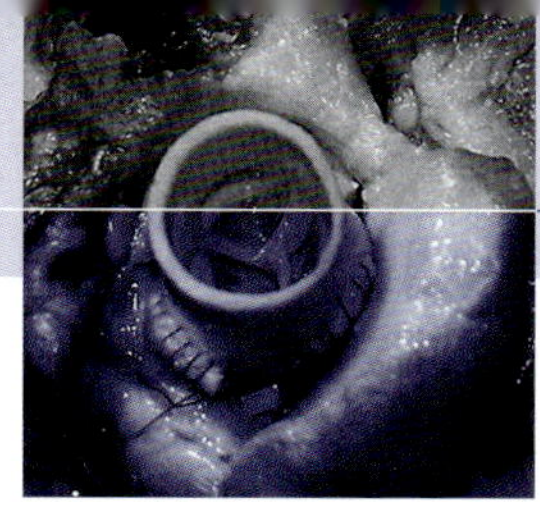

The distal anastomoses of inferior or lateral coronaries are performed first, and revascularisation of the LAD can follow at later time points. In case of using the right internal thoracic artery for the distal right coronary it is easier to perform this anastomosis following mitral valve replacement.
Also in combined mitral valve surgery, we prefer a regimen with all bypass grafts placed around the left ventricle.

On complete bypass, first assessment of the mitral valve is performed and the decision for either valve repair or replacement is made. If replacement is necessary, excision and decalcification of the valve are performed. A partial preservation of the posterior and anterior leaflets is preferred.
Sizing and decision for the valve prosthesis. In this patient a prolaps of the P2 segment and ruptured chordae can be seen.

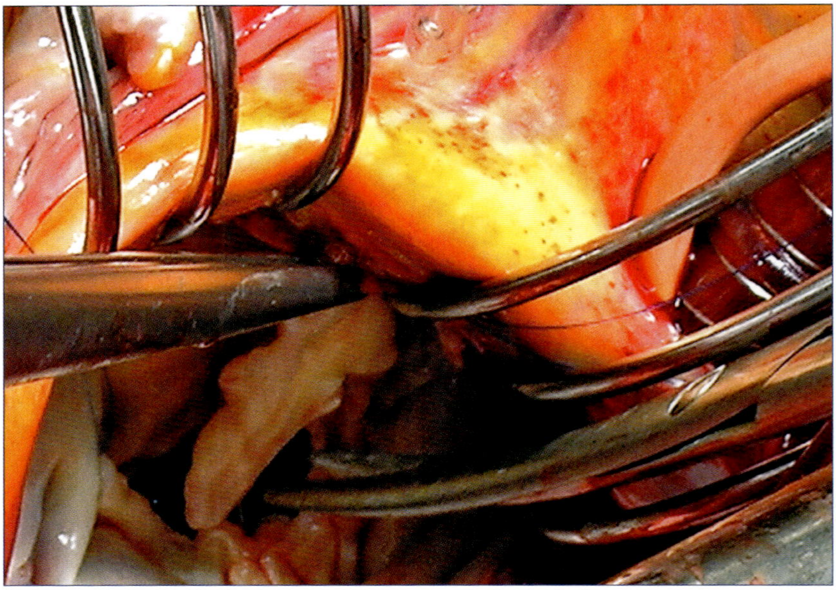

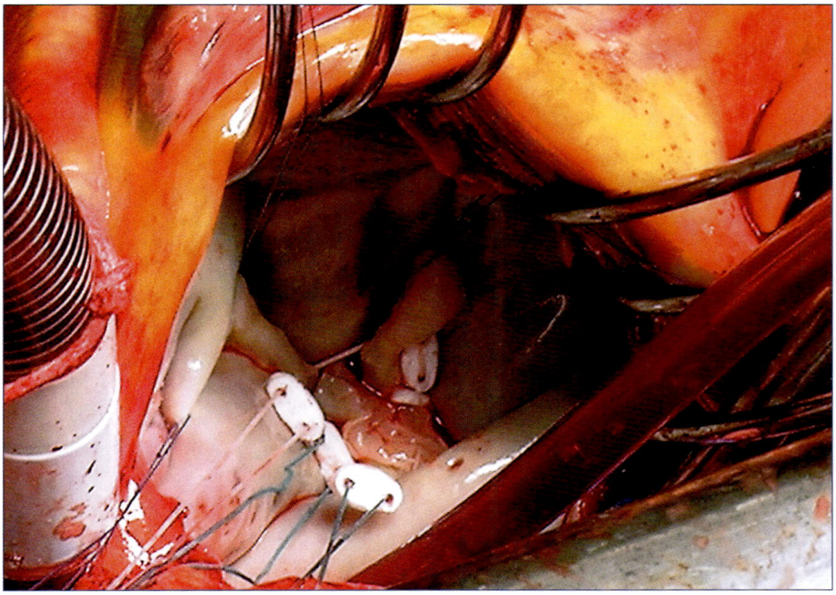

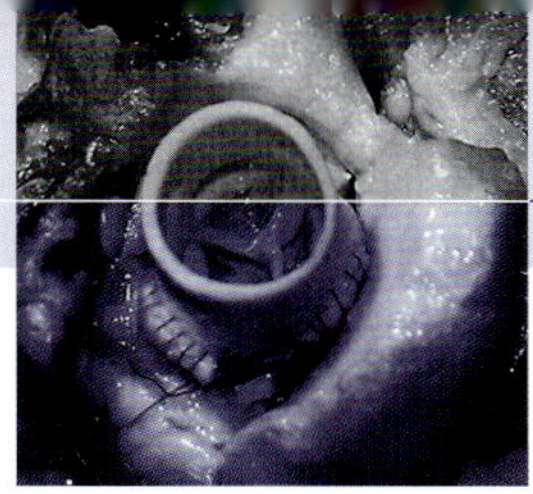

Quadrangular resection of the P2 segment.

First a reduction of the annulus with single U-stitch technique.

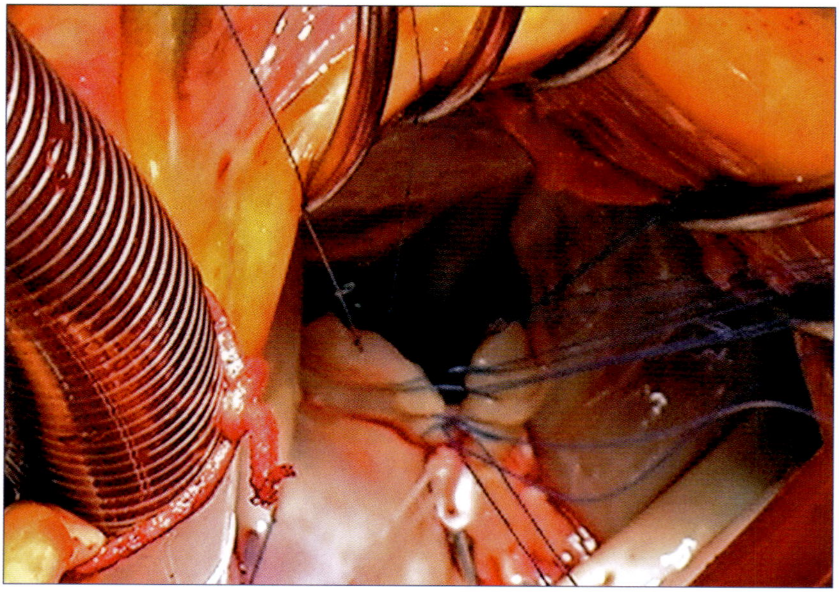

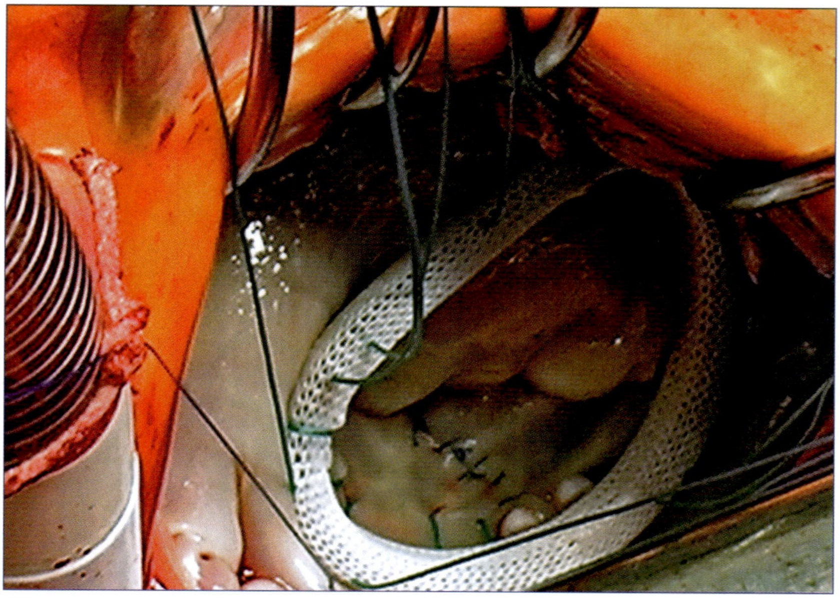

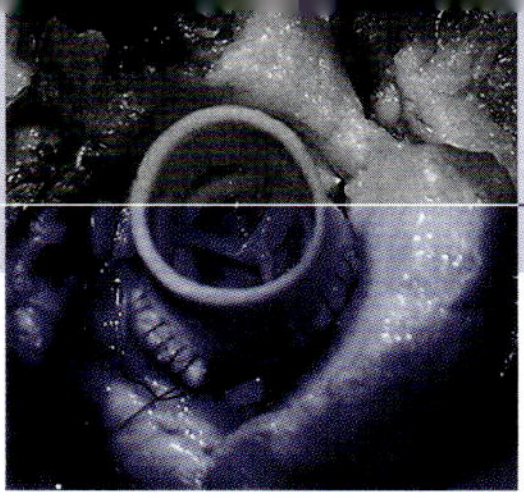

The leaflet edges are brought together with 5-0 prolene. The knot should lie on the ventricular side for an unobstructed coaptation of the leaflets. After reconstruction is completed coaptation of the valve can be tested with saline.

After sizing the annuloplasty-ring is implanted.

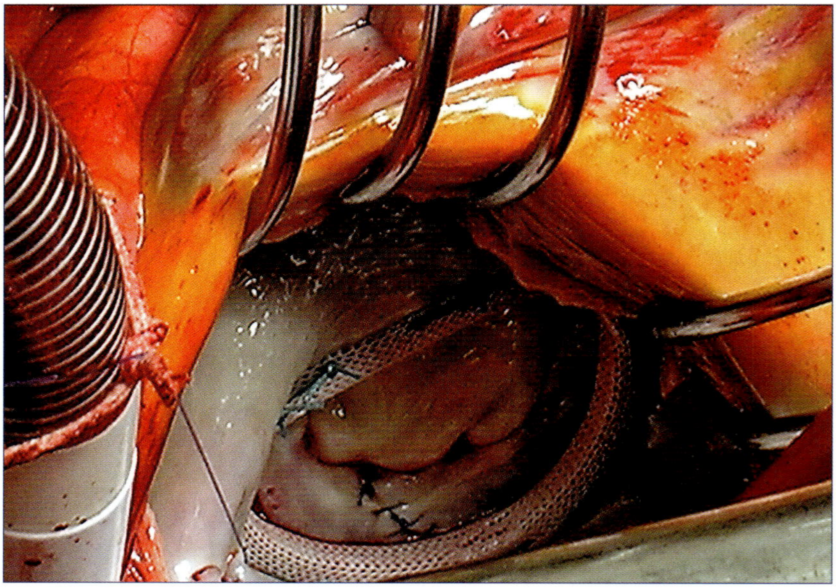

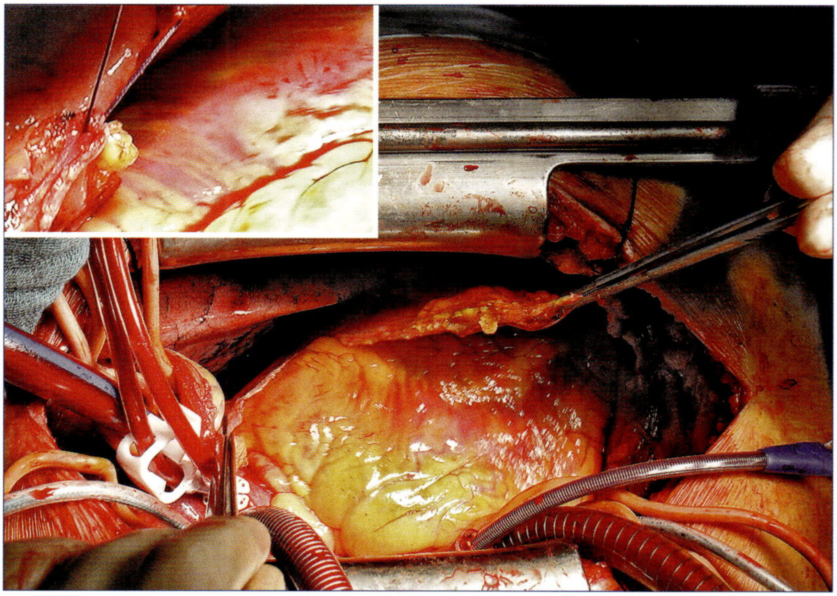

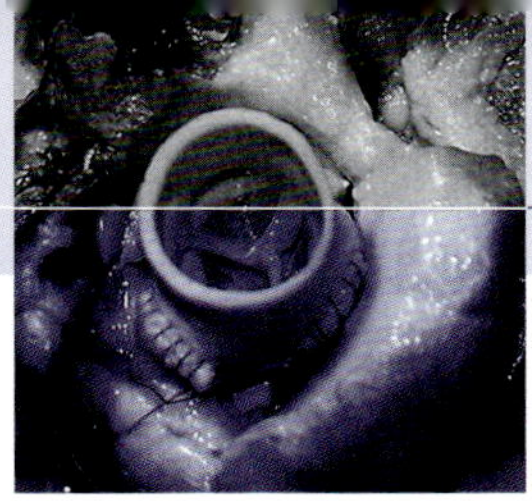

After implantation of the annuloplasty ring the saline test shows a competent closure of the mitral valve. Closure of left atriotomy is performed with a temporary left ventricular vent in situ, afterwards we proceed with the anastomosis of the LAD to the anterior wall, if this has not been done yet.

After de-airing the heart the aortic clamp is removed. De-airing is done usually through the ascending aorta. For complete judgement of complete de-airing the use of transoesophageal echocardiograpy is useful.

During reperfusion, partial clamping of the ascending aorta and proximal anastomosis of bypass grafts are performed. On partial bypass we control the anastomosis and all suture lines. Here it is advised to not dislocate the heart, in particular after valve replacement, to avoid atrioventricular rupture.

After extracorporeal circulation is finished, the LV vent is removed. LA catheters and Pacer wires are inserted in a standard way. A Swan-Ganz catheter can be placed after removal of the venous cannulae. It is recommended to place a Swan-Ganz catheter when there is a pre-existing pulmonary hypertension already before connection of to the heart lung machine.

Always we cover the In-Situ ITA graft with pericardium just before sternal closure in order to keep it lateral and away from the sternum

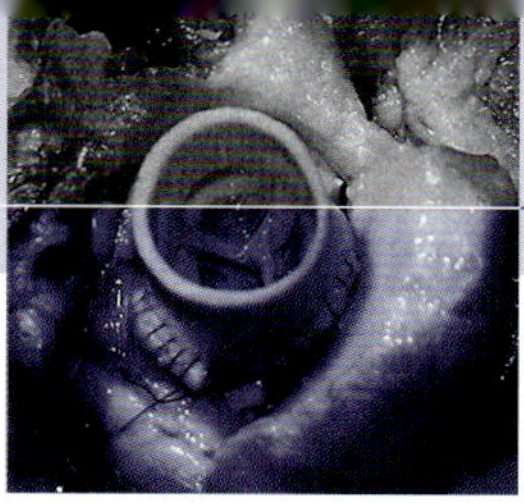

References

1. Akins CW, Hilgenberg AD, Vlahakes GJ, MacGillivray TE, Torchiana DF, Madsen JC. Results of bioprosthetic versus mechanical aortic valve replacement performed with concomitant coronary artery bypass grafting. Ann Thorac Surg. 2002 Oct; 74(4): 1098–106.
2. Akins CW, Buckley MJ, Daggett WM, Hilgenberg AD, Austen WG. Myocardial revascularization with combined aortic and mitral valve replacements. J Thorac Cardiovasc Surg. 1985 Aug; 90(2): 272–7.
3. Chitwood WR Jr, Wixon CL, Norton TO, Lust RM. Complex valve operations: antegrade versus retrograde cardioplegia? Ann Thorac Surg. 1995 Sep; 60(3): 815–8.
4. Dahlberg PS, Orszulak TA, Mullany CJ, Daly RC, Enriquez-Sarano M, Schaff HV. Late outcome of mitral valve surgery for patients with coronary artery disease. Ann Thorac Surg. 2003 Nov; 76(5): 1539–487; discussion 1547–8.
5. Flameng WJ, Herijgers P, Szecsi J, Sergeant PT, Daenen WJ, Scheys I. Determinants of early and late results of combined valve opera tions and coronary artery bypass grafting. Ann Thorac Surg. 1996 Feb; 61(2): 621–8.
6. Ibrahim MF, Paparella D, Ivanov J, Buchanan MR, Brister SJ. Gender-related differences in morbidity and mortality during combined valve and coronary surgery. J Thorac Cardiovasc Surg. 2003 Oct; 126(4): 959–64.
7. Szecsi J, Herijgers P, Sergeant P, Daenen W, Scheys I, Flameng W. Mitral valve surgery combined with coronary bypass grafting: multivariate analysis of factors predicting early and late results. J Heart Valve Dis. 1994 May; 3(3): 236–42.

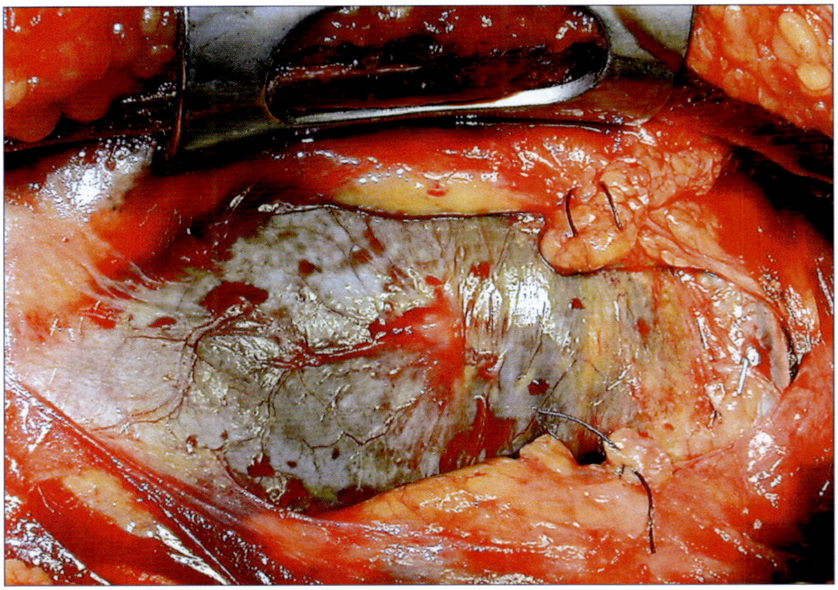

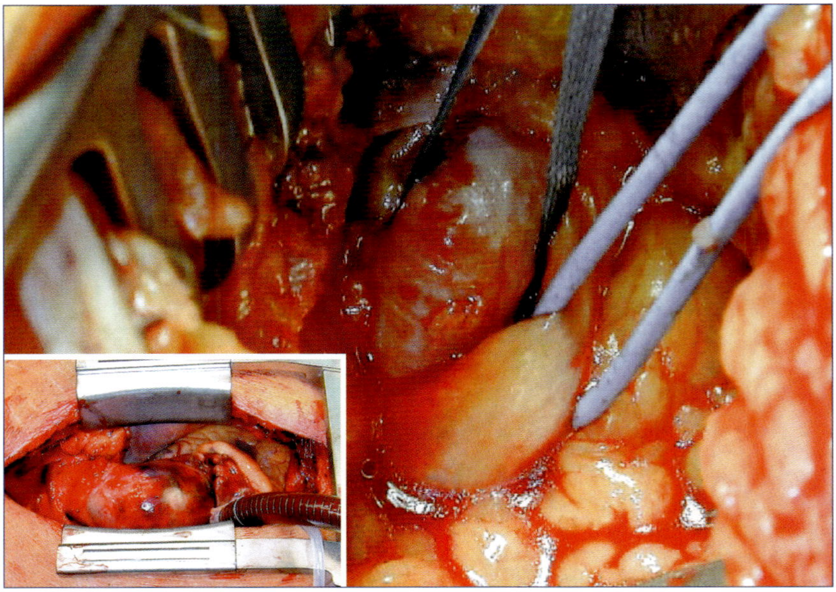

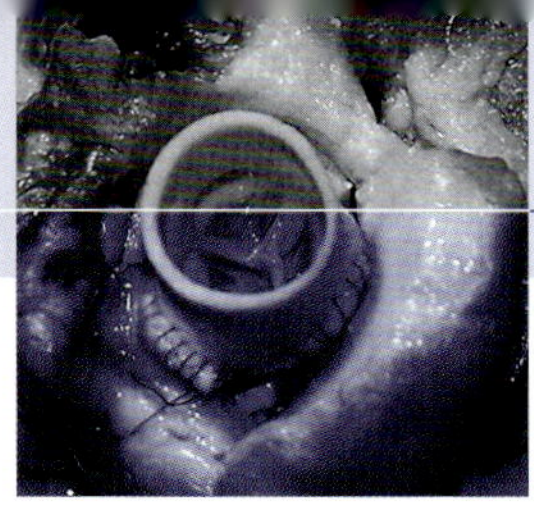

Acute Type A-Dissection:

Inspection of the Pericardium and Operative Strategy

Surgical treatment of acute Type A dissection necessitates cardiopulmonary bypass support. In general, the arterial cannulation site must be chosen carefully. Cannulation of the femoral artery, right axillary artery as well as the direct aortic cannulation are the most commonly used approaches. Antegrade perfusion provides the best perfusion conditions for the brain; hence, we generally cannulate the axillary artery in order to facilitate antegrade brain perfusion. All patients are cooled down to 25-28° C when isolated brain perfusion is planned, while all other patients are cooled down to 18° C for adequate brain protection. Fundamentally, the most significant step following the sternotomy is the verification of a pericardial hematoma and preparation of the arterial cannulation site. Heparin is administered after the sternotomy.

Cannulation of the Axillary Artery

Dissection and exposure of the axillary artery is made through an 8 cm incision below the right clavicle. The steps to be performed include dissection of the subcutaneous tissue and transection of the muscle tissue. Application of vessel loops for the brachiocephalic plexus (blue) and the axillary artery (green). Arterial cannulation is done using a 6.5-7.5 Fr angled cannula. Secure fixation of the arterial and of the venous line (small Figure).

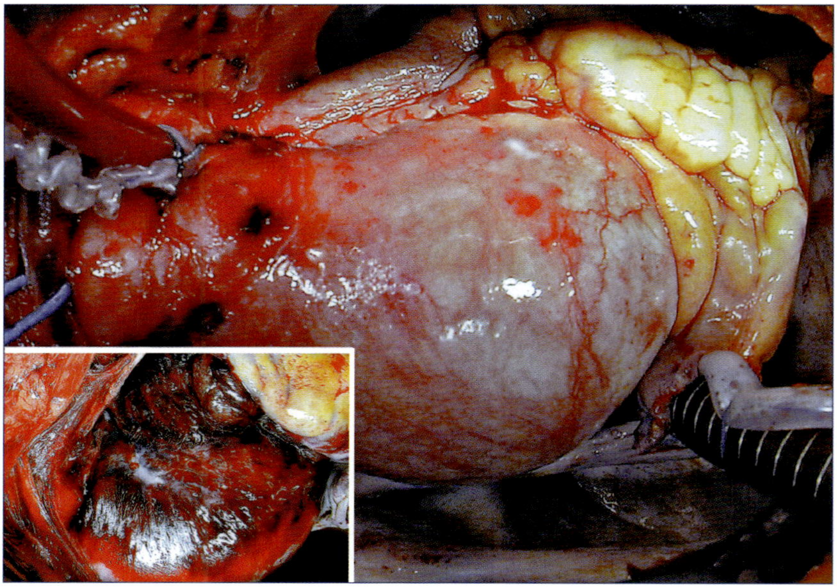

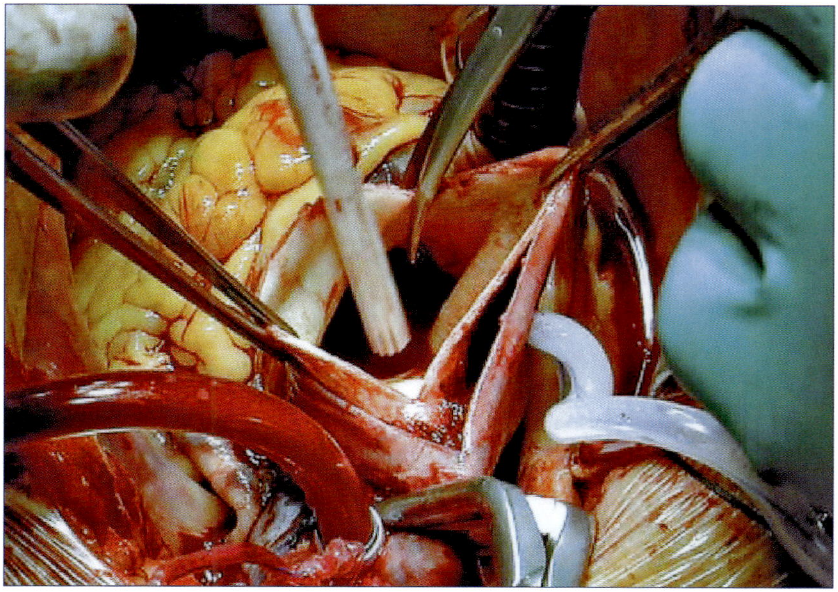

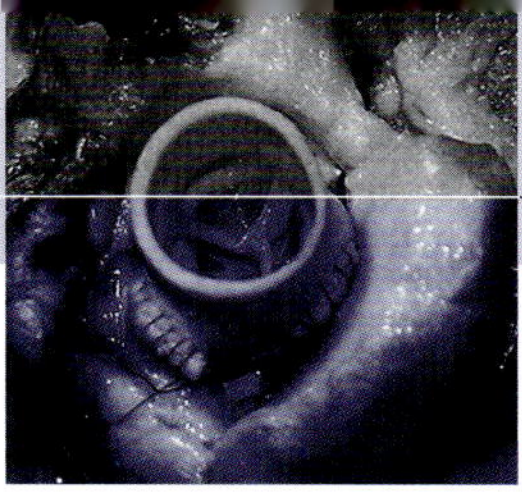

Cannulation of the Aortic Arch with an Intact Aortic Wall

Alternatively, conventional cannulation of the aortic arch in case of a local dissection can be performed by applying a doubled 3-0 prolene purse-string suture. In case of a significant wall hematoma, alternative cannulation is performed and the patient is cooled down. Subsequent planning of the cardioplegia strategy is necessary. The retrograde cardioplegia is advantageous as it shortens the total length of the operation and prevents manipulation of the coronary orifices.

Incision of the Aorta

Aortic cross-clamping and simultaneous check of the blood pressure in all available arterial lines (both radial arteries plus one femoral artery suggested) for exclusion of a malperfusion syndrome is done. When stable perfusion conditions are achieved, cooling of the patient and a longitudinal incision of the aorta below the aortic clamp are performed.

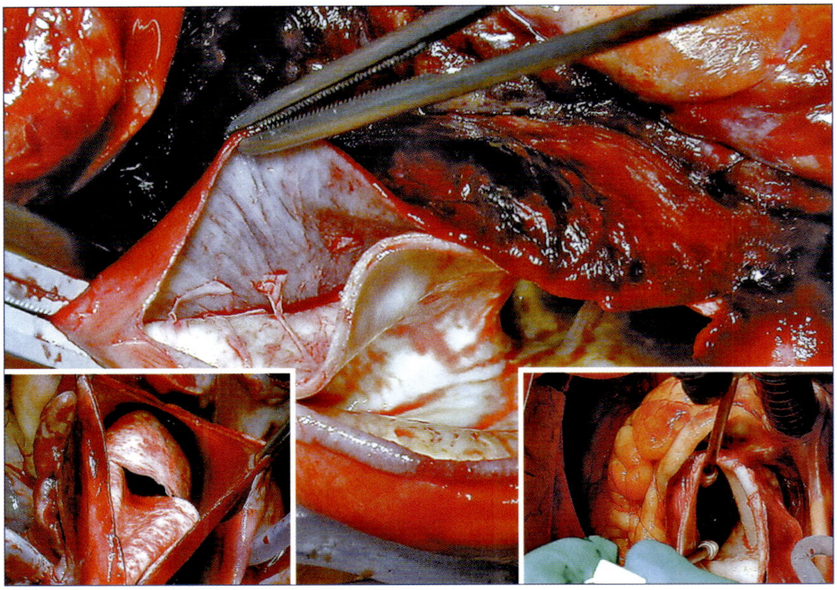

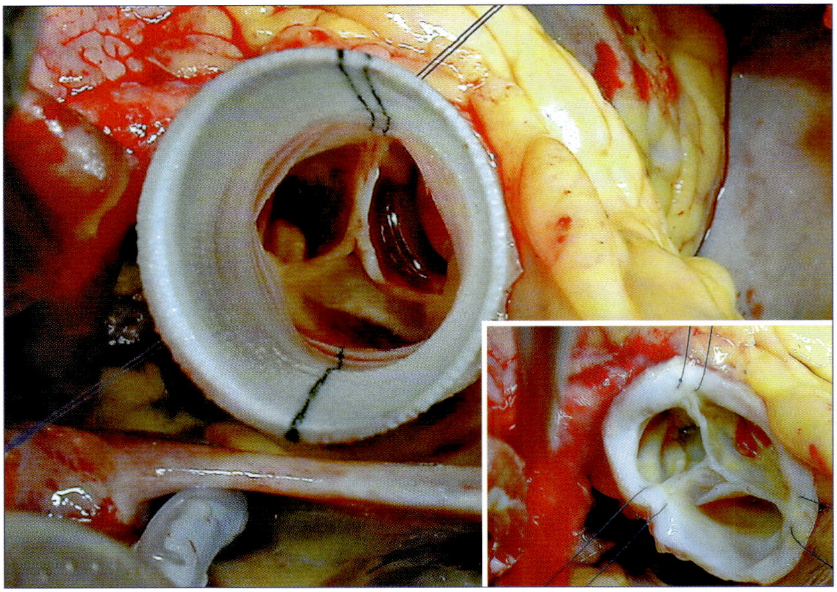

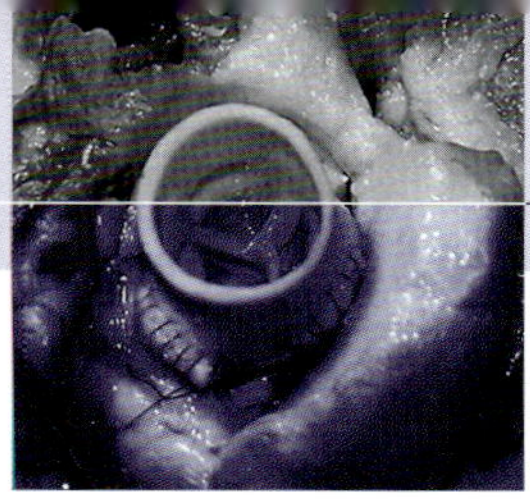

Analysis of the Aortic Dissection

Verification of the extent of the dissection is the first step. Examination of the aortic valve and coronary artery orifices is the second step. Administration of cardioplegia through the coronary orifices or, as preferred, alternatively via a previously introduced coronary sinus catheter will be the third step.

Proximal Anastomosis I

Administration of cardioplegia is completed. In case of an intact aortic base, establishment of a simple end-to-end anastomosis can be done. To achieve symmetric conditions, application of three separate 4-0 prolene sutures can be advantageous.

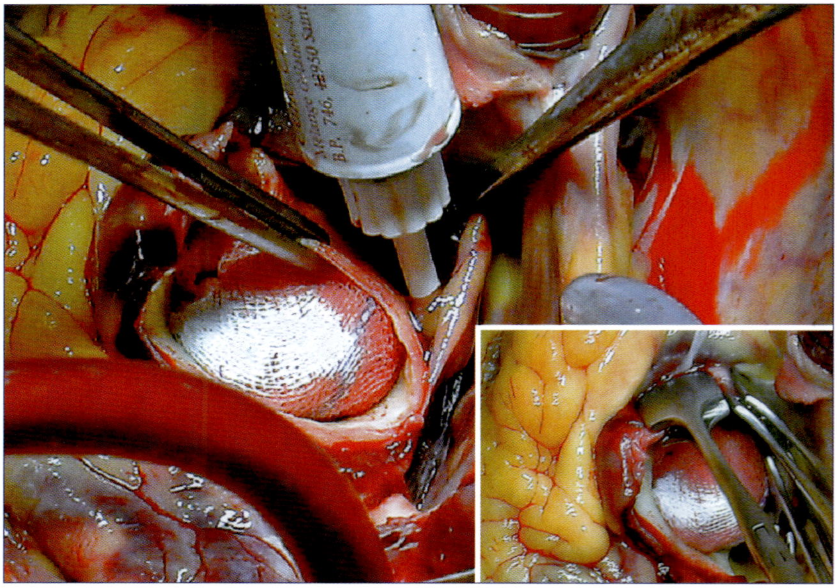

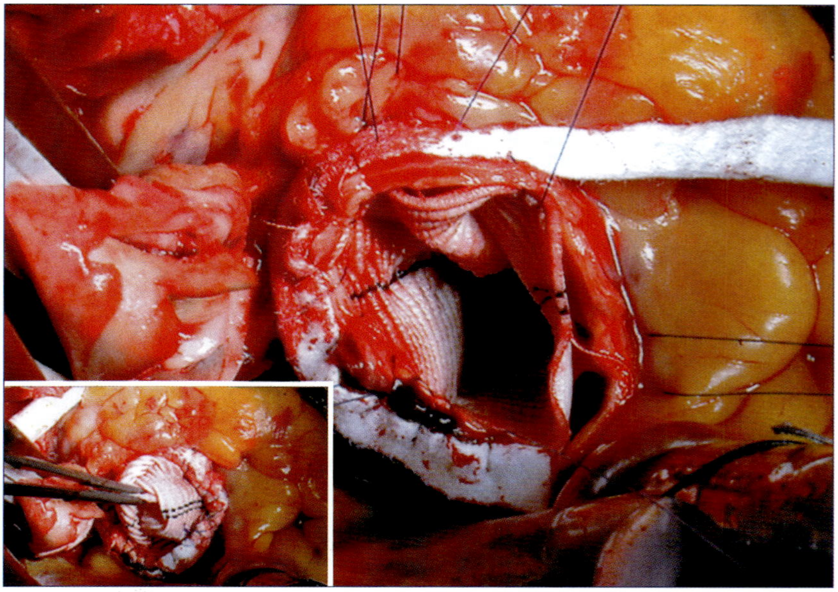

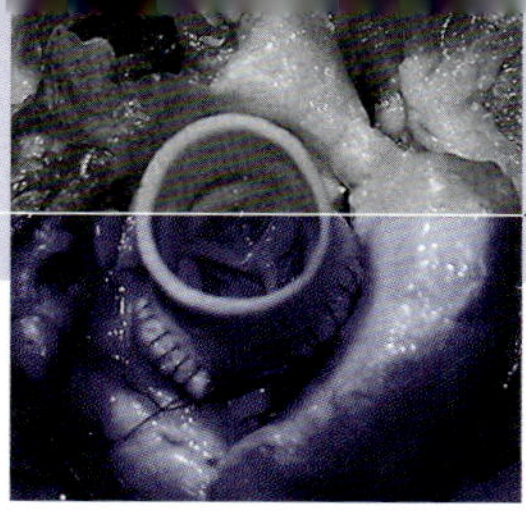

Proximal Anastomosis II

In the case of a dissection of the aortic base, reconstruction of the base applying a GRF-glue or an alternative glue is performed. However, necrosis, as a result of glue application, has been described in long term follow ups. As an alternative, a valve preserving repair technique, for example, by applying the David technique, should be considered. After applying the glue, the reconstructed aortic wall must be compressed for five minutes as a minimum.

Proximal Anastomosis III

Technical Trick:

Proximal anastomosis in case of an intact aortic valve: augmentation of the anastomosis line using Teflon strips (sandwich-technique).

Technical Trick: Inversion and insertion of the prosthesis into the left ventricular outflow track. Here, the prosthesis is folded and inserted using forceps.

After unfolding in the left ventricular outflow tract, the prosthesis can be anastomosed to the aortic base applying a running suture, optionally reinforced with a Teflon strip. In the last step the prosthesis is again everted from the LV into its anatomical position.

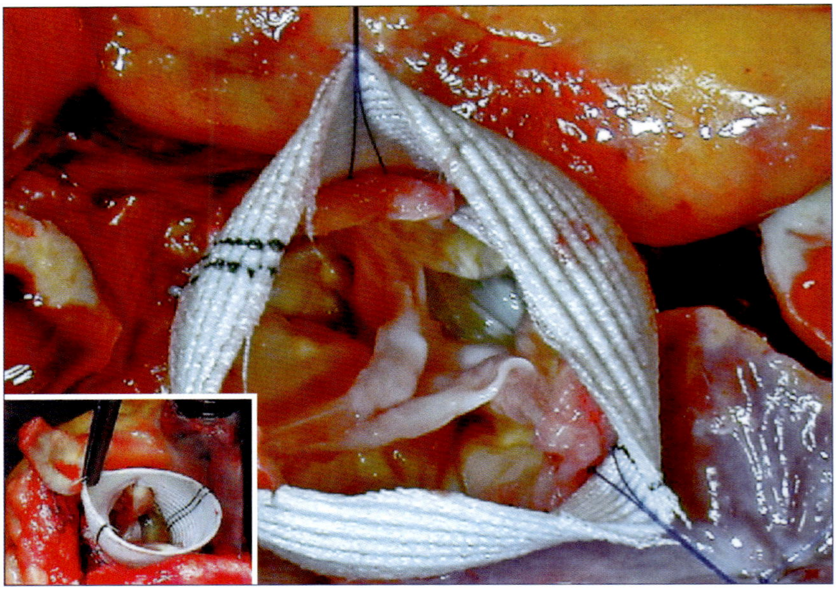

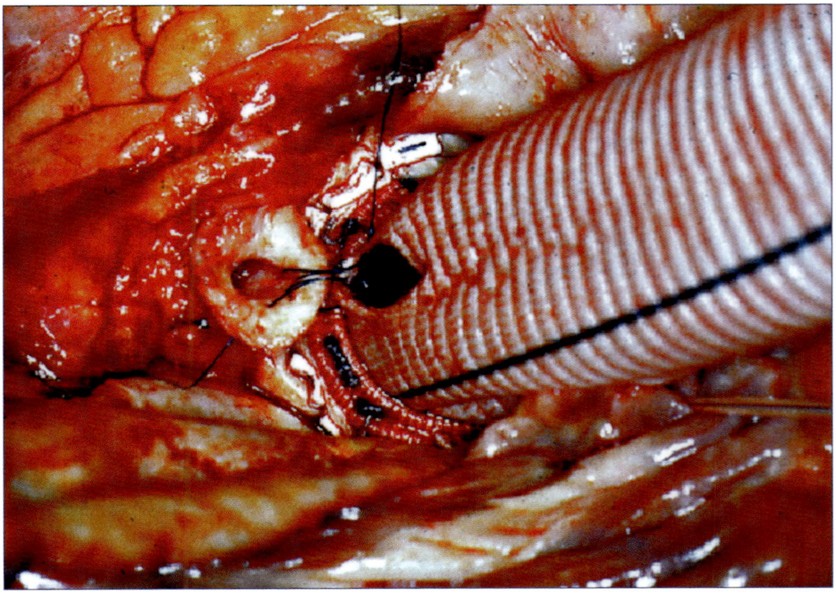

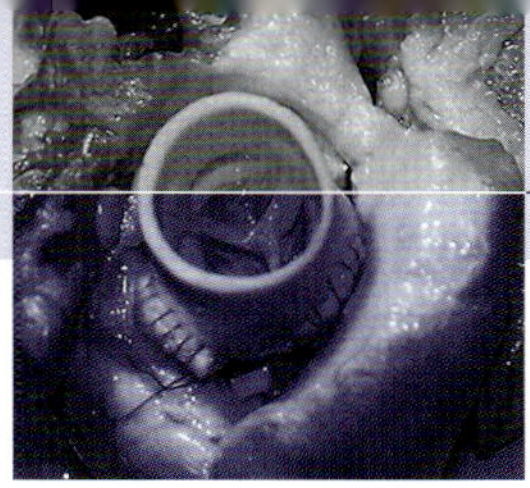

Repair of the Aortic Base I

In a Type-A dissection, the valve can be repaired by applying the David or Yacoub techniques as an alternative instead of an aortic valve replacement. The valve repair may be performed during the re-warming phase, following the completion of the aortic arch repair.

Repair of the Aortic Base with a Composite Replacement

In a composite replacement, as well as valve repair, the coronary arteries (button technique) are re-anastomosed using a 5-0 prolene running suture, and the anastomoses might be secured by application of fibrin glue.

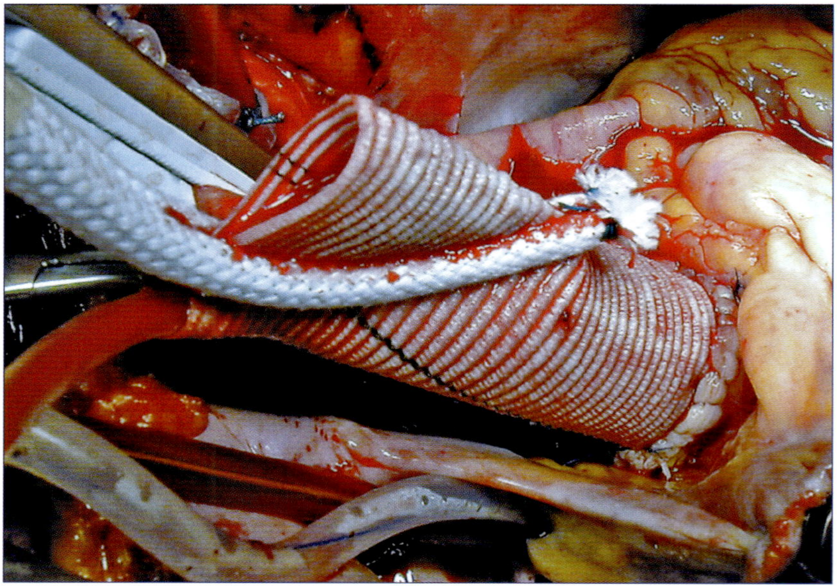

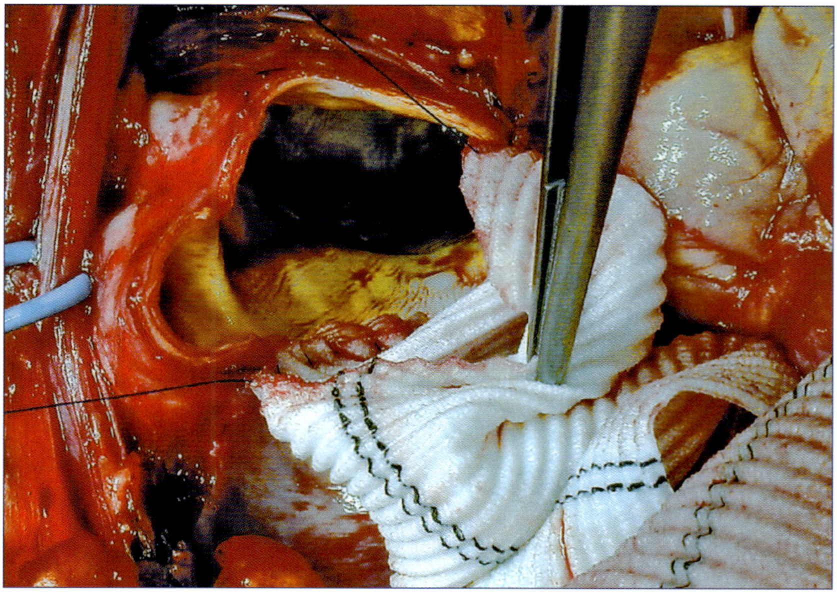

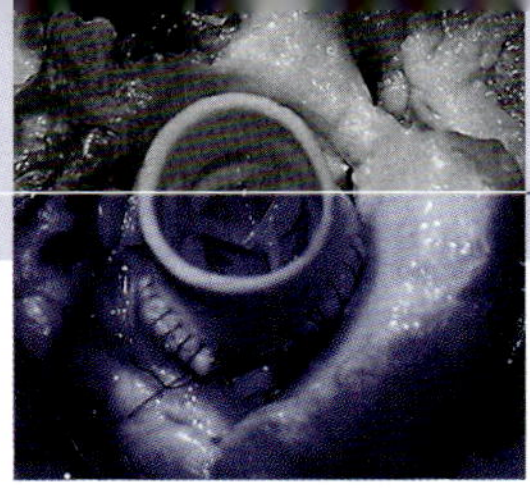

Testing of the Repaired Aortic Base

After completion of the proximal anastomosis, cardioplegia is administered antegradely into the prosthesis. This allows for detection of leakages which are easily treated using 4-0 prolene stitches. Cold blood cardioplegia is administered for at least 2 minutes using a covered Crawford clamp for clamping of the prostheses which is supported by an additional mosquito clamp in order to prevent leakage of cardioplegia.

Construction of the Arch Anastomosis I

After the patient is completely cooled down, the distal clamp is removed with the patient in Trendelenburg position. If the dissection is limited to the ascending aorta with resulting regular findings in the aortic arch, the prosthesis may be connected directly using a 3-0 or 4-0 prolene suture. In any case, the aorta is transected completely to facilitate the anastomosis. This figure illustrates a circulatory arrest without application of isolated cerebral perfusion. Today, continuous brain perfusion represents the gold standard.

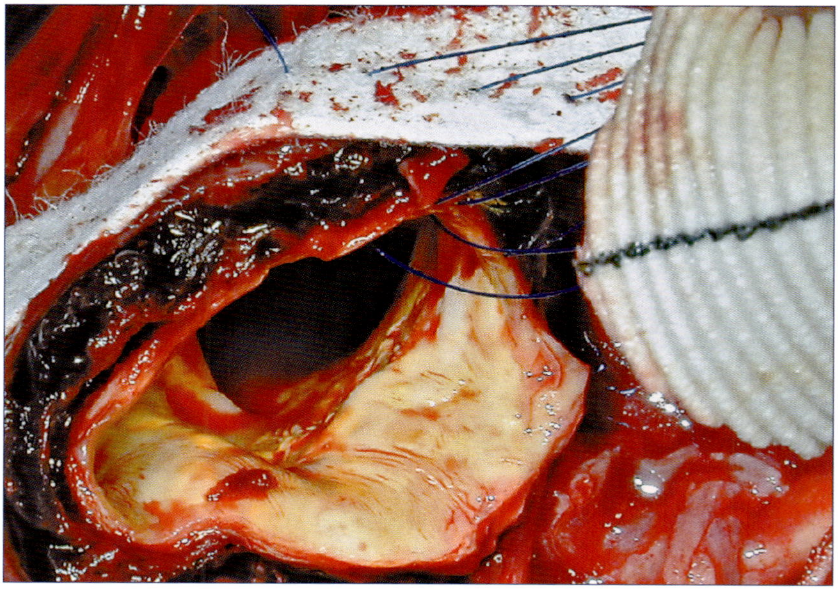

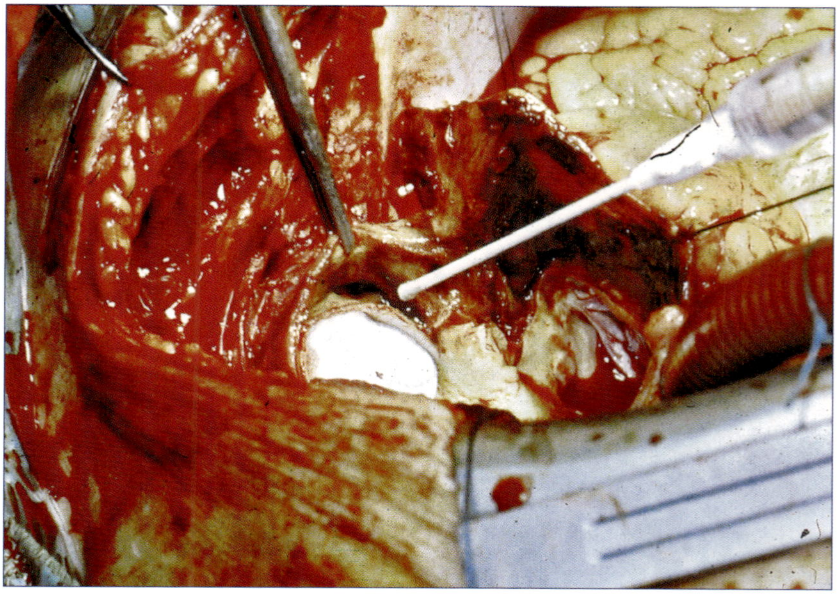

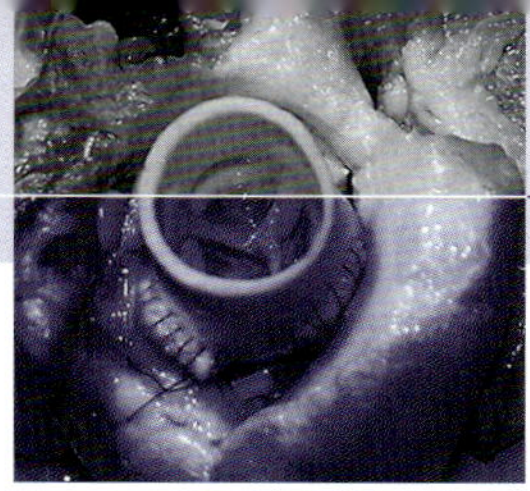

Construction of the Arch Anastomosis II

In analogy to the proximal repair, the distal anastomosis is constructed without glue or isolated selective brain perfusion. The anastomosis is augmented using a Teflon strip by applying the sandwich technique. The figure displays an intact intima layer, which can easily be sewn directly.

Construction of the Arch anastomosis III

In this case the aortic arch was entirely transected also. The false lumen is excluded by reconstruction of the aortic wall using the GRF glue. The glue components must be mixed with the utmost precision, given that the glue is toxic, and can cause cell necrosis, which however is less common for the aortic arch anastomoses .

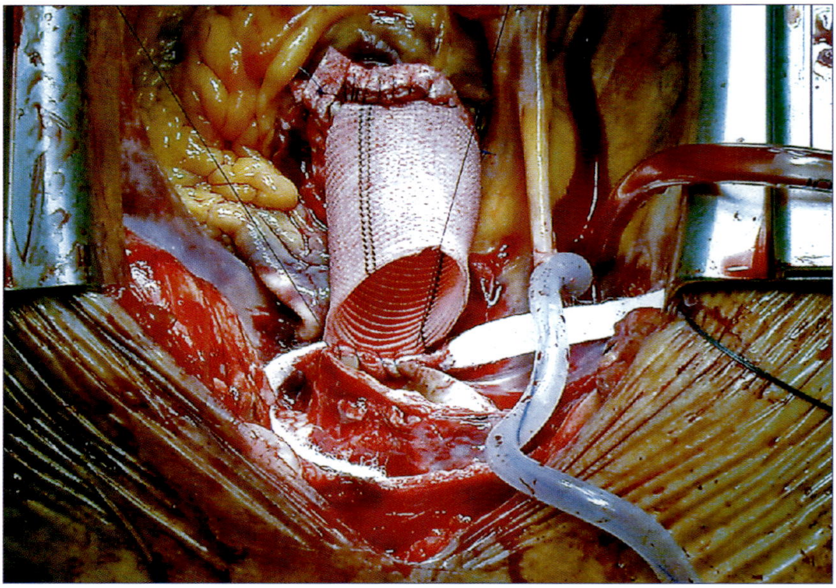

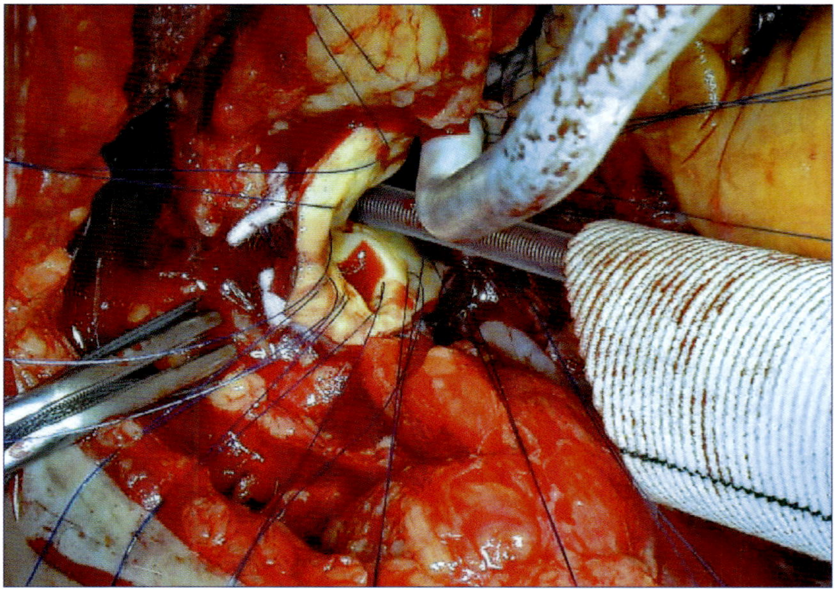

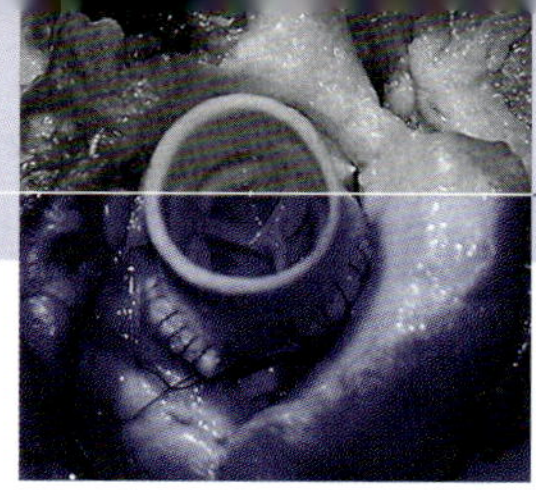

Construction of the Arch Anastomosis IV

As an alternative to the standard two-prosthesis technique, a single prosthesis was used in this case. The Teflon felt was positioned between the prosthesis and the aortic wall. With regard to the resulting wall thickness of his sandwich technique, a 3-0 prolene suture (SH-needle) was used. Possible drawbacks to the single prosthesis technique are difficulties in determination of optimal graft length and limited feasibility of de-airing. In the figure displayed, the patient was perfused in a retrograde fashion via the femoral artery at 18° C.

Construction of the Arch Anastomosis V

Establishment of the distal anastomosis. Continuous cerebral perfusion via the right axillary artery, retrogradely through the brachiocephalic trunk, then antegradely via the right carotid artery. The left carotid artery is directly perfused by the heart lung machine by an inserted coronary sinus catheter. For safety reasons, the anastomosis is performed using multiple Teflon armed 3-0 prolene U-sutures, where the stitches at the aorta are directed from "outside to inside". This method is a classical and time-consuming technique, however, it allows for the construction of a high-quality anastomosis with a low risk for leakage.

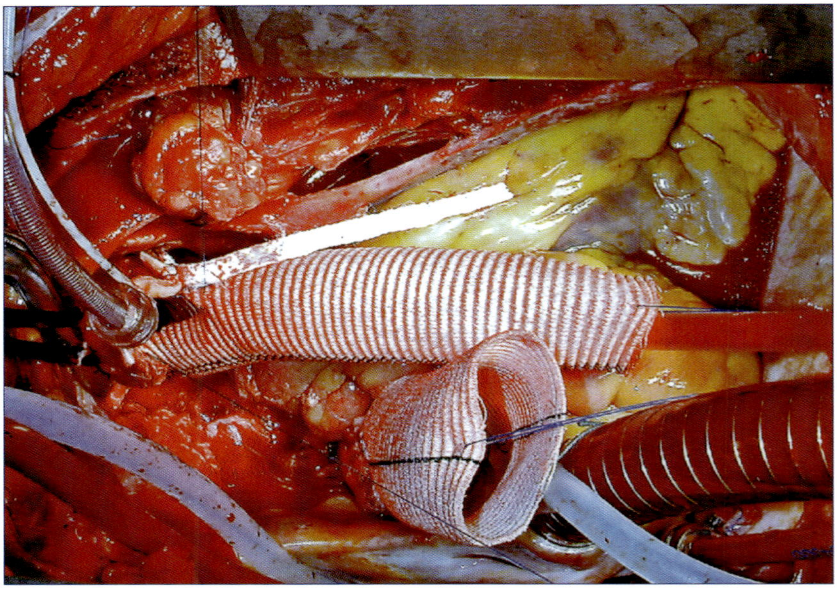

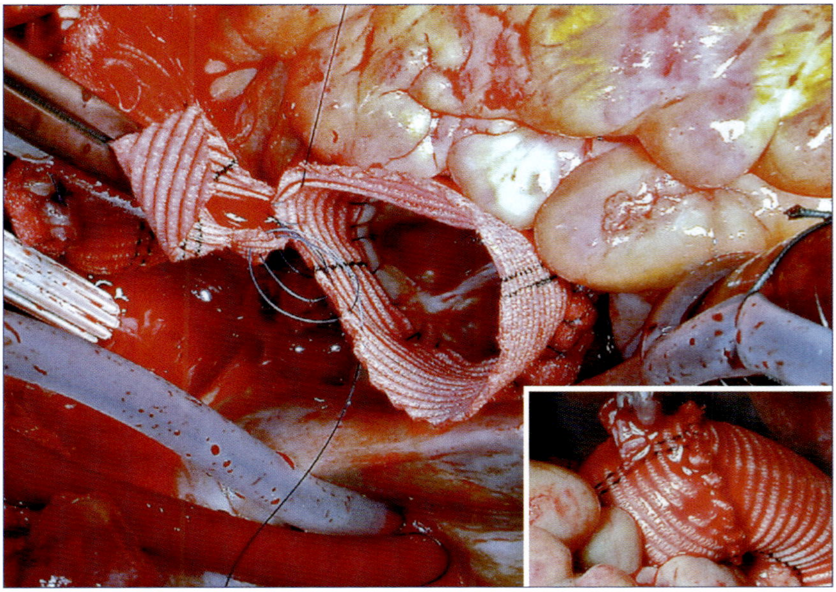

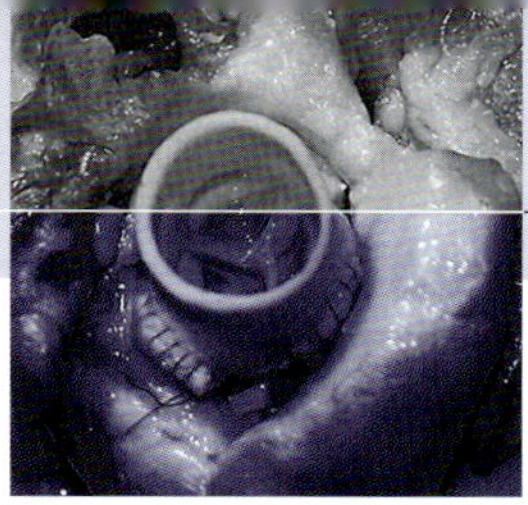

Complete Aortic Arch Replacement

Brain perfusion in a complete aortic arch replacement. The supra-aortic vessels are re-implanted as a single button. Prior to the completion of the anastomosis, the perfusion catheter is removed. The vessel clamp is removed from the brachiocephalic trunk and the arch is de-aired retrogradely. De-airing is completed by clamping the prosthesis far proximally which improves inspection of the distal anastomosis to control for blood leakage.

Two-Prosthesis Technique

Anastomosis of two prostheses using a 4-0 prolene suture (main figure). Optimal length estimation is important to prevent "neo-formations" (inlet).

1
2
3
4
5
6
7
8
9
10
11
12
13
14
15

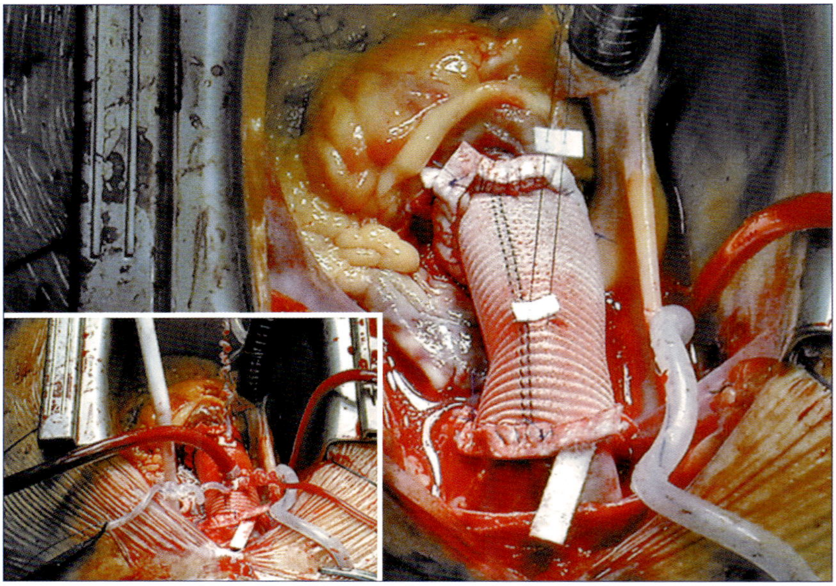

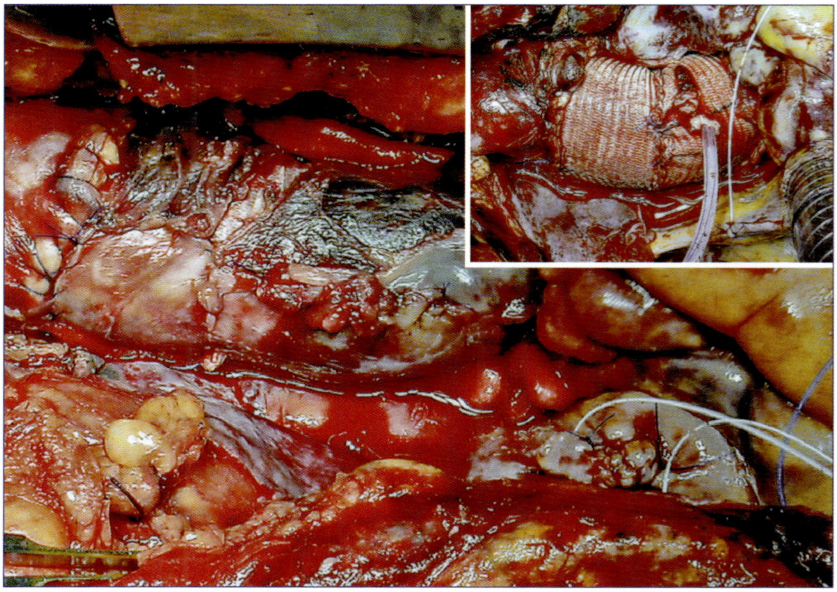

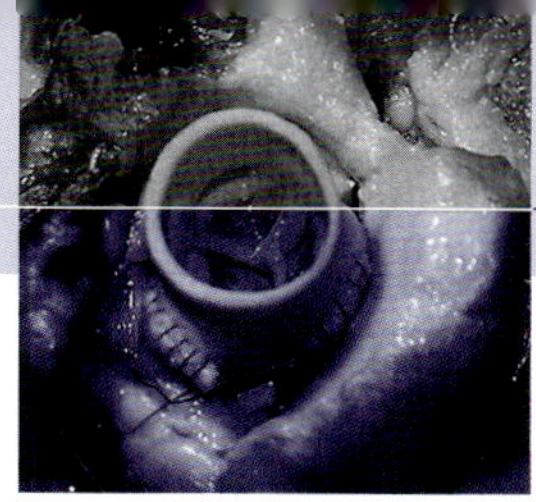

Antegrade Perfusion during Reperfusion

Principally, antegrade perfusion should be the aim when operating a Type-A dissection. In the displayed figure, primary perfusion was established via the femoral artery followed by a switch of the cannulation site into the aortic prosthesis. The purse string suture is supported by Teflon pledges in order to prevent leakage from the cannulation site. The small figure illustrates the antegrade perfusion during the re-warming phase.

Prosthesis Insertion

The small image displays the situs following the weaning of cardiopulmonary bypass. The venous cannula is still in position. The length estimation was correct. Inclusion plasty of the prosthesis using the former aneurysm material in order to reduce both the risk for infection and the risk of damage to the prosthesis in possible redo operations.

References

1. Chiappini B, Tan ME, Morshuis W, Kelder H, Dossche K, Schepens M. Surgery for acute type A aortic dissection: is advan ced age a contrain dication? Ann Thorac Surg. 2004; 78(2): 585–90.
2. Collins JS, Evangelista A, Nienaber CA, Bossone E, Fang J, Cooper JV, Smith DE, O'Gara PT, Myrmel T, Gilon D, Isselbacher EM, Penn M, Pape LA, Eagle KA, Mehta RH. International Registry of Acute Aortic Dissection (IRAD). Differences in clinical presentation, management and outcomes of acute type a aortic dissection in patients with and without previous cardiac surgery. Circulation 2004; 14: 110(11 Suppl 1): II237–42.
3. Crawford ES, Kirklin JW, Naftel DC, Svensson LG, Coselli JS, Safi HJ. Surgery for acute dissection of ascending aorta. Should the arch beincluded Journal of Thoracic & Cardiovascular Surgery 1992; 104(1): 46–59.
4. De Paulis R, Bassano C, Scaffa R, Nardi P, Bertoldo F, Chiariello L. Bentall procedures with a novel valved conduit incorporating "sinuses of Valsalva". Surgical Technologies International 2004; 12: 195–200.
5. Fusco DS, Shaw RK, Tranquilli M, Kopf GS, Elefteriades JA. Femoral cannulation is safe for type A dissection repair. Ann Thorac Surg. 2004; 78(4): 1285–9.
6. Hata M, Shiono M, Sezai A, Iida M, Negishi N, Sezai Y. Type A acute aortic dissection: immediate and mid-term results of emergency aortic replacement with the aid of gelatin resorcin formalin glue. Ann Thorac Surg. 2004; 78(3): 853–7; discussion 857.
7. Haverich A, Miller DC, Scott WC, Mitchell RS, Oyer PE, Stinson EB, Shumway NE. Acute and chronic aortic dissections-determi nants of long-term outcome for operative survivors. Circulation 1985; 72 (3 Pt 2): II 22–34.
8. Kallenbach K, Oelze T, Salcher R, Hagl C, Karck M, Leyh RG, Haverich A. Evolving strategies for treatment of acute aortic dissec tion type A. Circulation 2004; 14: 110(11 Suppl 1): II 243–9.

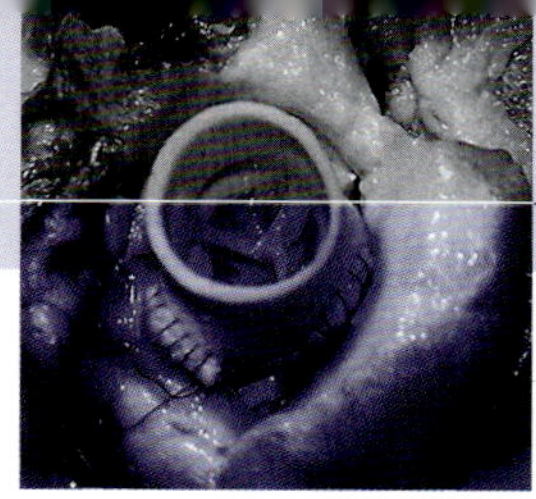

9. Obadia JF, Abdullatif Y, Henaine R, Chavanis N, Saroul C, Barthelet M, Andre-Fouet X, Raisky O, Robin J, Ninet J. Replacement of the ascending aorta with conservation of the aortic valve. Reults of 50 cases using the Tirone David procedure. Archives des Maladies du Coeur et des Vaisseaux 2004; 97 (12): 1183–7.
10. Raanani E, Georghiou GP, Kogan A, Wandwi B, Shapira Y, Vidne BA. 'BioGlue' for the repair of aortic insufficiency in acute aortic dissection. Journal of Heart Valve Disease 2004; 13 (5): 734–7.
11. Sabik JF, Nemeh H, Lytle BW, Blackstone EH, Gillinov AM, Rajeswaran J, Cosgrove DM. Cannulation of the axillary artery with a side graft reduces morbidity. Annals of Thoracic Surgery 2004; 77 (4): 1315–20.
12. Schachner T, Laufer G, Vertacnik K, Bonaros N,. Nagiller J, Bonatti J. Is the axillary artery a suitable cannulation site in aortic surgery? Journal of Cardiovascular Surgery 2004; 45 (1): 15–9.
13. Seike Y, Yamamoto S, Hosoda Y, Operation on acute type A aortic dissection using transapical aortic cannulation. Kyobu Geka – Japanese Journal of Thoracic Surgery 2004; 57 (10): 945–8.
14. Sugita T, Matsumoto M, Nishizawa J, Matsuyama K, Kawanishi Y, Tokuda Y, Yoshida K, Uehara K, Matsuo T. Management for type A acute dissection. Kyobu Geka – Japanese Journal of Thoracic Surgery 2004; 57 (3): 201–6.
15. Trimarchi S, Nienaber CA, Rampoldi V, Myrmel T, Suzuki T, Mehta RH, Bossone E, Cooper JV, Smith DE, Menicanti Frigiola A, Oh JK, Deeb MG, Isselbacher EM, Eagle KA. Contemporary results of surgery in acute type A aortic dissection: The International Registry of Acute Aortic Dissection experience. Journal of Thoracic & Cardiovascular Surgery 2005; 129 (1): 112–22.

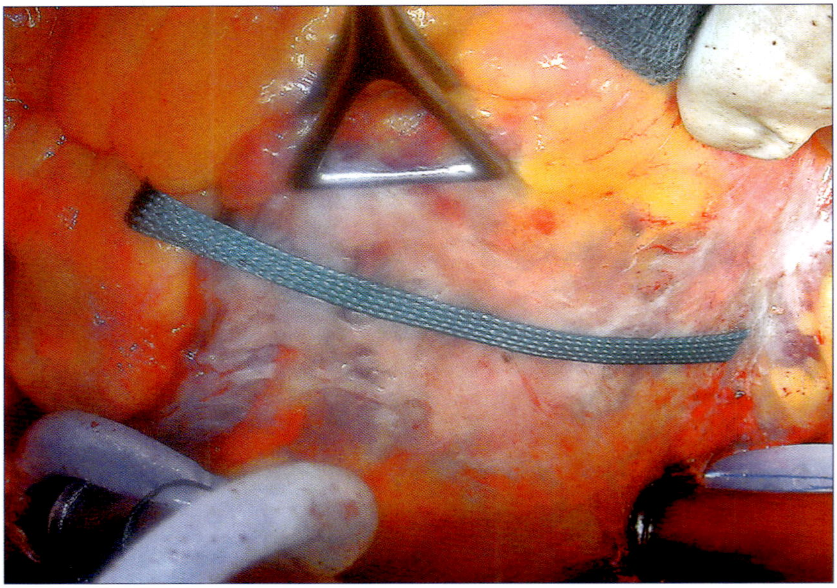

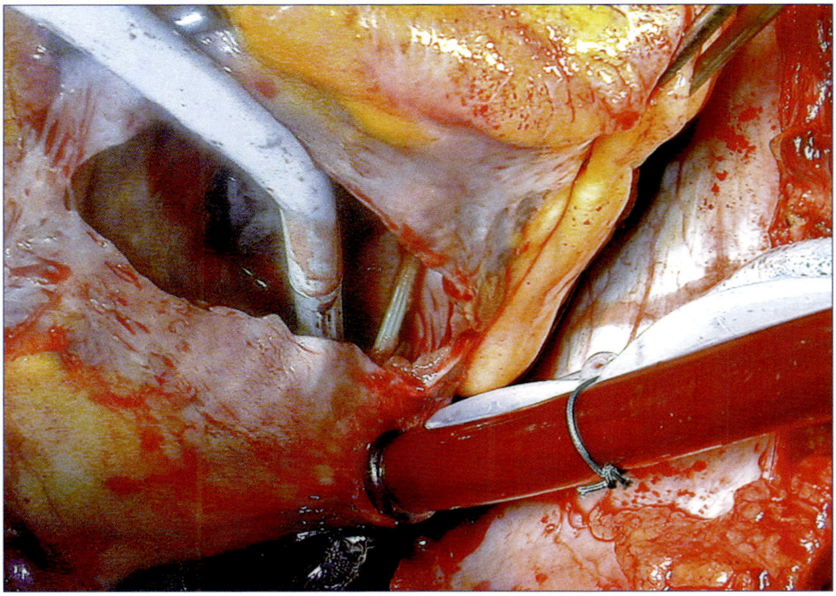

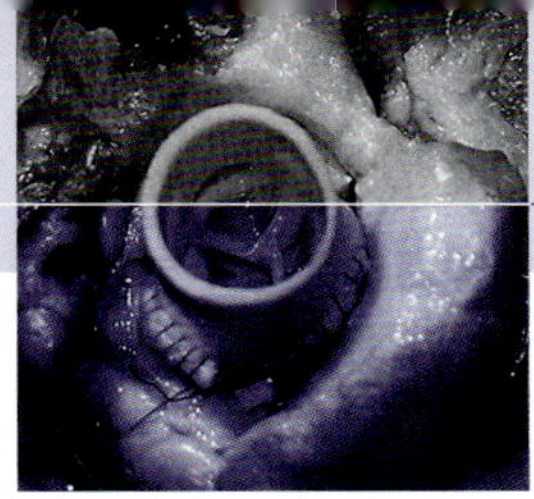

Subsequent to sternotomy, pericardiotomy and cannulation of the distal ascending aorta (in redo cases cannulation of the axillary artery or femoral artery might be preferred), the bicaval venous cannulation is performed. Following the standard transplantation technique describedby Lower and Shumway (1, 2) both venae cava are cannulated separately, where the inferior vena cava (IVC) is cannulated as lateral as possible. In order to establish a total cardio-pulmonary bypass, both venae cava are secured additionally by a tourniquet. After aortic cross-clamping, the explantation of the recipient's heart starts with an incision of the right atrium. This figure illustrates the incision line with a green ribbon (the right atrial appendage is retracted by a lung forceps). Note that a sufficient width between the incision and the IVC is available for the right atrial anastomosis!

The initial incision of the right atrium is extended caudally close to the atrioventricular groove into the coronary sinus. The coronary sinus, which marks the atrioventricular borderline at the posterior wall of the heart, can be intubated with the pericardial suction line for improved orientation. Cranially, the incision is extended to immediately below the aortic root.

1 2 3 4 5 6 7 8 9 10 11 12 13 14 15

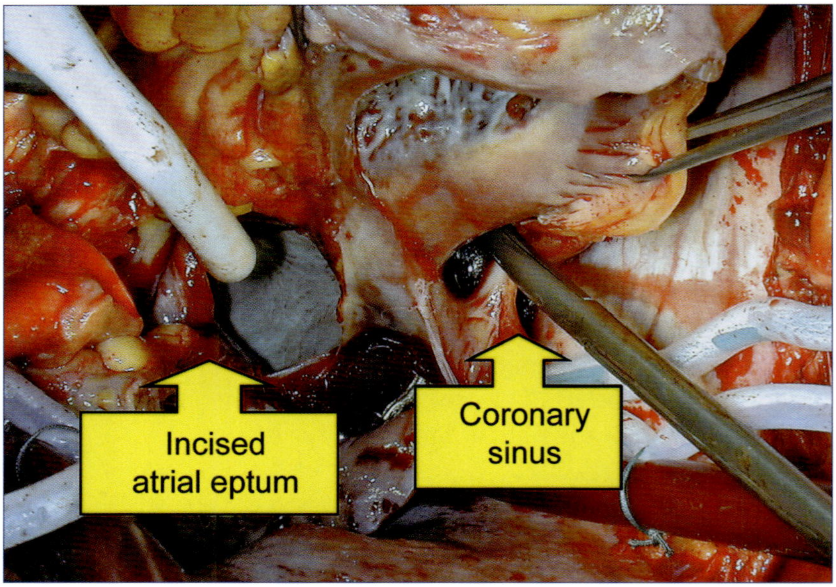
Incised
atrial eptum
Coronary
sinus

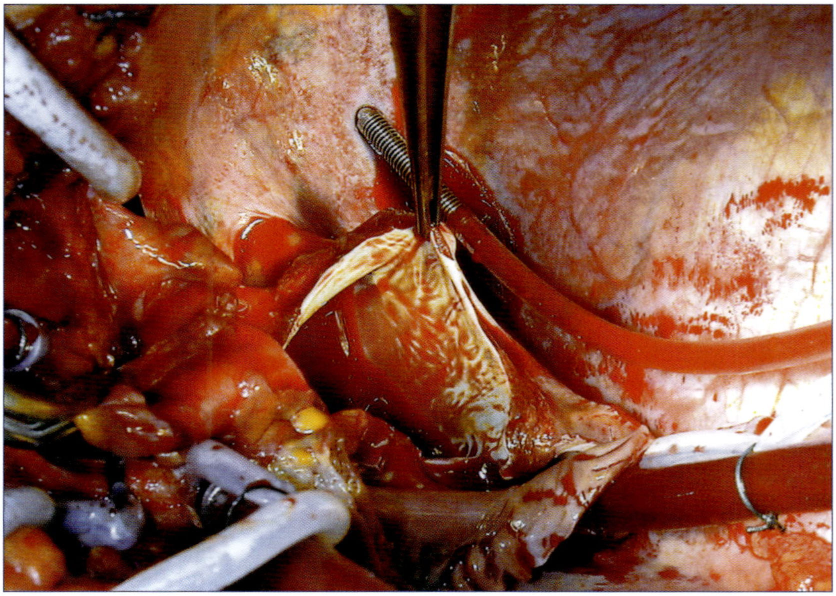

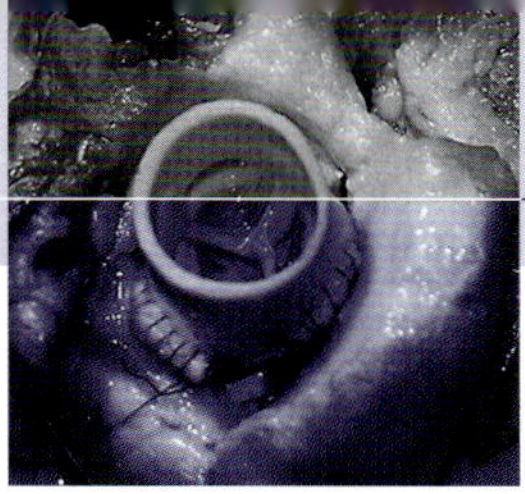

The interatrial septum is incised at the fossa ovalis (intubated with the pericardial suction line) and extended caudally towards the existing incision line of the coronary sinus (marked with scissors). For further expansion of the incision towards the posterior wall, the heart is displaced cranially.

The incision of the left atrium follows the coronary sinus at the posterior wall in cranial direction towards the left atrial appendage. Attention: To avoid injury to the pulmonary veins, the incision should be made within a safe distance ventrally from these structures. To facilitate a better orientation, some trabecular tissue of the left atrial appendage may be left temporarily. Following this preparation, the heart is repositioned into the situs.

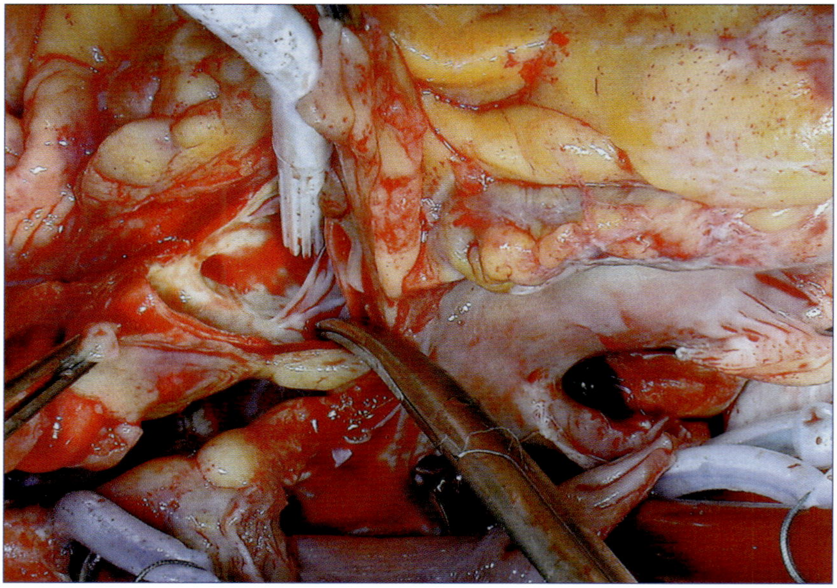

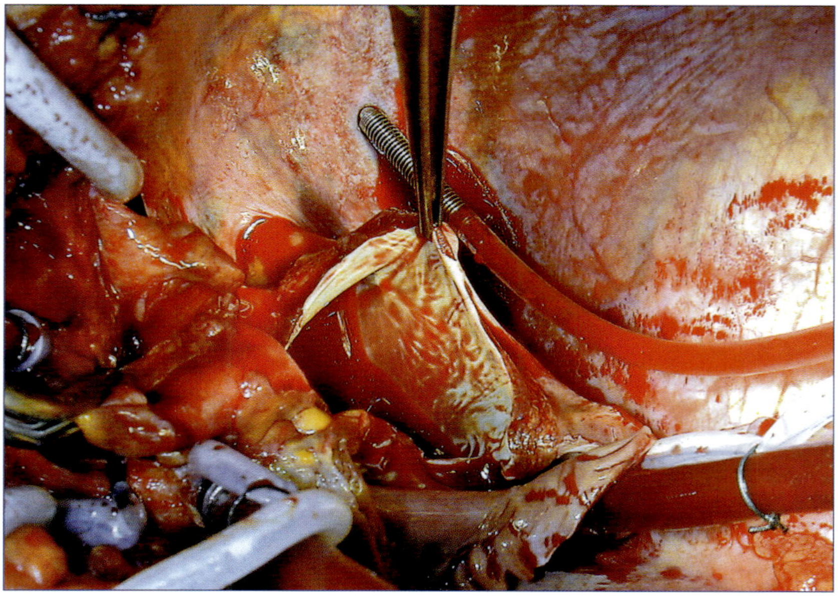

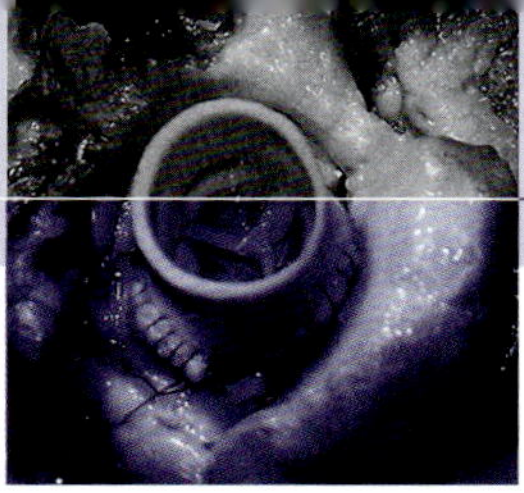

The transection of the aorta and the pulmonary artery is performed with both maximal length of the remaining recipient vessels and preservation of the aortic and pulmonary valve which may be used for later homograft preparations. Thereafter, the previous incision line of the right atrium is extended underneath the aortic base and into the roof of the left atrium, towards the left atrial appendage.

This figure illustrates the situation following complete excision of the recipient heart with the remaining cuffs of the left (held with forceps) and right atrium (bottom portion of the picture) and the distal ends of the aorta (aortic clamp) at the pulmonary artery (intubated with the ECC suction).

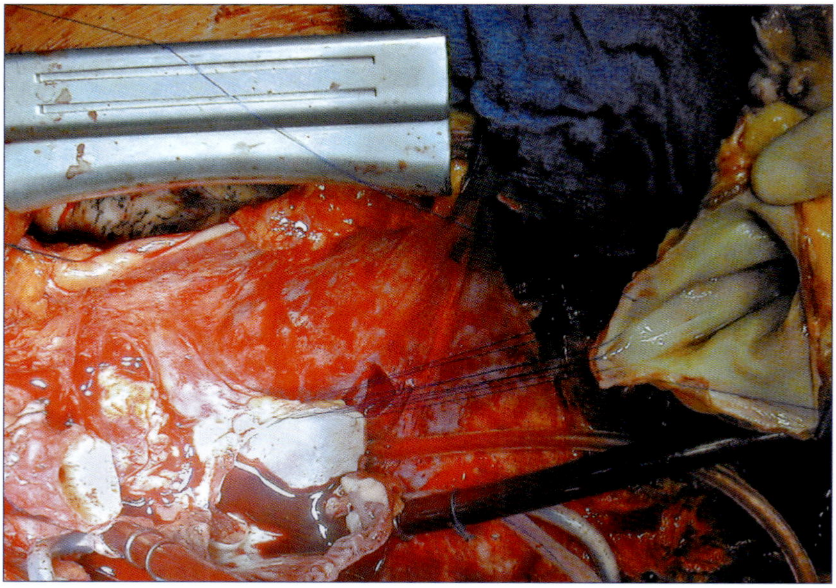

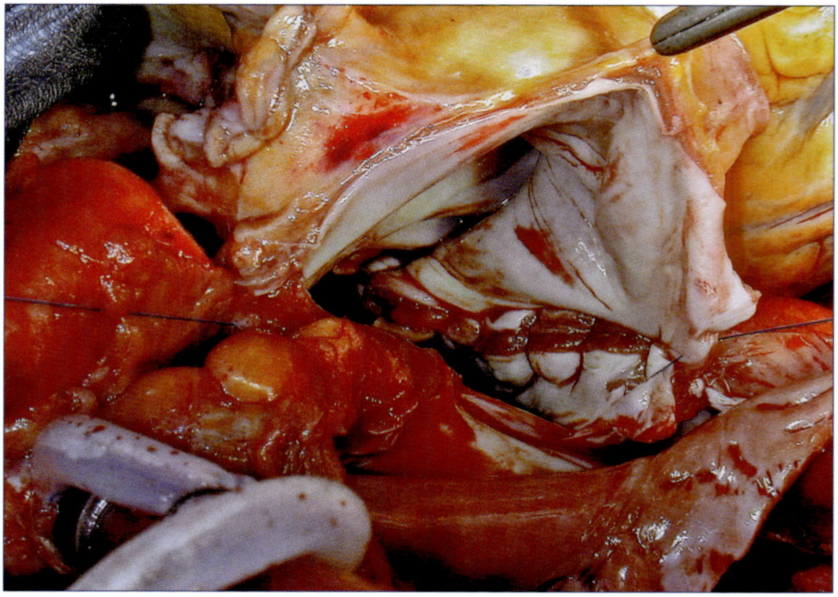

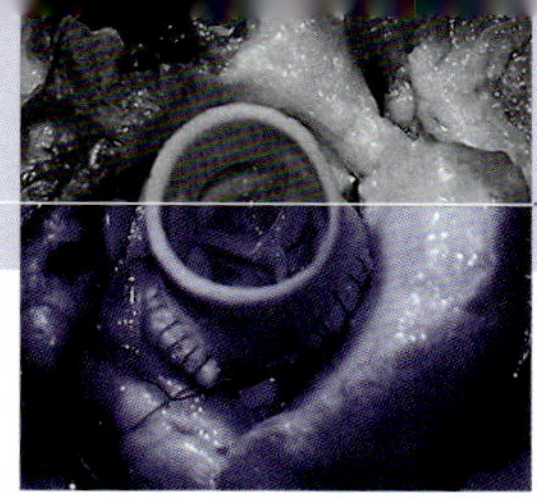

The donor organ is meticulously inspected. The left atrium is opened crosswise connecting the pulmonary veins, followed by adequate resection of left atrial excess tissue. The preparation includes: separationof the aorta and pulmonary artery; testing and closure of a patent foramen ovale, respectively, as well as inspection and palpation of the heart valves and coronary arteries in order to exclude pathology of those relevant structures.

The implantation starts with the left atrial anastomosis at the base of the left atrial appendage (marked by the remaining trabecular tissue) using a prolene 3-0 SH suture with 3–4 parachute-technique stitches (direction of the stitches: donor "inside to outside", recipient "outside to inside").

With traction to the suture, the donor organ is carefully positioned into the situs. To alleviate the anastomosis, cold gauzes might be placed underneath the graft. The suture line is continued caudally along the free atrial wall towards the septum. Cranially, the anastomosis is completed towards the roof of the atrium and the interatrial septum, respectively.

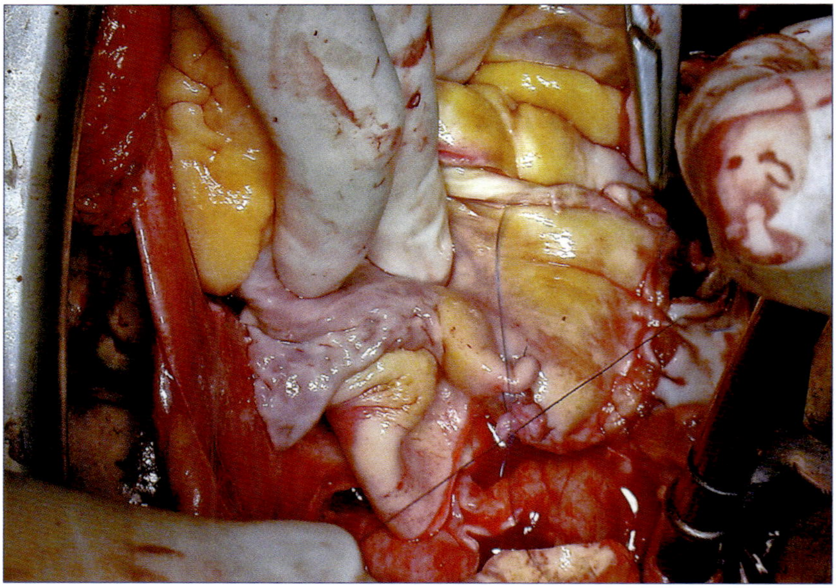

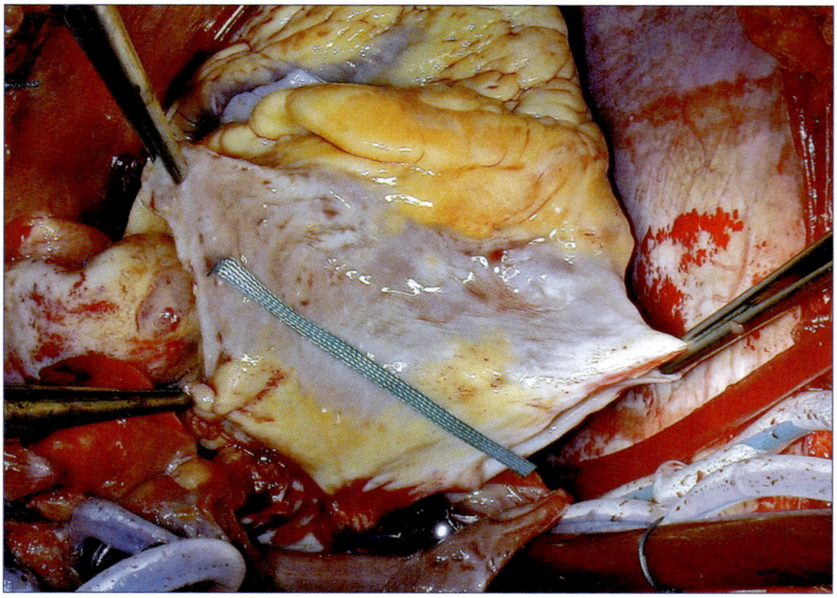

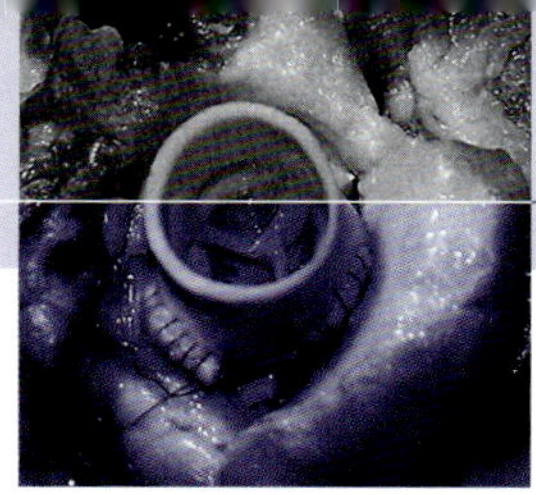

(Cranial view into the situs).
The left atrial anastomosis is completed at the interatrial septum, where both suture ends are tied. To facilitate the suture line, the first assistant retracts the right atrium and the right atrial appendage towards the left.

The right atrial anastomosis is initiated at the graft with an incision of the right atrium which starts at the IVC (right forceps) and which is extended towards the right atrial appendage (left forceps, incision line marked with a green ribbon).

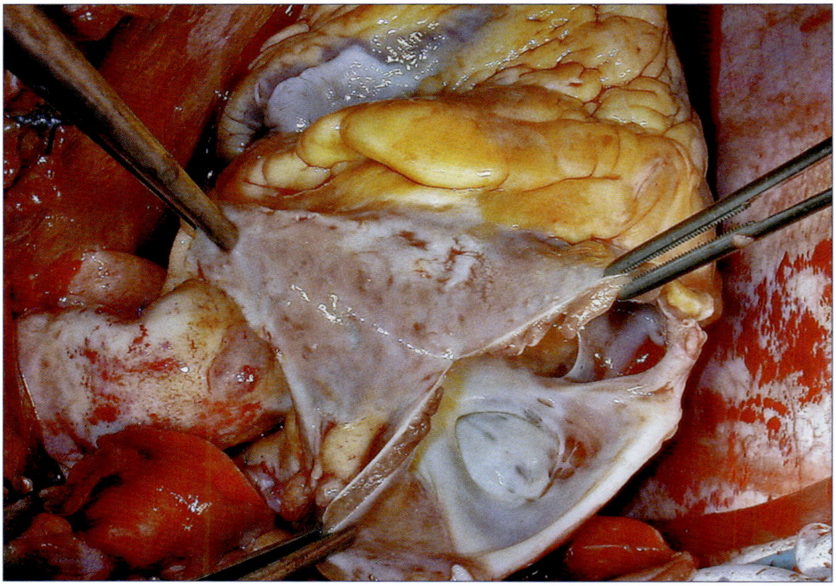

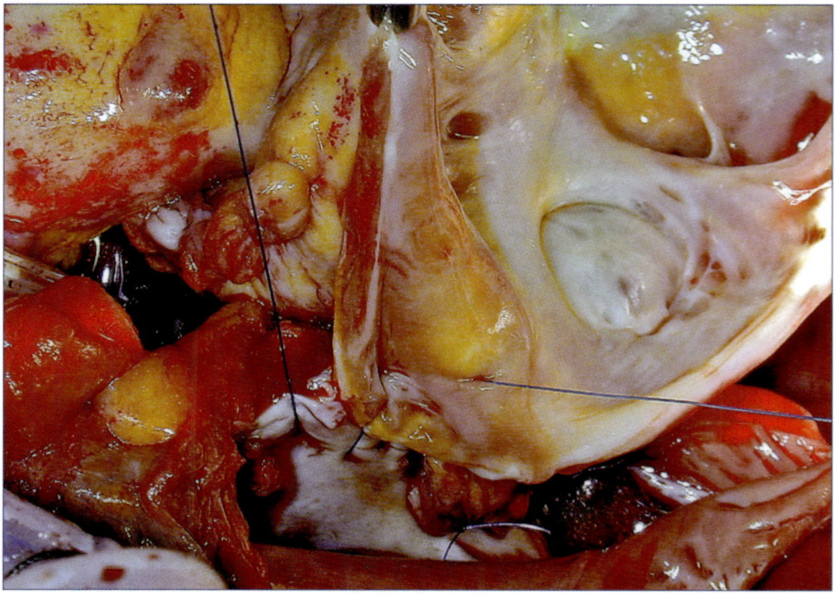

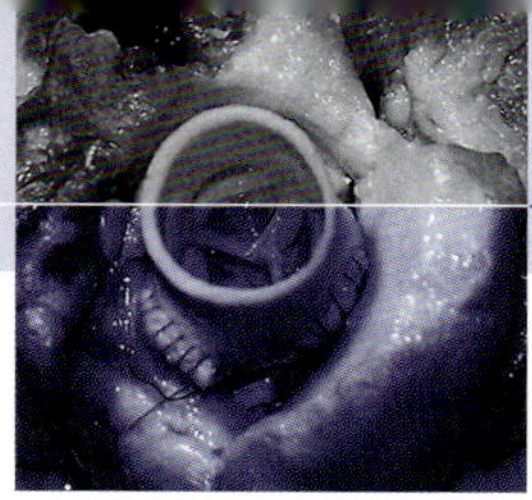

In order to achieve optimal congruence, the length of the right atrial incision is dependent on specific anatomical characteristics and has to be performed with the intention of carefully preserving the sinus node and the coronary sinus orifice.
With this "Shumway"-technique, a relative risk of resulting tricuspid valve incompetence exists due to slight distortion despite careful anastomotic technique. In our experience, this risk is extremely low but might be minimised by a concomitant tricuspid valve annuloplasty (3) or by choosing a "bicaval anastomotic technique" with separate anastomosis of both caval veins ([4, 5], not described in detail).

The right atrial anastomosis also starts with a prolene 3-0 SH suture with the intention of creating a "double-plication" of the interatrial septum: the donor right atrium is anastomosed to the existing suture line of the left atrial anastomosis (stitch direction: donor: "inside to outside", recipient: "outside to inside").

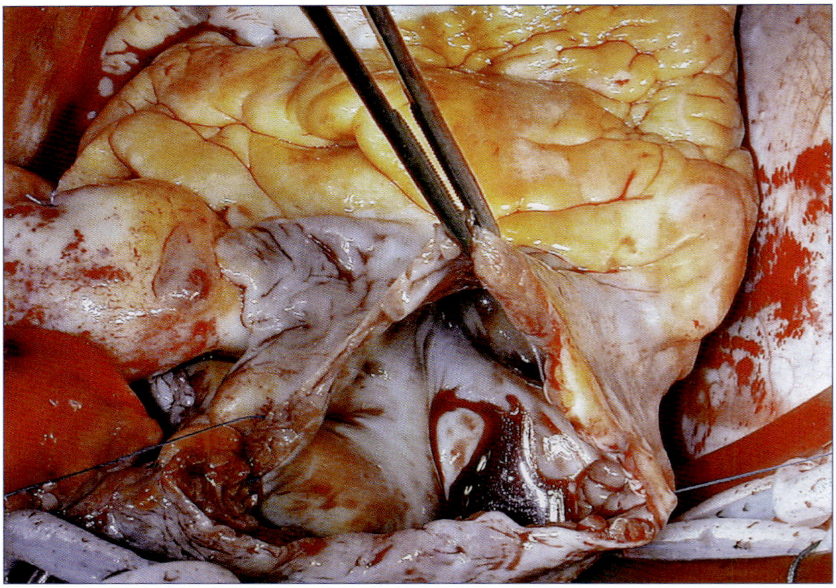

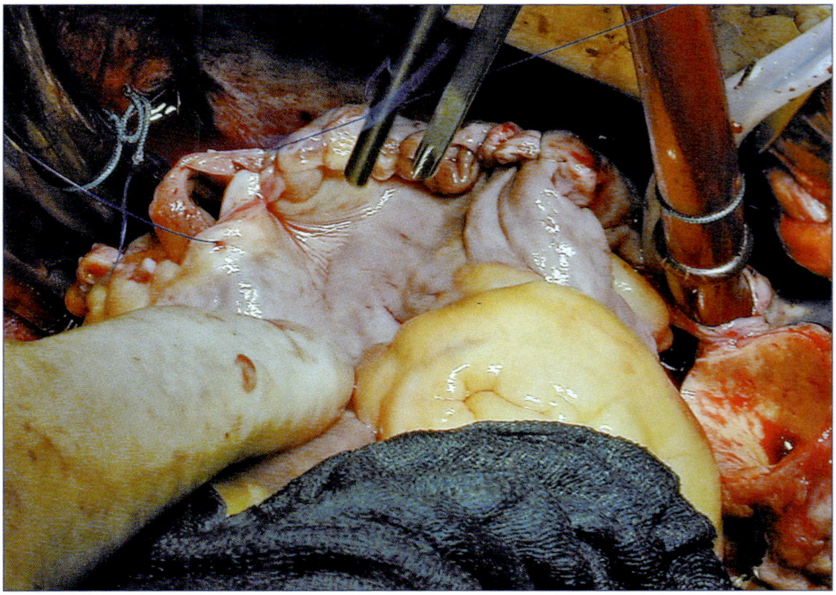

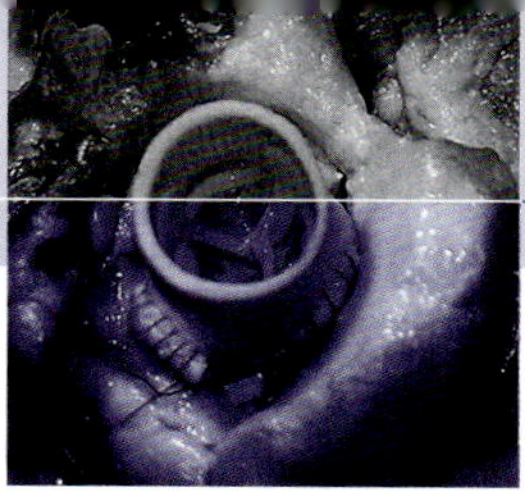

The anastomosis is continued caudally across the inferior circumference (attention: avoid injury of the coronary sinus!) and cranially towards the free wall of the right atrium.

(Perspective from the first assistant)
Continuing the suture line across the cranial circumference completes the right atrial anastomosis at the free wall.

1 2 3 4 5 6 7 8 9 10 11 12 13 14 15

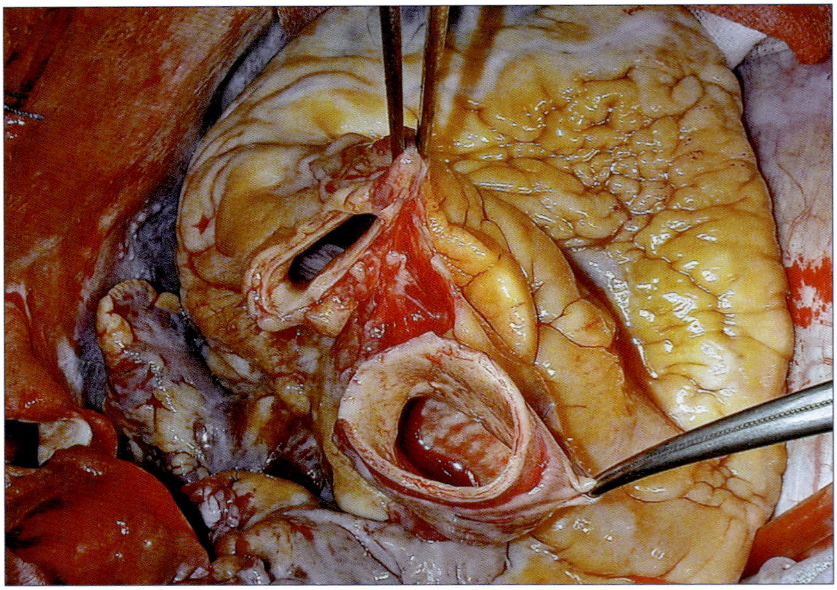

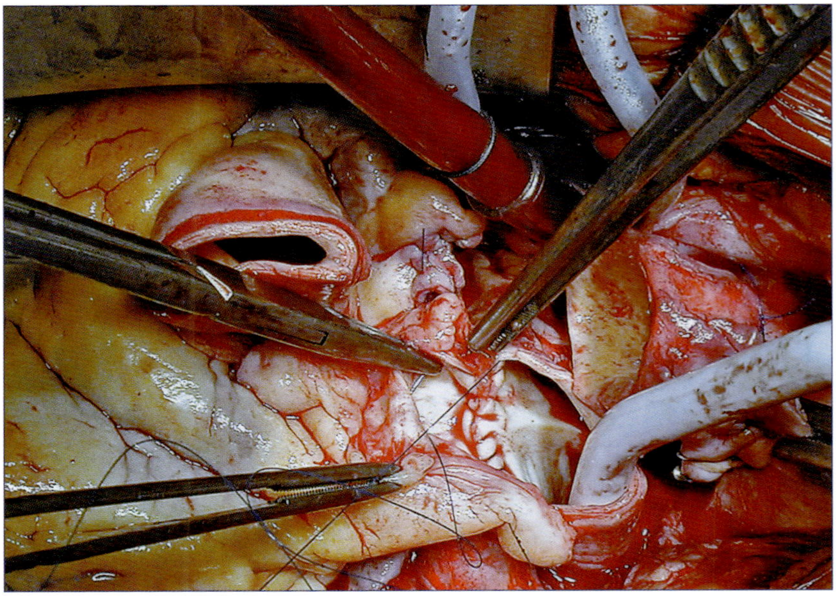

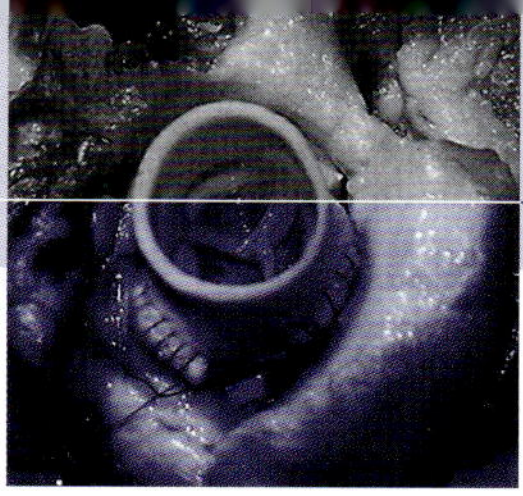

Anastomosis of the large vessels starts with the pulmonary artery while the aorta might be retracted using a long vessel clamp. One must pay special attention to acquiring the optimal length. A pulmonary artery that is too short may cause tension on the anastomosis, and excessive length may cause kinking, which usually results in right heart failure.

(Perspective of the first assistant).
The pulmonary artery anastomosis is performed with a prolene 4-0 SH suture line which begins at the left atrial circumference and is continued across the posterior wall as an everting suture. To obtain optimal hemostasis, the stitches are placed closely (stitch direction: recipient "outside to inside", donor "inside to outside").
With avoidance of any distortion or significant size mismatch, the anastomosis is completed ventrally.

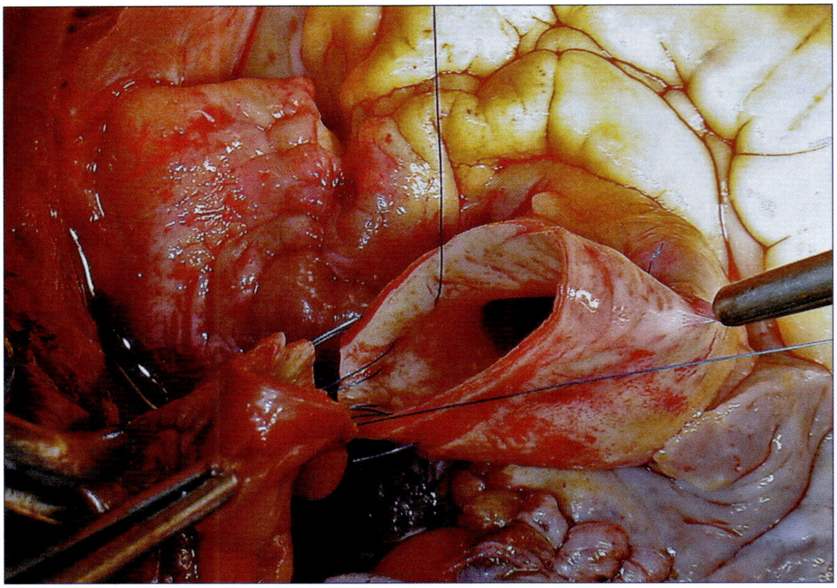

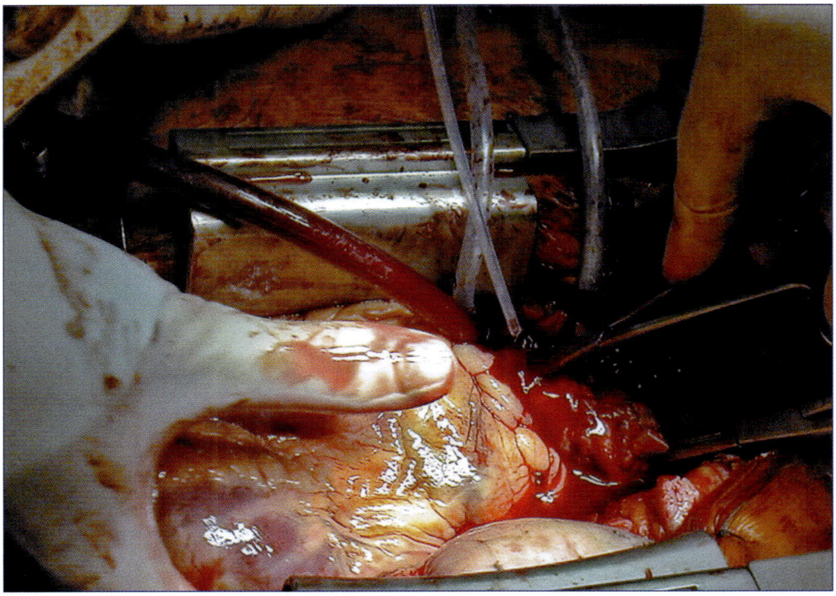

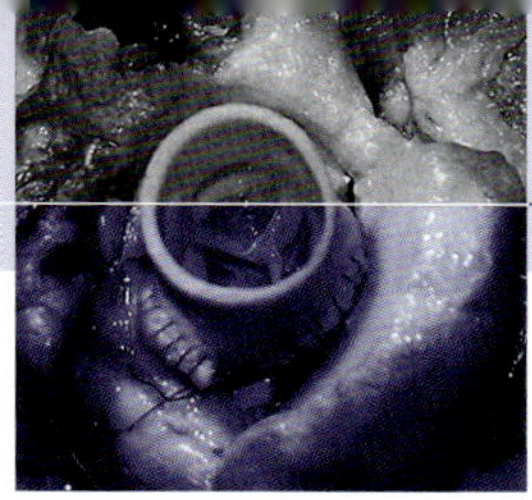

While separating donor aorta and pulmonary artery, it is of significant importance to leave sufficient adventitia tissue on the aorta. Furthermore, the correct estimation of the length of the donor aorta is crucial in order to prevent tensile stress on the aortic anastomosis. A slightly longer aorta might even serve as an augmentation to the pulmonary artery and may reduce the risk of pulmonary artery kinking. A prolene 4-0 SH suture is used for the aortic anastomosis. A compensation of a slight size mismatch may be achieved by a v-shaped incision into the smaller vessel.

(Perspective of the first assistant).
Subsequent to the completion of the anastomosis, the ascending aorta is incised additionally for de-airing, followed by initiation of partial cardio-pulmonary bypass.
With slight volume load of the heart, moderate lung ventilation and repetitive Trendelenburg maneuvers for de-airing of heart and aorta, the aortic clamp is removed and reperfusion of the graft is established.

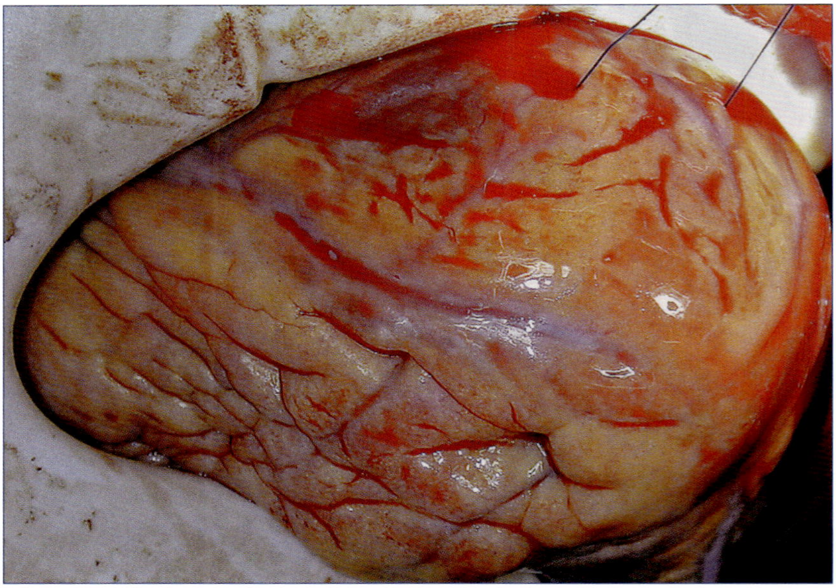

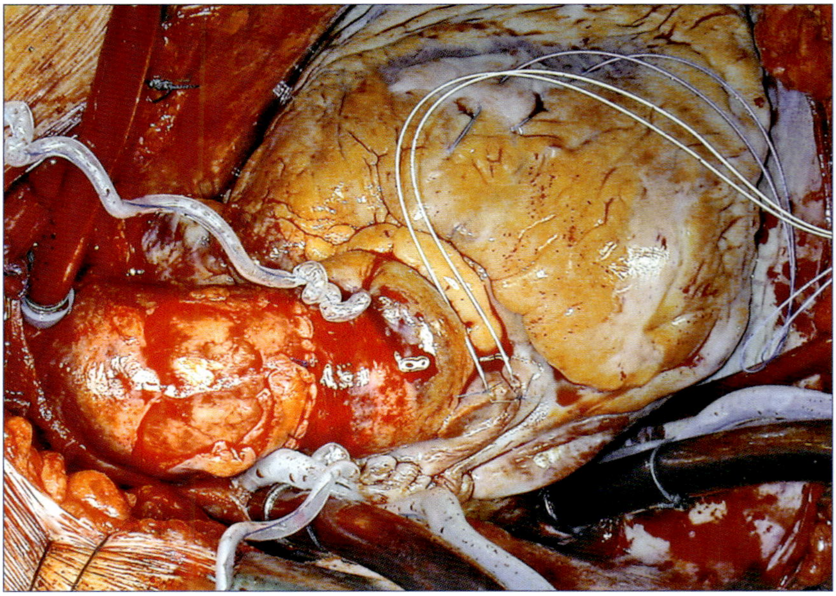

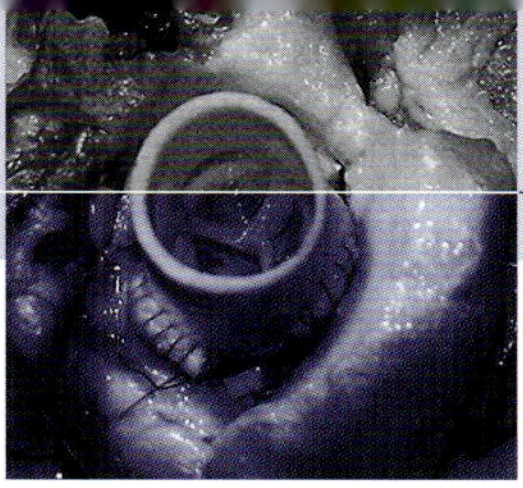

1 2 3 4 5 6 7 8 9 10 11 12 13 14 15

In addition, de-airing might be optimized through the apex with subsequent closure of the puncture site (prolene 3-0).

Graft reperfusion is performed for approximately 60 minutes. A volume overload of the right ventricle should be absolutely avoided (if necessary, complete cardio-pulmonary bypass has to be re-estalished). For invasive hemodynamic monitoring, a Swan-Ganz catheter and a left atrial pressure line is introduced, and epicardial pacing wires are applied.
The weaning from the ECC is performed after implementation of epinephrine infusion (0.1–0.3 μg/kg/min) under restricted volume load. In selected cases with significant right heart insufficiency, concomitant NO-ventilation and/or aerosolisation of Iloprost might be necessary.

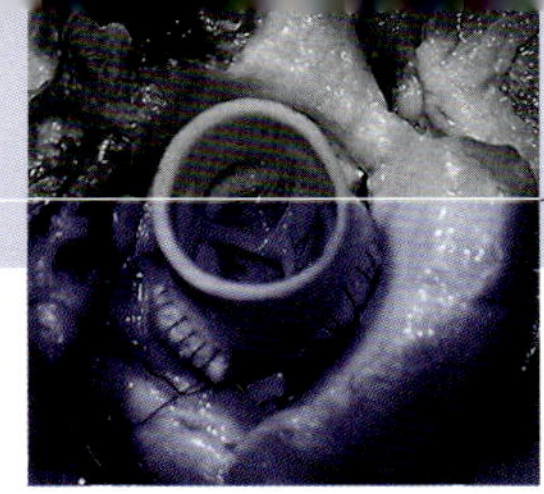

References

1. Shumway NE. Way is clear for heart transplantation. JAMA 1967; 202: 31–32
2. Lower RR, Shumway NE. Studies on orthotopic homotransplantations of the canine heart. Surg Forum 1960; 11: 18–19
3. Brown NE, Muehlebach GF, Jones Phil, Gorton ME, Stuart RS, Borkon AM. Tricuspid Annuloplasty Significantly Reduces Early Tricuspid Regurgitation after Biatrial Heart Transplantation. J Heart Lung Transplant 2004; 23: 1160–2
4. Aziz T, Burgess M, Khafagy R. et al. Bicaval and standard techniques in orthotopic heart transplantation: medium-term experience in cardiac performance and survival. J Thorac Cardiovasc Surg 1999; 118: 115–122
5. Grande AM, Rinaldi M, D'Armini AM, Campana C, Traversi E, Pederzolli C, Abbiate N, Klersy C, Vigano M. Orthotopic heart transplantation: standard versus bicaval technique. Am J. Cardiol 2000; 85: 1329–33.
6. Schwilden ED, van Dongen RJAM. Technik der Gefäßchirurgie. In: Heberer G, van Dongen RJAM (Hrsg.). Gefäßchirurgie. Springer Verlag, Berlin, 2004: 47–72

1 2 3 4 5 6 7 8 9 10 11 12 13 14 15

Support modes:

"serial":

Inlet → Apex
Outlet → Great vessels
Better filling – larger pump volume/time: Reduction of ventricular diameter and wall tension

"parallel":

Inlet → Atrium
Outlet → Great vessels

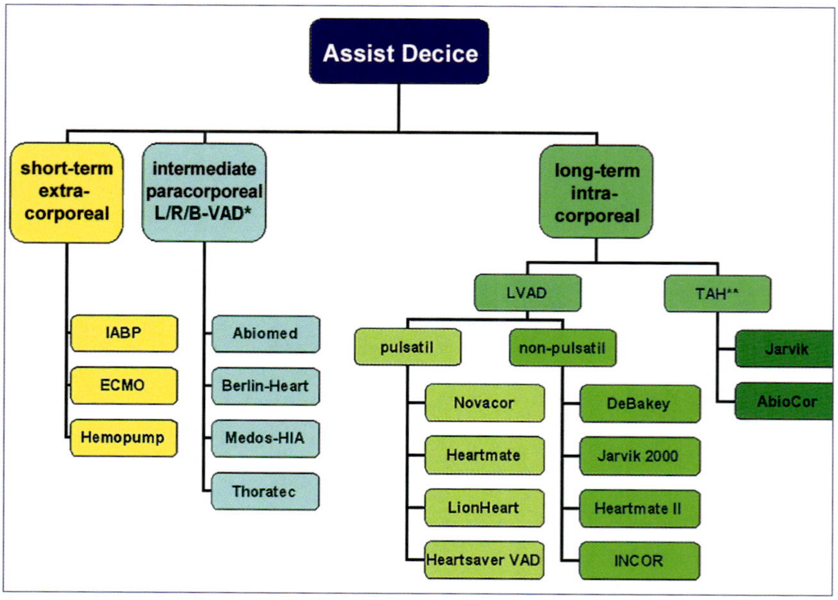

* VAD: ventricular assist device ** TAH: Total artificial heart

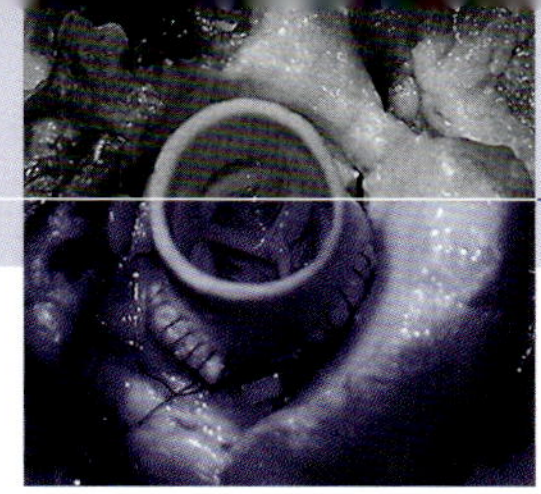

Mechanical pump chambers can be implanted serially or in parallel with regard to their function. The serial LVAD implant has proven advantageous, as there is a better filling of the VAD and a superior unloading of the native ventricle.

Overview:
Overview on the mechanical circulatory support and artificial heart systems. Apart from the IABP and ECMO mainly paracorporeal pneumatic and intracorporeal electric systems are used.

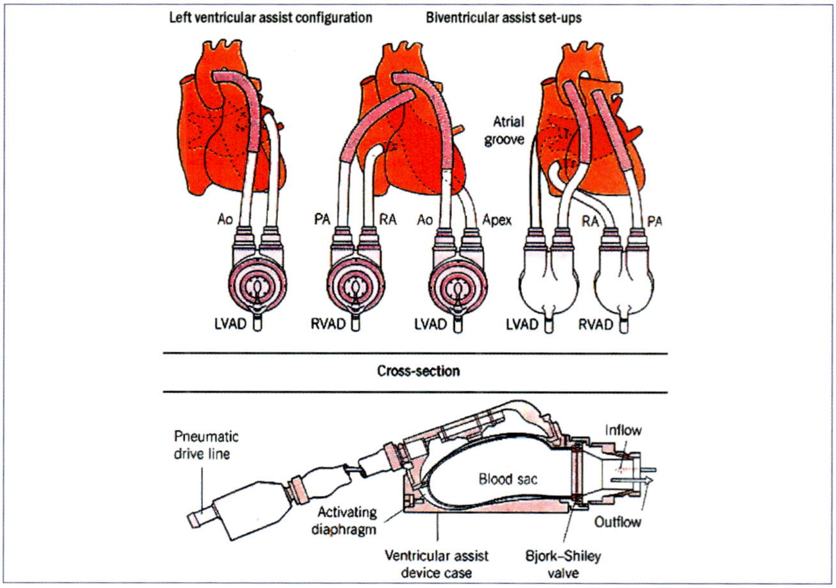
Left ventricular assist configuration
Biventricular assist set-ups
Atrial groove
Ao
PA
RA
Ao
Apex
RA
PA
LVAD
RVAD
LVAD
LVAD
RVAD
Cross-section
Pneumatic drive line
Activating diaphragm
Blood sac
Inflow
Outflow
Ventricular assist device case
Bjork–Shiley valve

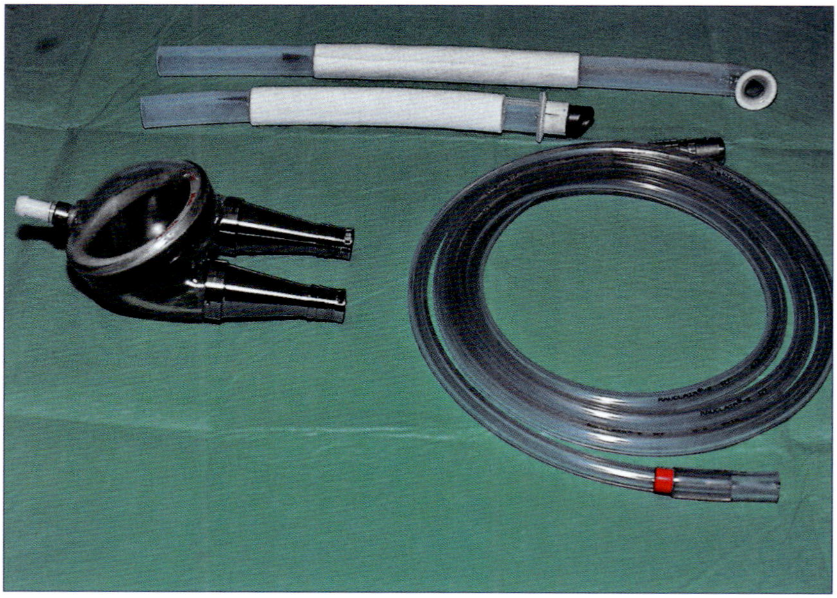

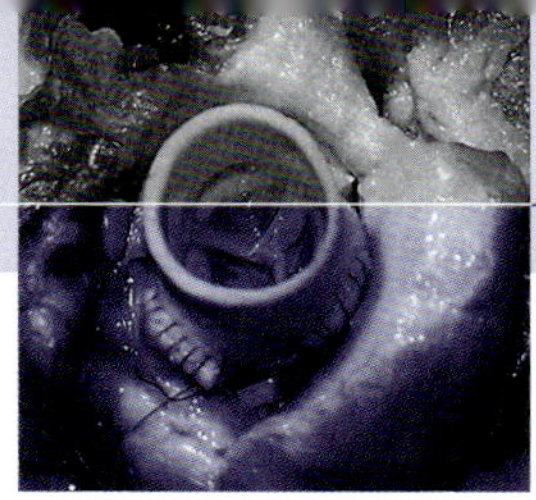

Paracorporeal pulsatile:
Paracorporeal pneumatic systems can be used for a variety of indications for left-sided and right-sided circulatory support, in adults as well as in children.

Components of the Berlin Heart Excor system

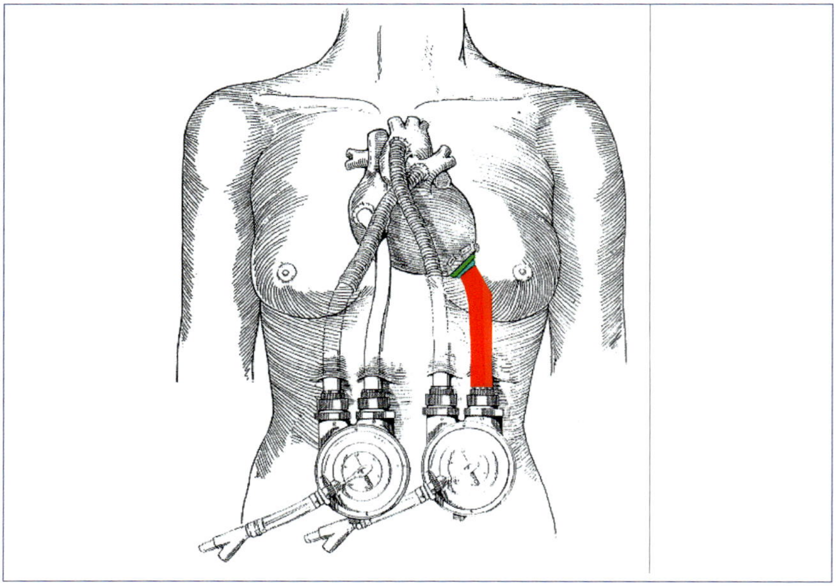

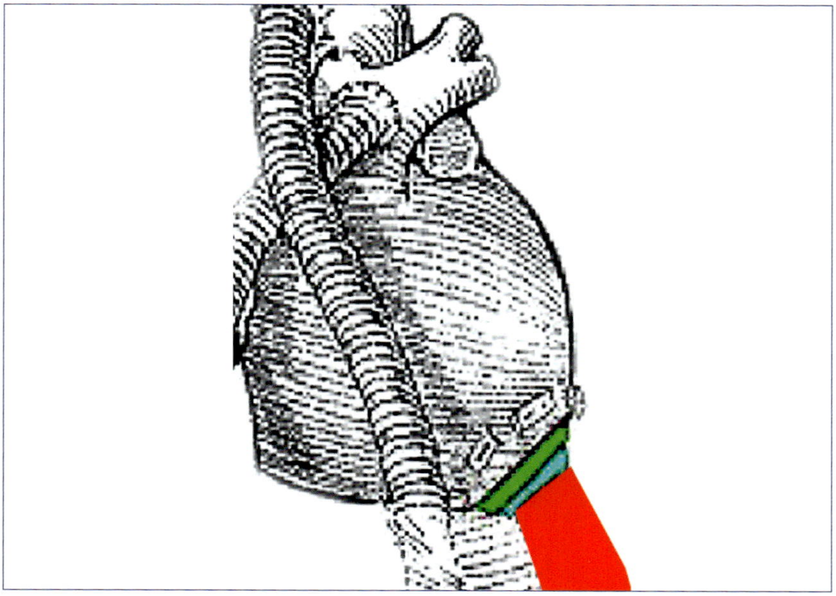

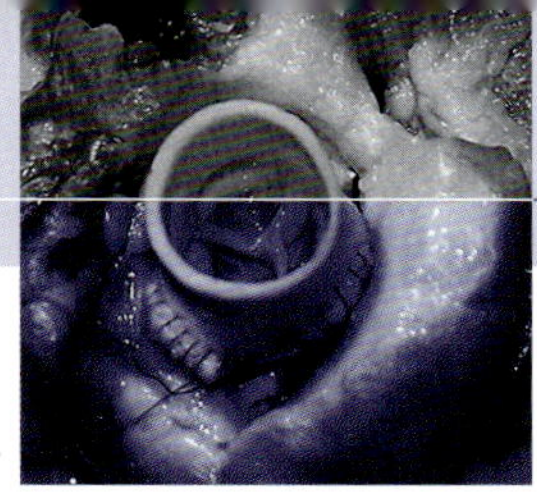

Ventricular cannulation offers excellent flow through the conduit and superior unloading of the native heart, but subsequent decannulation, i.e. after weaning due to recovery of myocardial pump function, is more difficult.

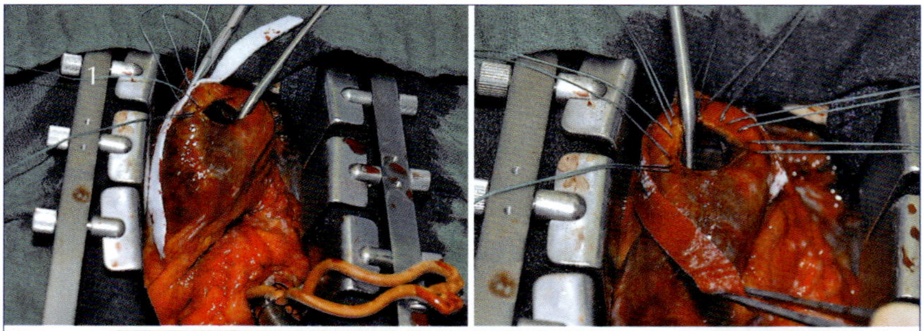
1

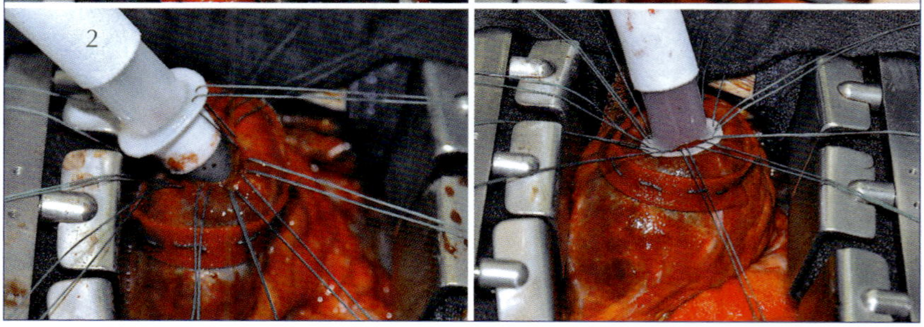
2

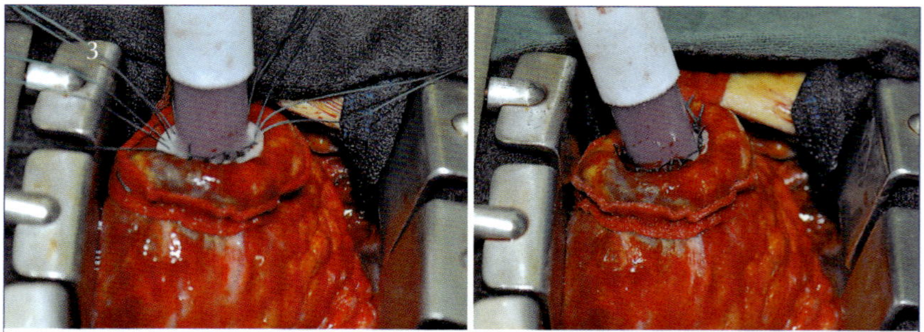
3

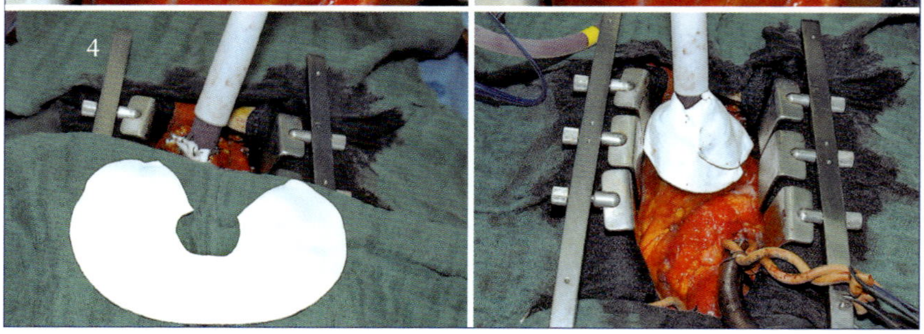
4

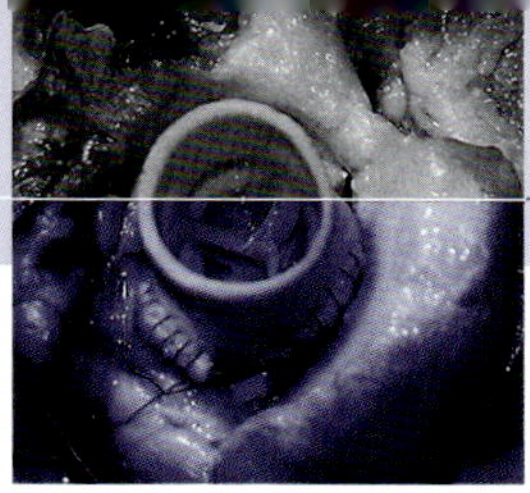

Excor

Multiple sutures are placed over a strip of PTFE felt as abutment (1st). The sutures are guided through the sutures ring of the inflow cannula (2nd) and tied (3rd). Wrapping of the apex with a sheet of PTFE prevents strong adhesion (4th).

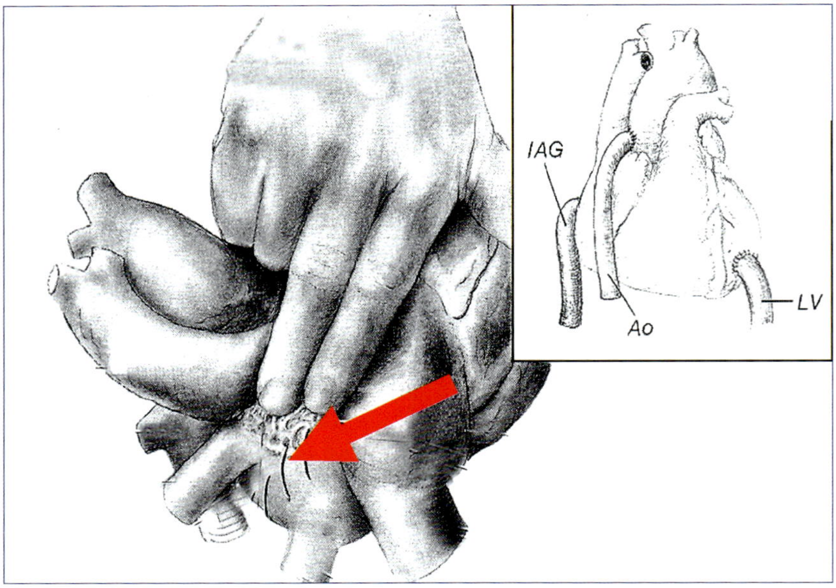
IAG
Ao
LV

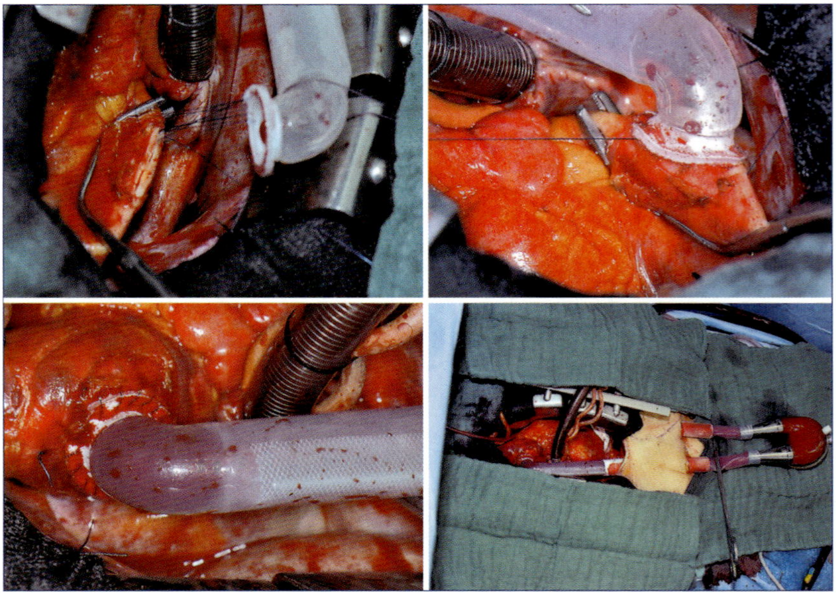

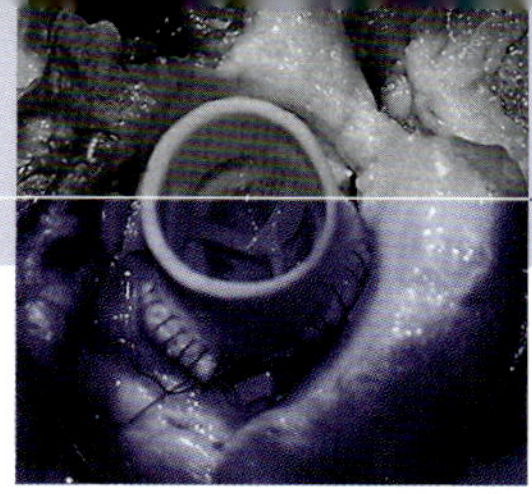

Inflow cannula

Atrial cannulation at the interatrial groove is much simpler. However, decompression of the native heart is worse. A purse-string suture suffices to fix the cannula in place and to secure hemostasis. PTFE felts prevent tearing.

End-to-side-anastomosis of the outflow conduit (BerlinHeart Excor) with the side-clamped aorta.

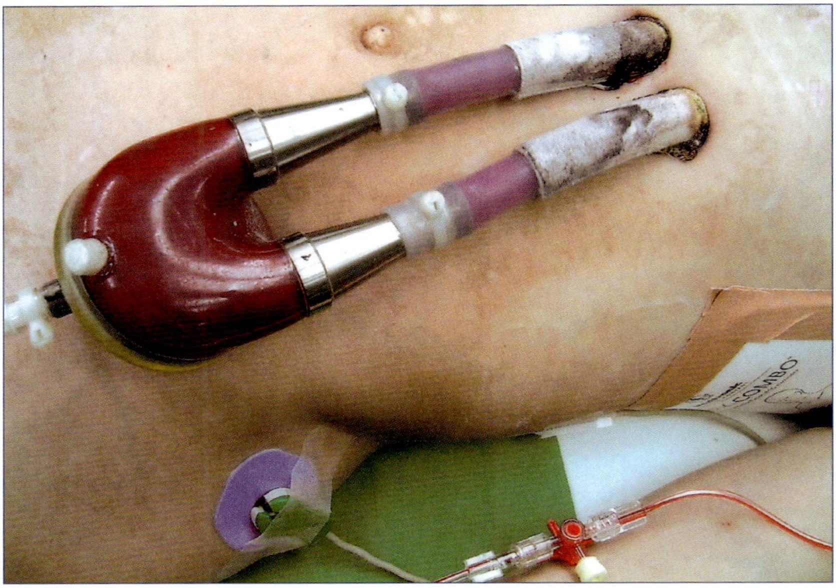

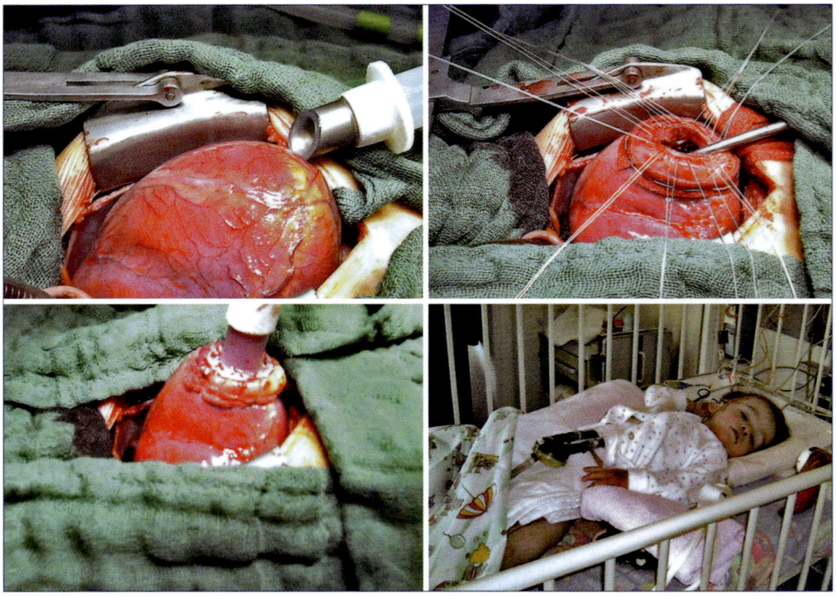

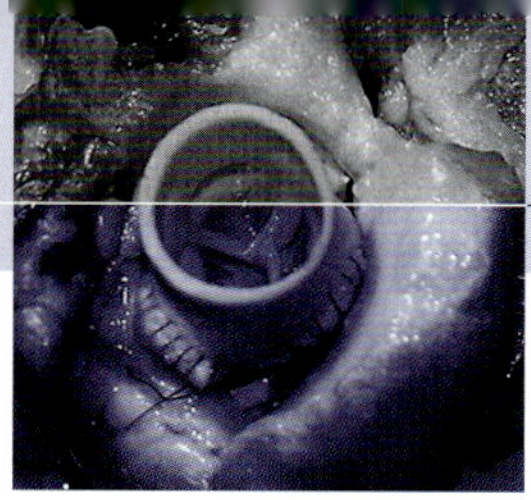

VAD position adults

In adults the paracorporeal pump chambers are directed to the side (not towards the midline) to avoid problems during sitting and bending forward.

VAD – children

In children, the same technique is used for VAD implantation. However, cannulas are placed in a way that the pump chambers lie in a midline position.

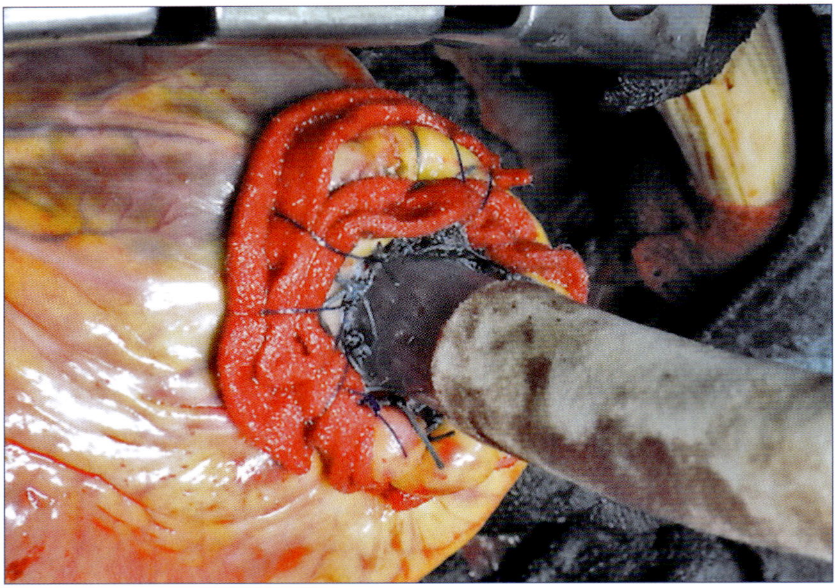

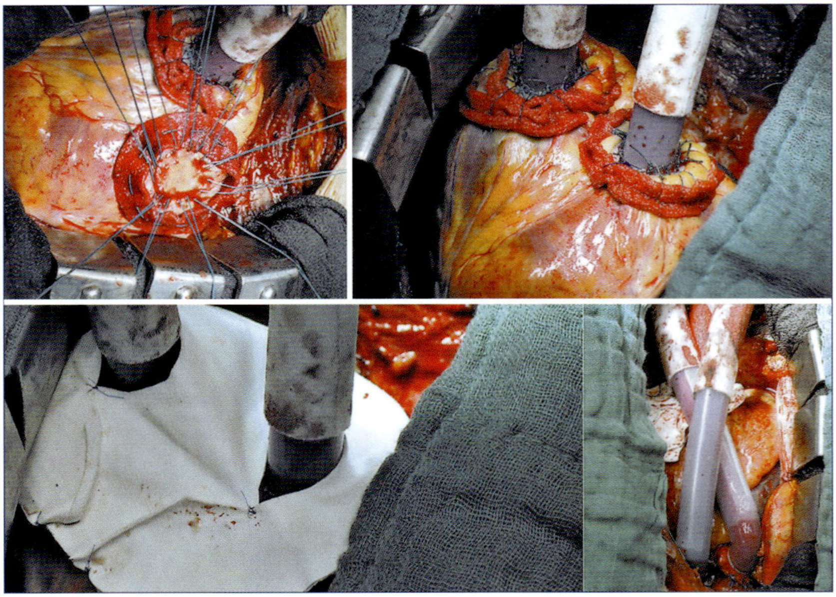

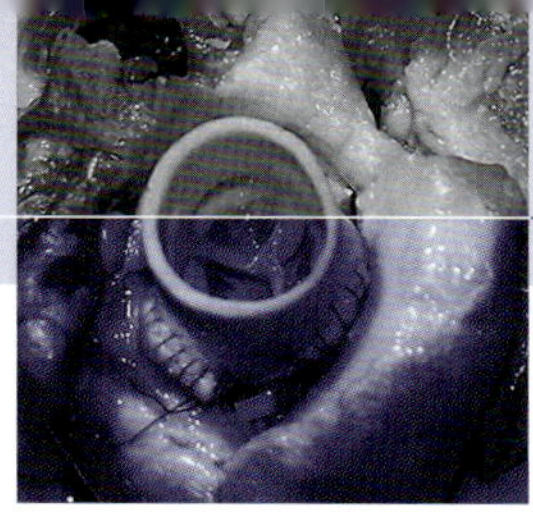

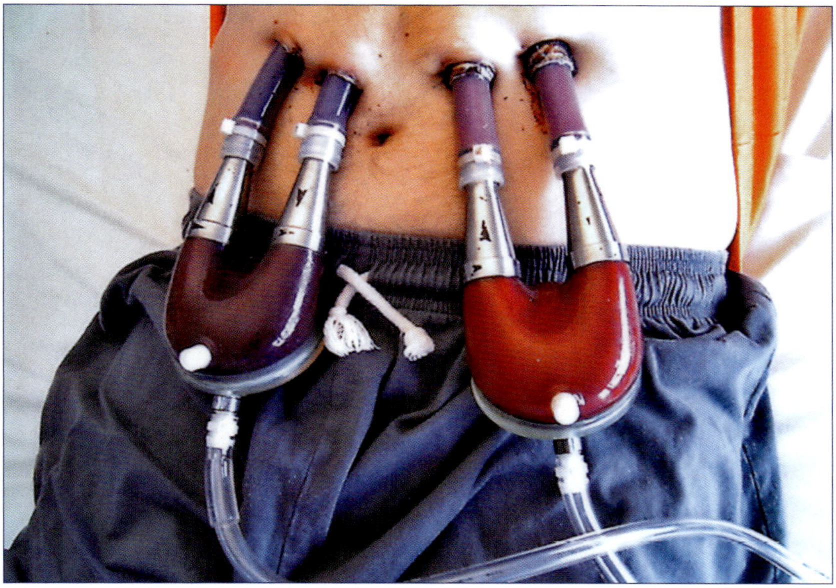

Excor – BiVAD – ventricular cannulas

For BiVADs, the right-sided cannulation is also accomplished via the ventricular apex in Muenster – identical to the left-sided implantation technique. Cannulas always cross inside (not outside) the thoracic cavity which allows a better positioning of the pump chambers.

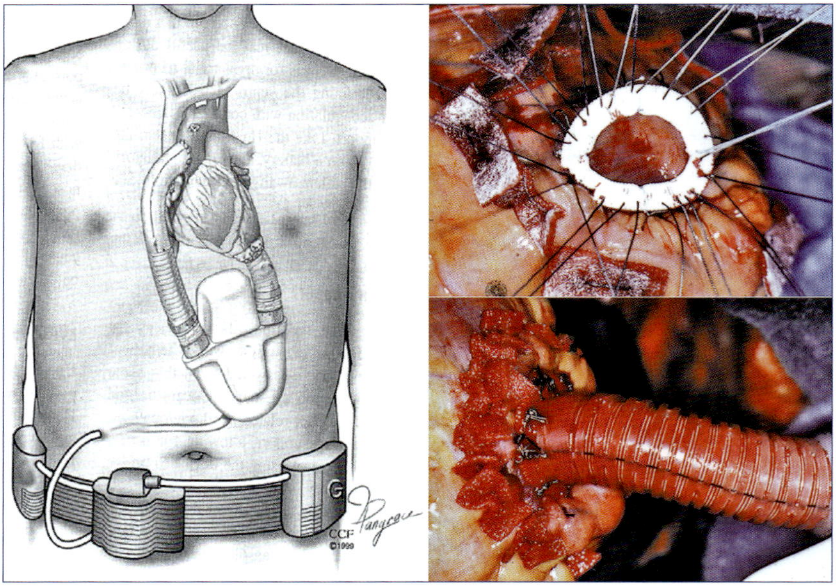
CCF

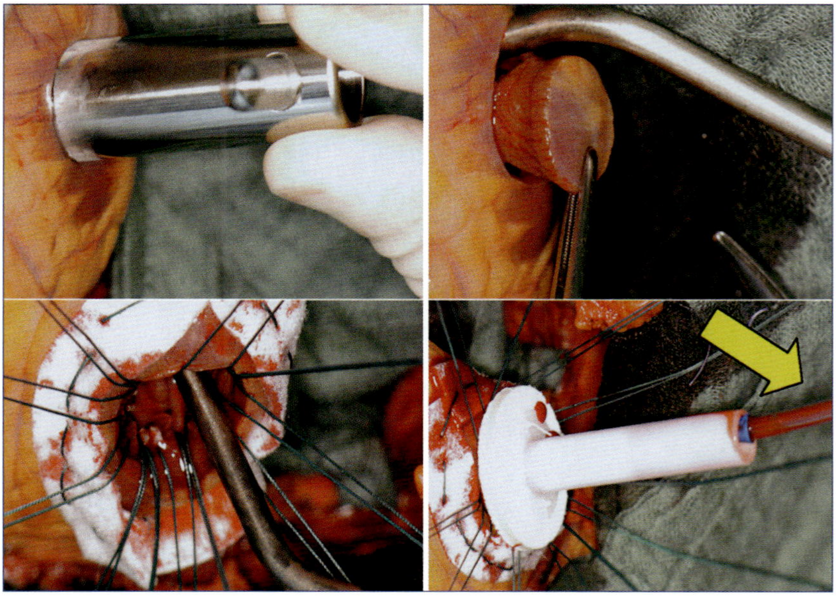

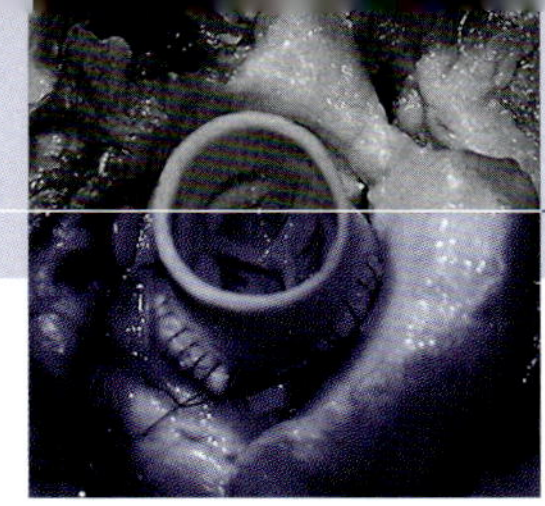

Intracorporeal, pulsatile support system (Novacor LVAD)

Intracorporeal LVADs like the Novacor are especially suitable for long-term support, since patients can be well treated on an ambulatory basis. However, the bulky systems of the first generation are still prone to infectious and thromboembolic complications.

Intracorporeal, non-pulsatile support system (INCOR)

For implantation of an Incor-LVAD, access to the left-ventricular cavity is provided with a coring knife. Afterwards, single sutures are placed over a strip of PTFE, and later guided through the fixation ring for the inflow conduit.

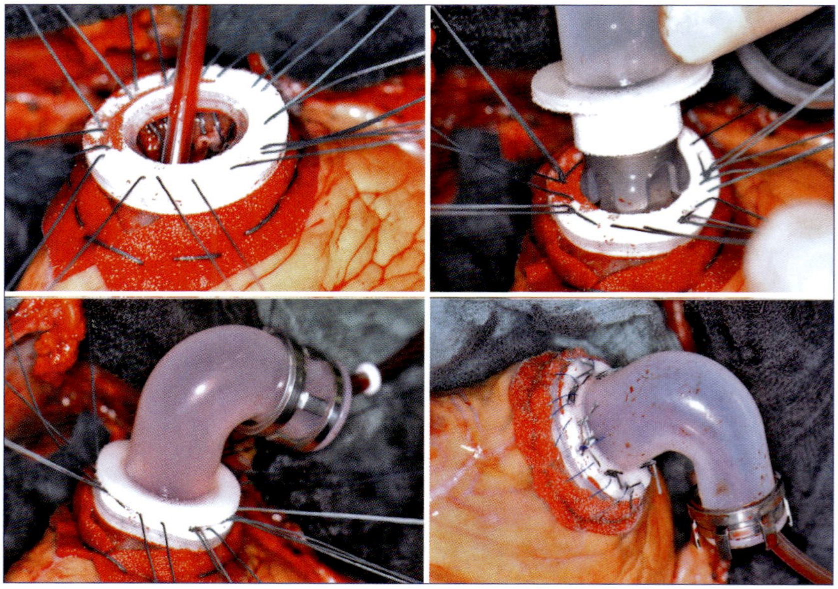

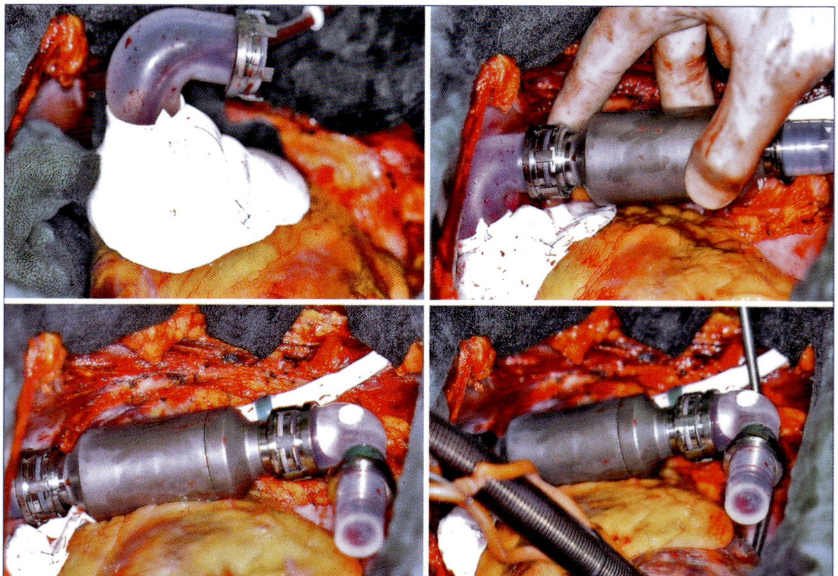

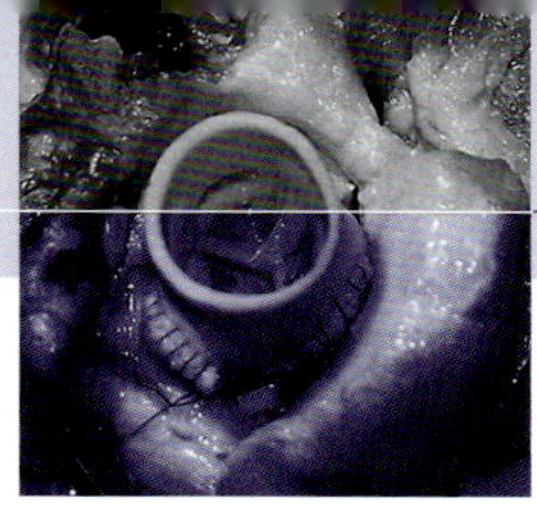

The sutures are no yet tied, but additionally guided through the cuff of the inflow cannula. Now all sutures are tied. An additional running suture may provide better hemostasis.

The ventricular apex is covered with a sheet of PTFE to prevent excessive adhesions, and the pump is placed intrapericardially. There is no need for a pump pocket.

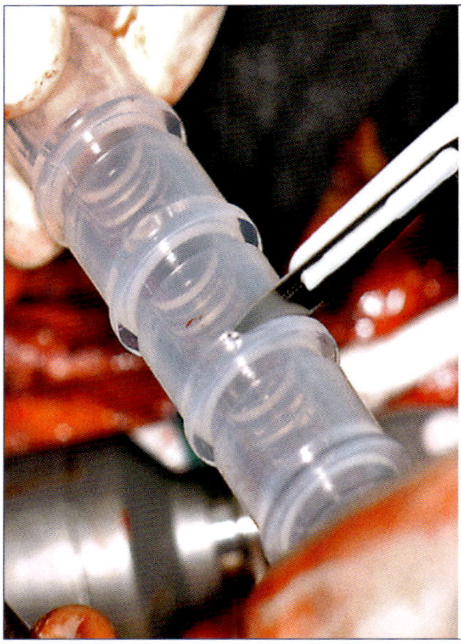

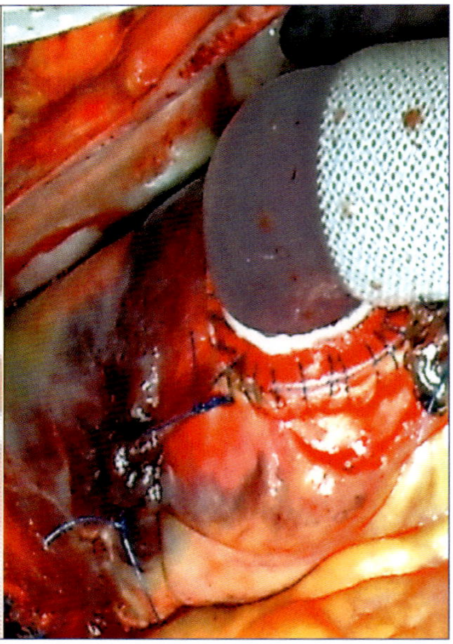

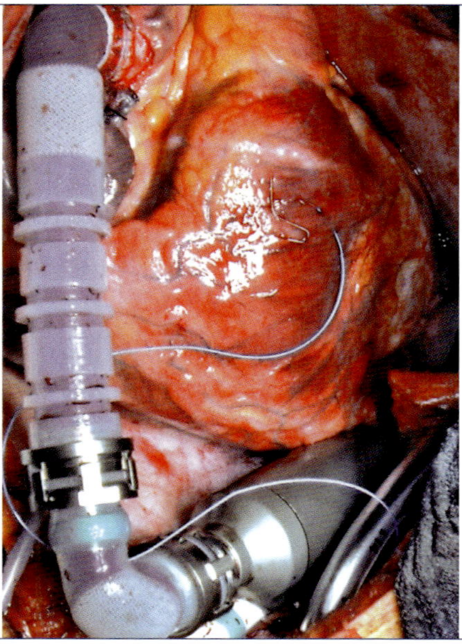

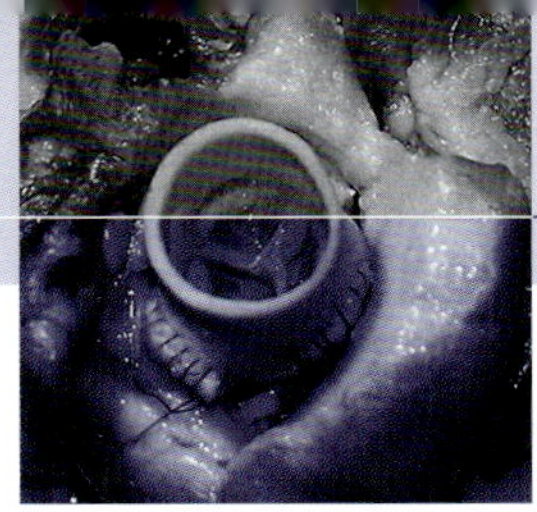

The outflow conduit is adequately shortened and anastomosed to the ascending aorta end-to side.

Completed implantation of the Berlin Heart Incor system.

References

1. El-Banayosy A, Arusoglu L, Kizner L, tendrich G, Minami K, Inuoe K, Körfer R. Novacor left ventricular assist system versus HeartMate vented electric left ventricular assist system as a long term mechanical circulatory support device in bridging patients: a prospective study. J Thorac Cardiovasc Surg 2000; 119: 581–587
2. McCarthy PM, Portner PM, Tobler HG, Starnes VA, Ramasamy N, Oyer PE. Clinical experience with the Novacor ventricular assist system. Bridge to transplantation and the transition to permanent application. J Thorac Cardiovasc Surg 1991; 102: 578–586
3. Schmid C, Weyand M, Nabavi DG, Hammel D, Deng M, Ringelstein E, Scheld HH. Cerebral and systemic embolization during left ventricular support with the Novacor N100 device. Ann Thorac Surg 1998; 65: 1703–1710
4. Frazier OH, Rose EA, Macmanus Q, Burton NA, Lefrak EA, Poirier VL, Dasse KA. Multicenter clinical evaluation of the Heart Mate 1000 IP left ventricular assist device. Ann Thorac Surg 1992; 53: 1080–1090
5. McCarthy PM, Smedira NO, Vargo RL, Goormastic M, Hobbs RE, Starling RC, Young JB. One hundred patients with the Heartmate left ventricular assist device: evolving concepts and technology. J Thorac Cardiovasc Surg 1998; 115: 904–912
6. Minami K, El-Banayosy A, Sezai A, Arusoglu L, Sarnowsky P, Fey O, Koerfer R. Morbidity and outcome after mechanical ventricular support using Thoratec, Novacor, HeartMate for bridging to heart transplantation. Artif Organs 2000; 24: 421–426
7. Noon GP, Hetzer R, Loebe M, Wolner E, Wiesethaler G, Schima H, Fabiani JN, D'Attellis N, DeBakey ME. Clinical experience with the DeBakey VAD axial flow pump. Cardiovasc Engineering 2000; 5: 30–32
8. Vitali E, Lanfranconi M, Ribera E, Bruschi G, Colombo T, Frigerio M, Russo C. Successful experience in bridging patients to heart transplantation with the MicroMed DeBakey ventricular assist device. Ann Thorac Surg 2003; 75: 1200–1204

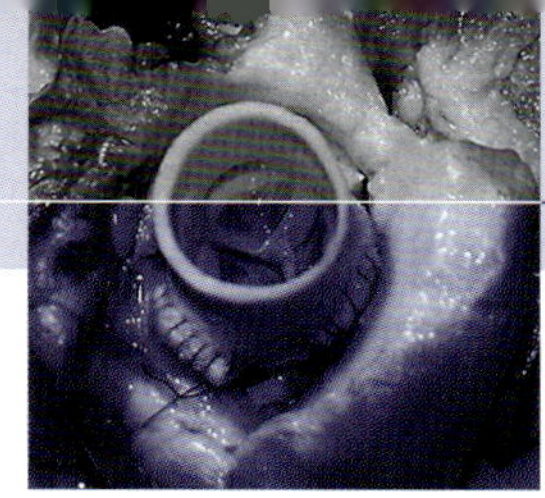

9. Weyand M, Kececioglu D, Kehl H, Schmid C, Loick H, Vogt J, Scheld H. Neonatal bridging to total orthotopic heart transplantation. Ann Thorac Surg 1998; 66: 519–522
10. Schmid C, Hammel D, Deng MC, Weyand M, Baba H, Tjan TDT, Drees G, Roeder N, Schmidt C, Scheld HH. Ambulatory care of patients with left ventricular assist devices. Circulation 1999; 100: II–224, II–228
11. Schmid C, Tjan TDT, Etz C, Wilhelm MJ, Schmidt Ch, Wenzelburger F, Rothenburger M, Drees G, Scheld HH. First clinical experience with the Incor left ventricular assist device. J Heart Lung Transplant (in press)

David H. Adams, MD, PhD
Professor and Chairman
Department of Cardiothoracic Surgery
Mount Sinai Medical Center
One Gustave L. Levy Place
1190 Fifth Avenue, New York, NY 10029, USA
eMail: david.adams@mountsinai.org

Johannes M. Albes, MD, PhD, MBA
Professor and Chairman
Department of Cardiovascular Surgery
Heart Center Brandenburg, Bernau
Ladeburger Stasse 17, 16321 Bernau, Germany
e-mail: j.albes@immanuel.de

Matthias Bechtel, MD, PhD
Department of Cardiac Surgery
University of Luebeck
Ratzeburger Allee 160 • 23538 Luebeck, Germany
eMail: m.bechtel@herzchirurgie-luebeck.de

Jochen Cremer, MD, PhD
Professor and Chairman
Department of Cardiac and Vascular Surgery
Christian-Albrechts-University Kiel
Arnold Heller Str. 7 • 24105 Kiel, Germany
eMail: jcremer@kielheart.uni-kiel.de

Ashraf El-Essawi, MD
Department of Cardiothoracic and Vascular Surgery
Staedtisches Klinikum Braunschweig
Salzdahlumer Strasse 90 • 38126 Braunschweig, Germany
eMail: a.el-essawi@klinikum-braunschweig.de

Ulrich F. W. Franke, MD, PhD
Chairman
Department of Cardiac and Vascular Surgery
Robert Bosch Hospital Stuttgart
Auerbachstrasse 110 • 70376 Stuttgart, Germany
eMail: ulrich.franke@rbk.de

Jan F. Gummert, MD, PhD
Professor and Chairman
Department of Cardiothoracic Surgery
Friedrich-Schiller University Jena
Erlanger Allee 101 • 07740 Jena, Germany
eMail: gummert@med.uni-jena.de

Wolfgang Harringer, MD, PhD
Chairman
Department of Cardiothoracic and Vascular Surgery
Staedtisches Klinikum Braunschweig
Salzdahlumer Strasse 90 • 38126 Braunschweig, Germany
eMail: w.harringer@klinikum-braunschweig.de

Parwis Rahmanian, MD
Department of Cardiothoracic Surgery
Mount Sinai Medical Center
One Gustave L. Levy Place
1190 Fifth Avenue, New York, NY 10029, USA
eMail: parwis.rahmanian@uk-koeln.de

Chanaka Rajakaruna, MD
Department of Cardiothoracic Surgery
King´s College Hospital
Denmark Hill
London SE5 9RS, Great Britain
eMail: Chanaka.Rajakaruna @kingsch.nhs.uk

Hans H. Scheld, MD, PhD
Professor and Chairman, Department of
Cardiothoracic and Vascular Surgery
Westfaelische Wilhelms-University of Muenster
Albert-Schweitzer-Str. 33 • 48149 Muenster, Germany
eMail: h.h.scheld@ukmuenster.de

Felix Schoeneich, MD
Department of Cardiac and Vascular Surgery
Christian-Albrechts-University Kiel
Arnold Heller Str. 7 • 24105 Kiel, Germany
eMail: fschoeneich@kielheart.uni-kiel.de

Hans H. Sievers, MD, PhD
Professor and Chairman
Department of Cardiac Surgery/University of Luebeck
Ratzeburger Allee 160 • 23538 Luebeck, Germany
eMail: h.sievers@herzchirurgie-luebeck.de

Thorsten Wahlers, MD, PhD
Professor and Chairman, Department of
Cardiothoracic Surgery/Heart Center
University of Cologne
Kerpener Str. 62 • 50924 Cologne, Germany
eMail: thorsten.wahlers@uk-koeln.de

Olaf Wendler, MD PhD FRCS
Clinical Director of Cardiology & Cardiac Surgery
Consultant Cardiothoracic Surgeon
King's College Hospital
Denmark Hill • London
SE 22 8ST
United Kingdom
olaf.wendler@kingsch.nhs.uk

Thorsten Wittwer, MD, PhD, MA
Professor of Cardiac Surgery, Department of
Cardiothoracic Surgery/Heart Center
University of Cologne
Kerpener Str. 62 • 50924 Cologne, Germany
eMail: thorsten.wittwer@uk-koeln.de

Hans R. Zerkowski, MD, PhD
Professor of Surgery
Auf der Bischofshoehe 6 • 4125 Riehen, Switzerland

Gerhard Ziemer, MD, PhD
Head, Dept. Thoracic, Cardiac and Vascular Surgery
Tuebingen University Hospital
Professor of Surgery
Eberhard-Karls-University Tuebingen
eMail: gerhard.ziemer@med.uni-tuebingen.de

Index